You Don't Know Sh*t!

Until You Read This Book

Volume One

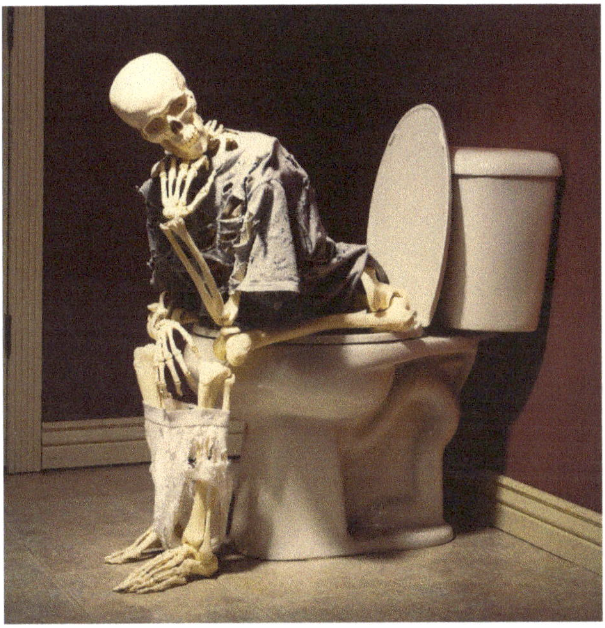

Joseph Weiss MD, FACP, FACG, AGAF
Clinical Professor of Medicine,
Gastroenterology
University of California, San Diego

SmartAsk Books
Rancho Santa Fe, California, USA
www.smartaskbooks.com

ISBN-13: 978-1-943760-22-0 (Volume One)
ISBN-13: 978-1-943760-23-7 (Volume Two)
ISBN-13: 978-1-943760-04-6 (Combined Volumes)

Last digit is the print number: 9 8 7 6 5 4 3

Dedication

This volume is dedicated to correcting misperceptions, and enhancing our appreciation of all aspects of nature. Natural processes that society has denigrated are as valuable and necessary as those that have been praised and elevated.

I am indebted to my loved ones Nancy, Danielle, Jeremy, Courie, Lizzy, & Indy, who have offered their insights, suggestions, comments, and unwavering support throughout the writing process of a volume on an underappreciated subject commonly considered a waste.

Preface

The Scoop on Poop! Flush with Knowledge is a uniquely informative, entertaining, illustrated volume that is full of it! The 'it' being information, knowledge, eccentricities, and peculiarities of the remains of the digestive process. Although these remains are more politely described as feces or excrement, it is more commonly and properly known as poop. We all generate it, carry it around with us in our bowels and eliminate it on a regular basis.For the purists who prefer to use the official terminology, the original word from Old English was shyte or shite, and in the modern form of the English language the correct word is shit. For those ready to embrace proper English the same book content is available under the cheeky title: **You Don't Know Sh*t, Until You Read This Book.** It covers everything you ever wanted to know about this primitive but most ubiquitous of subjects. Whether you disdain it or appreciate it, it is part of the human experience of nature. The purpose of this volume is to inform the public that there is a lot more to know about it, and that the information can be helpful, possibly lifesaving, and downright entertaining. The trivia in this volume can sustain a long conversation, or cut it short abruptly. Reading this volume will offer a newfound appreciation that the title actually reflects the state of knowledge of those who have not yet read the book.

The process of diet and digestion from a food source to the elimination of digestive waste is information worth acquiring and understanding. This information allows one to enhance healthful aspects of diet and nutrition, and to reduce the risk of harmful practices that increase being exposed to disease and toxins. The subjects covered in this book range from the traditional and expected to the offbeat, bizarre, and downright unbelievable. The saying that the truth is often stranger than fiction is unquestionably true when it comes to nature, the digestive tract, and humans in particular. The volume is structured as an alphabetical compendium of topics scatological in nature.

For those interested in more scatological subject matter ***To 'Air' is Human, Everything You Ever Wanted to Know About Intestinal Gas*** covers everything you ever wanted to know about the burp, belch, bloat, fart and everything digestive, but were either too afraid or too embarrassed to ask. A companion volume is ***Artsy Fartsy, Cultural History of the Fart*** is a fascinating and factually correct review of the common fart through human culture and history. ***How Do You Doo? Everybody Pees & Poops!*** A delightfully informative, entertaining, and colorfully illustrated volume with valuable practical insights on toilet training. Tasteful color photographs of animals answering the call of nature allows the child to understand that every body does it!

Table of Contents - Volume One

Introduction 5
Digestion 8
Anal Canal 20
Anal Columns 23
Anal Expulsiveness 24
Anal Glands 25
Anal Glands, Musk 26
Anal Glands, Skunk 27
Anal Hygiene 28
Anal Hygiene, Toilet Contamination 41
Analingus 44
Anal Reflex 45
Anal Retentive 47
Anal Sex 51
Anal Sphincter, External 48
Anal Sphincter, Internal 49
Anal Stimulation 51
Anal Valves 52
Anal Wink 53
Anoscopy 53
Aroma, Feces 54
Assume 75
Autointoxication 75
Ayurveda 75
Barium Enema 78
Bashful Bowel 78
Bidet 79
Bismuth 81
Blue Ice Fall 83
Bowel 84
Bowel Management 84
Bowel Movement 85
Bowel Sounds 88
Bristol Stool Scale 88
Bullshit 89
Cathartic 90
Chamber Pot 91
Chickenshit 92
Close (Night) Stool 92
Coffee, Kopi Luwak 278
Clyster 161
Colon 93, 286
Colonic Hydrotherapy, Proctoclysis 94
Colonography 95

Colonoscopy 98
Composting Toilet 102
Constipation 103
Constitutional 108
Continence, Fecal 108
Coprolith 113
Coprographia 115
Coprolalia 117
Coprology 117
Coprophagia 118
Coprophilia 128
Copropraxia 128
Defecation 129
Defecography 134
Dentate Line 135
Deoxyribonucleic Acid (DNA) 136
Diarrhea 137
Dietary Fiber 144
Digestion 8, 148
Dung 155
Dung Beetle 155
Dung Fuel 157
Dysbiosis 223, 310
Encopresis 160
Enema 161
Enema, Coffee 171
Enteric Nervous System 175, 241
Epigenetics 178
Eproctophilia 182
Evacuative Dysfunction 182
Excrement 183
Exercise 185
Fart 185
Fecal Continence 108
Fecal Impaction 188
Fecal Incontinence 191, 265
Fecalith 197
Fecal Occult Blood 196
Fecaloma 197
Fecal Oral Contamination Route 198
Fecal (Microbiota) Transplant 200
Feces 201
Feces, Aroma 202
Feces, Density 214
Feces Waste Management 215

Fiber 144, 269
Flora, Gastrointestinal 223, 310
Afterword 231
Appendix A (Foreign Languages – Feces/Shit) 235
Appendix B (Euphemisms - Feces/ Shit) 237
Index 241

Table of Contents - Volume Two

Gastrocolic Reflex
Gastroenteritis
Gastroenterology
Gastrointestinal Motility
Gastrointestinal Nervous System
Genetics
Genome
Gong Farmer
Groom of the Stool
Guano
Gut-Brain-Microbiome-Food Axis
Gut Feeling
Gut Flora
Hemorrhoid
Honey Bucket & Honey Wagon
Horseshit
Hydrogen
Hydrogen Sulfide
Ileum
Incontinence, Fecal
Indole
Insoluble Fiber
Intestinal Fortitude
Irritable Bowel Syndrome
Jejunum
Keriorrhea
Klismaphilia
Kopi Luwak Coffee
Lactose Intolerance
Large Bowel (Large Intestine)
Laxative
Laxative Abuse & Dependence
Levator Ani
Malabsorption & Maldigestion
Manure
Mass Movements
Meconium

Melena
Methane
Microbiome, Gut
Mucoid Plaque
Mucus
Night Soil
Night Stool
Olestra
Orlistat
Outhouse
Panchagavya
Perineal Body
Peristalsis
Pit Toilet
Prebiotic
Probiotics
Proctology
Proctoscopy
Pruritis Ani
Pubococcygeus Muscle
Puborectalis Muscle
Rectal Bleeding
Rectal Examination
Rectum
Runner's Trots
Scatology
Scybalum
Septage (Septic Field & Tank)
Sewer
Shart
Shit
Shrimp Coprophagia
Sigmoidoscopy
Skatole
Small Intestine
Steatorrhea
Stinkbug
Suppository
Toilet
Toilet Gods
Toilet (Potty) Training
Transverse Folds of Houston
Traveler's Diarrhea
Valsalva Maneuver
Villi

You Don't Know Sh*t! Volume One

Introduction

The subject of this book is a human necessity, but rarely discussed in an informative manner. As a physician and educator in the field of gastroenterology, the end product of the digestive process is ubiquitous. The Old English word 'shyte' or 'shite' may sound a bit politer, but the modern equivalent of 'shit' is a perfectly acceptable and proper word in the English language vocabulary. The word 'shit' appears often in this book along with its synonyms and alternates of feces, excrement, bowel movement, and others. Shit seems to be a particularly popular word in the adolescent vocabulary, and in the common day language of nearly all languages as listed in Appendix A. The alternative words and euphemisms are numerous, and a partial list is provided in Appendix B.

The word shit, a proper term for a natural and universal human and animal activity and product, has a reputation that frequently raises embarrassment and offense. This attitude leads to avoidance of discussion, with the result that most people have very limited knowledge about the material that is produced by their own body. The fact of the matter is that lack of basic information and knowledge is unfortunately the norm and contributes to avoidable health problems. One of the main purposes of this book and its companion volumes is to provide information that is interesting, understandable, valuable, and entertaining. Visual images can aid in understanding, and this volume uses them liberally. Many people find that a visual image often imparts more understanding and information than the written word alone. This is particularly true when dealing with human health and physiology.

The process of digestion, besides a remarkable demonstration of biology and physiology, carries a lot of psychological aspects and considerations. It is animal-like in its primal role of being an absolute requirement to stay alive. It is primitive in that we are following the same activity as our prehistoric ancestors. We have to hunt, forage, barter, steal or accept the charity of others for our sustenance. Many of our most basic cultural taboos are intimately involved with the process of digestion, from the spitting of saliva to the abhorrence of vomit and feces. Digestion and bodily sounds, smells, and excretions are often associated with repugnance and revulsion. In spite of the base nature of the process, we recognize its critical importance to health, wellness, satisfaction, and happiness.

Selecting and maintaining a healthy diet is essential to eating, just as staying away from smog and pollution is to breathing. Humans have some interesting, yet very dangerous and self-acquired habits. These include smoking tobacco to assure that we breathe in grossly polluted air with cancer causing particles. It also includes eating junk food with disease inducing contents. As with alcohol and drugs, many of us seem to be pre-wired to be at risk for self-destructive habits that exchange short-term pleasures for long-term harmful effects. As primitive as eating and digestion may seem, especially to those with an eating disorder, it is a natural and healthy requirement of life in general and our species in particular. Humans have the ability to learn from the lessons of others, especially about how the body works and the best way to maintain it for maximal efficiency, longevity, and enjoyment. For many, the anticipation, preparation, and ingestion of food and drink are one of their greatest pleasures in life. Although the wise saying is that we should eat to live, it is apparent that a significant portion of the population embraces its mirror image, in that they live to eat.

The process of diet and digestion from a food source to the elimination of digestive waste is information worth acquiring and understanding. This information allows one to enhance healthful aspects of diet and nutrition, and to reduce the risk of harmful practices that increase being exposed to disease and toxins. The subjects covered in this book range from the traditional and expected to the offbeat, bizarre, and downright unbelievable. The saying that the truth is often stranger than fiction is unquestionably true when it comes to nature, the digestive tract, and humans in particular. The volume is structured as an alphabetical compendium of topics scatological in nature. There is much information and knowledge to share about human health, and subjects historically considered too sensitive for public discussion are especially ripe for attention. The book you are holding, ***The Scoop on Poop! Flush with Knowledge*** is one of several volumes that aim to accomplish this goal. There are several companion volumes that may also be of interest, that provide an in-depth discussion of subjects closely related to this book.

To 'Air' is Human, Everything You Ever Wanted to Know About Intestinal Gas is a uniquely informative, entertaining, and well-illustrated volume. Useful knowledge about the physiology and science of the fart, burp, and bloat often associated with the digestive process is clearly explained. It covers everything you ever wanted to know about farts and digestion, but were either too afraid or too embarrassed to ask. More for entertainment and historical value is its companion volume, ***Artsy Fartsy, Cultural History of the Fart***. This book provides a fascinating and factual overview of the common fart through human culture and history. The cough, sneeze, hiccup, stomach rumble, burp, belch, and other bodily sounds simply cannot compete with the notoriety of the fart. ***How Do You Doo? Everybody Pees & Poops!*** is a delightfully informative, entertaining, and colorfully illustrated volume with valuable practical insights on toilet training. Tasteful color photographs of animals answering the call of nature allows the child to understand that everybody does it! Additional informative relevant content to entertain the adult while the child is 'on the potty' is included.

AirVeda: Ancient & New Medical Wisdom, Digestion & Gas covers the remarkable advances in the understanding of digestive health and wellness. New information about the critical role of genomics, epigenetics, the gut microbiome, and the gut-brain-microbiome-diet axis are opening new avenues to optimal whole body health and wellness. Although intestinal gas, basic bodily functions, and feces have been topics culturally suppressed, knowledge and understanding are needed to achieve and maintain optimal health.

"Ayurveda is a 5,000 year old system of natural healing that reminds us that health is the balanced and dynamic integration between our environment, body, mind and spirit. In Dr. Joseph Weiss' book, AirVeda, he provides an informative and entertaining approach to sharing insights about our digestive system and wellbeing by applying the ancient wisdom of Ayurveda to everyday life." **Deepak Chopra, MD**

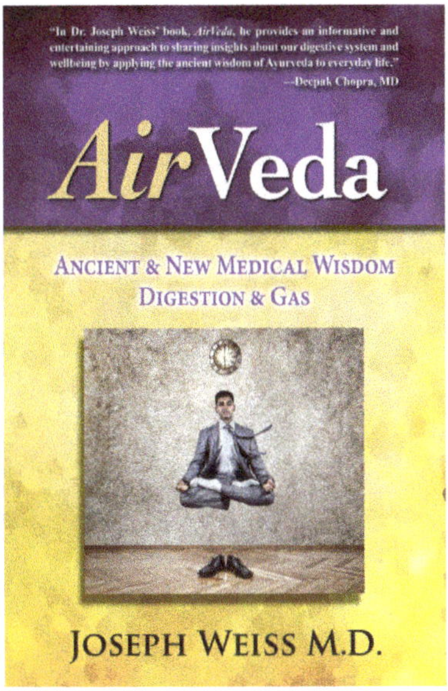
"In Dr. Joseph Weiss' book, AirVeda, he provides an informative and entertaining approach to sharing insights about our digestive system and wellbeing by applying the ancient wisdom of Ayurveda to everyday life."
—Deepak Chopra, MD
AirVeda
Ancient & New Medical Wisdom
Digestion & Gas
Joseph Weiss M.D.

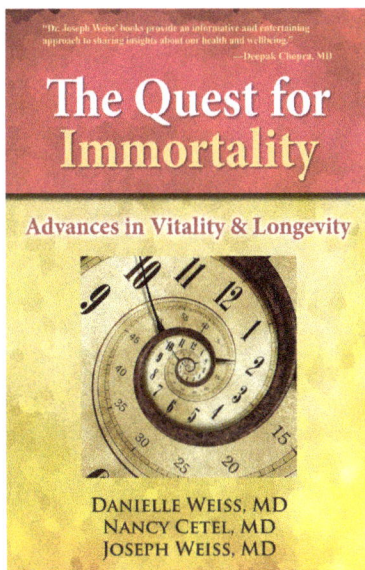
"Dr. Joseph Weiss' books provide an informative and entertaining approach to sharing insights about our health and wellbeing."
—Deepak Chopra, MD
The Quest for Immortality
Advances in Vitality & Longevity
Danielle Weiss, MD
Nancy Cetel, MD
Joseph Weiss, MD

The Quest for Immortality, Advances in Vitality & Longevity provides an informative and enlightening overview of the remarkable advances in science and medicine that are dramatically enhancing human health and lifespan. The volume is written in clear, understandable, and engaging language with striking colorful illustrations. From groundbreaking nanotechnology to genomics and stem cells, the secrets of vitality and longevity are being uncovered along with more traditional advances and practical insights into disease prevention and health enhancement.
The website www.smartaskbooks.com has a complete list of books and programs.

Digestion

Perhaps the best analogy is to think of the digestive tract as the reverse of an assembly line; it serves as a disassembly line. A factory has a goal to be efficient and profitable, and may not win too many awards for architecture and beauty. So too with the digestive tract, the process has been refined over eons of evolution, yet still has its primitive origin and end products.

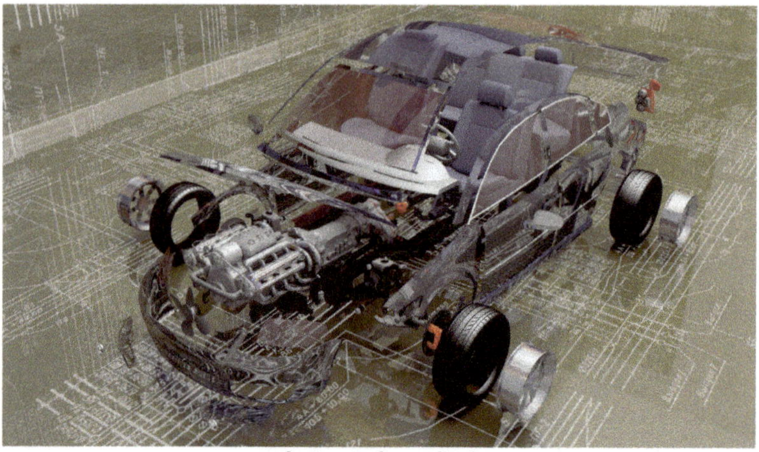

shutterstock.com/iurii

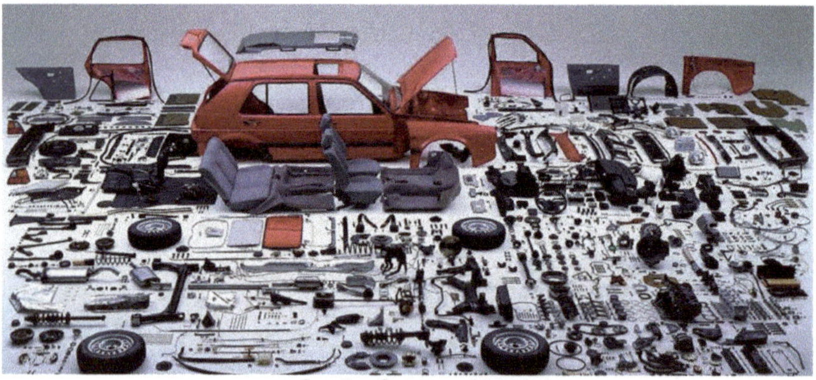

Creative Commons License

We begin the factory tour with a view much like you would get sitting in your car going through a car wash. Before you even go to the car wash, your brain has to make the conscious decision that that is what it wants to do. In the same manner, the brain begins the digestive process with the decision to satisfy its hunger call, or because an appetizing opportunity presents itself. When thinking about food and eating, the brain may release hormones and neurotransmitters, activate the secretion of saliva, and prime the release of gastric acid and digestive enzymes to prime and initiate the process of digestion.

Much like the water hoses and spray that greet your vehicle as you enter the beginning of the car wash tunnel, the entrance of food to the mouth receives a similar welcome. Jets of saliva are secreted from the ducts of the salivary glands located strategically around the oral cavity of the mouth. Saliva that is in the resting mouth is viscous and coats and protects the teeth and the inner surface of the mouth. The secreted saliva associated with eating or drinking is of a thinner more watery consistency. It has digestive enzymes including amylase to digest carbohydrates and lipase to digest fats.

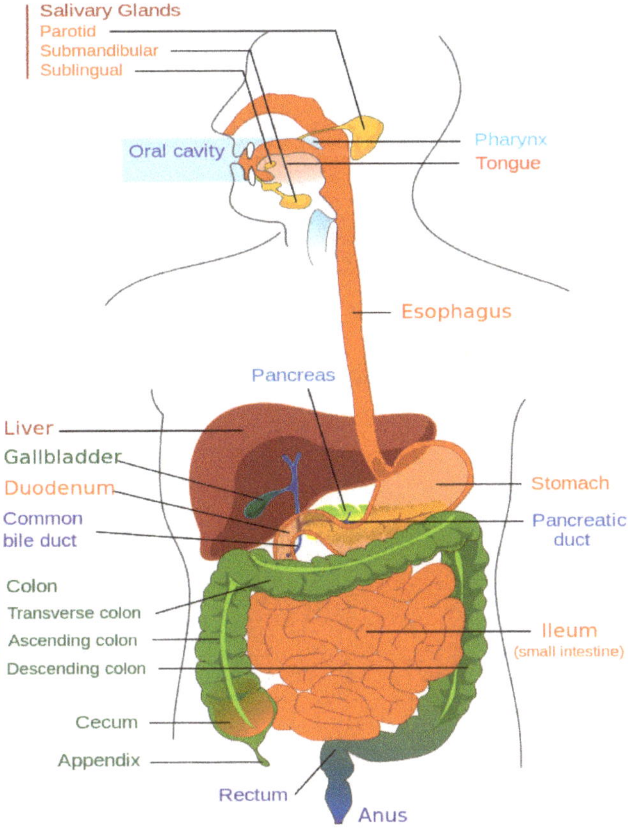
Salivary Glands
Parotid
Submandibular
Sublingual
Oral cavity
Pharynx
Tongue
Esophagus
Pancreas
Liver
Gallbladder
Duodenum
Common bile duct
Stomach
Pancreatic duct
Colon
Transverse colon
Ascending colon
Descending colon
Ileum
(small intestine)
Cecum
Appendix
Rectum
Anus

Mariana Ruiz LadyofHats, edited by Joaquim Alves Gaspar Creative Commons License

If your carwash is as sophisticated as your digestive tract, it will have a crew to make sure your side mirrors are tucked in, and a prewash scrub of your tires and residue that would otherwise be difficult for the machinery to access. The teeth, jaws, and tongue work together in a remarkable and powerful dance with very few of the missteps that would be the dance equivalent of stepping on toes, the biting of the tongue.

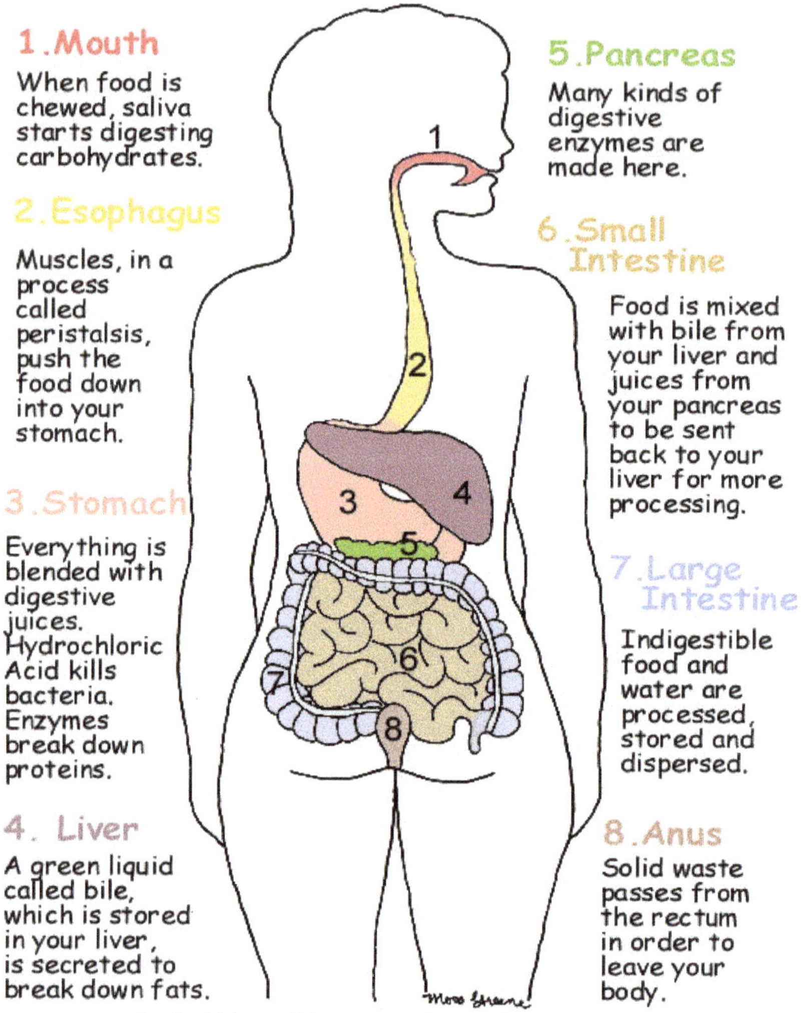
1. Mouth
When food is chewed, saliva starts digesting carbohydrates.
2. Esophagus
Muscles, in a process called peristalsis, push the food down into your stomach.
3. Stomach
Everything is blended with digestive juices. Hydrochloric Acid kills bacteria. Enzymes break down proteins.
4. Liver
A green liquid called bile, which is stored in your liver, is secreted to break down fats.
5. Pancreas
Many kinds of digestive enzymes are made here.
6. Small Intestine
Food is mixed with bile from your liver and juices from your pancreas to be sent back to your liver for more processing.
7. Large Intestine
Indigestible food and water are processed, stored and dispersed.
8. Anus
Solid waste passes from the rectum in order to leave your body.
1
2
3
4
5
6
7
8

hawkesbiology.wikispaces.com Creative Commons License

The food has to be processed into smaller more manageable portions than what is found on your plate. Your dining utensils are just the preliminary, as the teeth do the real work in preparing food for the process of digestion. The teeth are subdivided into specific categories that have unique functions.

The incisors cut the food as you bite into an apple, the canines tear the food apart as you dig into your pastrami sandwich, and your molars crush and grind the salad and crunchy vegetables you have as a side dish. The grinding and crushing break the plant cell walls apart that would otherwise protect its internal nutritious content. They also increase the surface area for food to be exposed to digestive acid and enzymes.

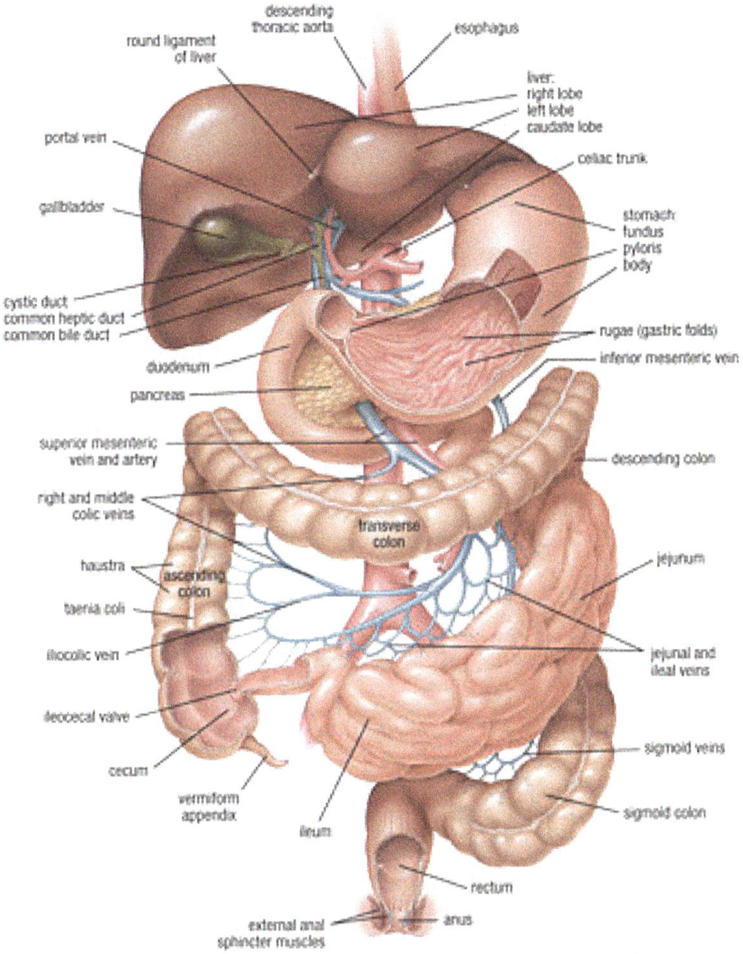
descending thoracic aorta
esophagus
round ligament of liver
liver:
right lobe
left lobe
caudate lobe
portal vein
celiac trunk
gallbladder
stomach:
fundus
pyloris
body
cystic duct
common hepatic duct
common bile duct
rugae (gastric folds)
inferior mesenteric vein
duodenum
pancreas
superior mesenteric vein and artery
descending colon
right and middle colic veins
transverse colon
jejunum
haustra
ascending colon
taenia coli
ileocolic vein
jejunal and ileal veins
ileocecal valve
sigmoid veins
cecum
vermiform appendix
ileum
sigmoid colon
rectum
external anal sphincter muscles
anus
Openstax College courses.candelalearning.com Creative Commons License

The chewing process assures that the saliva and its active enzymes are well mixed with the increased surface area of the food. They begin the process of breaking down the carbohydrates and lipids into their essential components to ready them for further digestion and absorption. The saliva also moistens the food and lubricates it for the coordinated motion of the tongue, teeth, palate, and pharynx.

These muscles and organs work together to roll it into an easy to swallow food bolus. The muscles of the swallowing process include those that protect the larynx and airway. By having the epiglottis close off the passageway to the trachea, bronchi, and lungs, it prevents aspiration into the airways as the food and saliva swallows take place. The coordinated action is developed with age, which is why small children should avoid foods, such as nuts, grapes, and larger oval or rounded candies. These foods, if misdirected into the airway, can lead to fatal choking episodes. Tragically a number of children die because the oval or rounded shape can completely block the airway. An irregular shaped object, which can still be life threatening, rarely completely obstructs the airway and usually allows some air to pass.

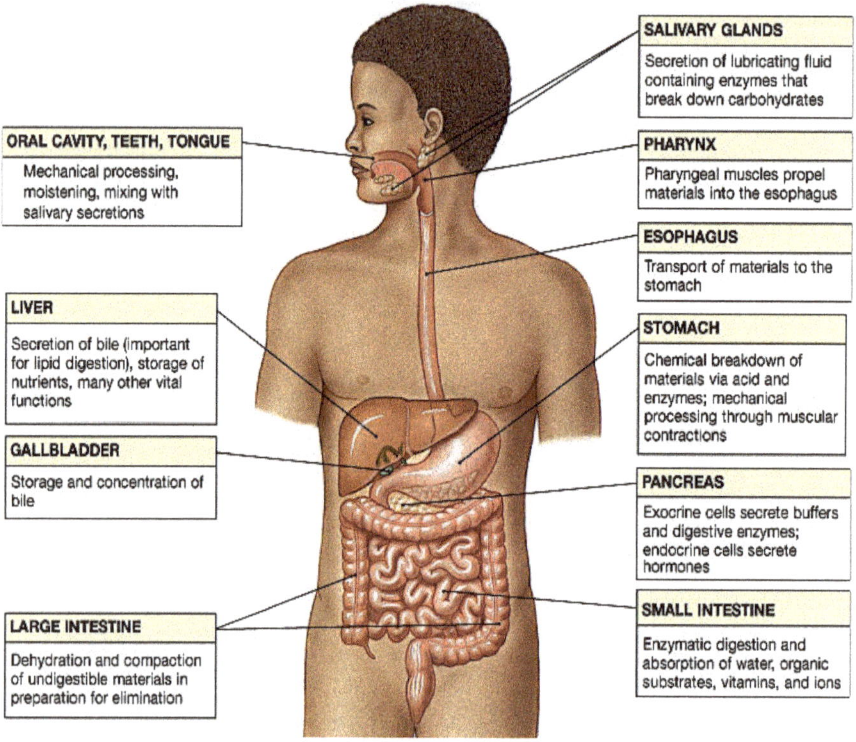
SALIVARY GLANDS
Secretion of lubricating fluid containing enzymes that break down carbohydrates
ORAL CAVITY, TEETH, TONGUE
Mechanical processing, moistening, mixing with salivary secretions
PHARYNX
Pharyngeal muscles propel materials into the esophagus
ESOPHAGUS
Transport of materials to the stomach
LIVER
Secretion of bile (important for lipid digestion), storage of nutrients, many other vital functions
STOMACH
Chemical breakdown of materials via acid and enzymes; mechanical processing through muscular contractions
GALLBLADDER
Storage and concentration of bile
PANCREAS
Exocrine cells secrete buffers and digestive enzymes; endocrine cells secrete hormones
SMALL INTESTINE
Enzymatic digestion and absorption of water, organic substrates, vitamins, and ions
LARGE INTESTINE
Dehydration and compaction of undigestible materials in preparation for elimination
Creative Commons License

The complicated swallowing neuromuscular coordination can also be affected by neurological disorders, stroke, surgery or other conditions, which may increase the risk of aspiration. Once swallowed, the food bolus is propelled down the esophagus by a coordinated snakelike muscular action called peristalsis. It is not recommended, but peristalsis is powerful enough that you can swallow against gravity while standing on your head.

The muscular valve at the junction of the esophagus and stomach is called the lower esophageal sphincter. The lower esophageal sphincter is designed to allow food and fluid to enter the stomach, with the door closed behind them once they leave the esophagus. If the valve opens at the wrong time, gastric acid, digestive enzymes, and food can flow back into the esophagus. This can lead to symptoms of heartburn or mucosal damage. If it occurs frequently gastroesophageal reflux disease (GERD) can predispose to a change in the tissue lining of the esophagus. The growth of intestinal type tissue is called a Barrett esophagus and is at a higher risk of cancer development than the normal tissue lining.

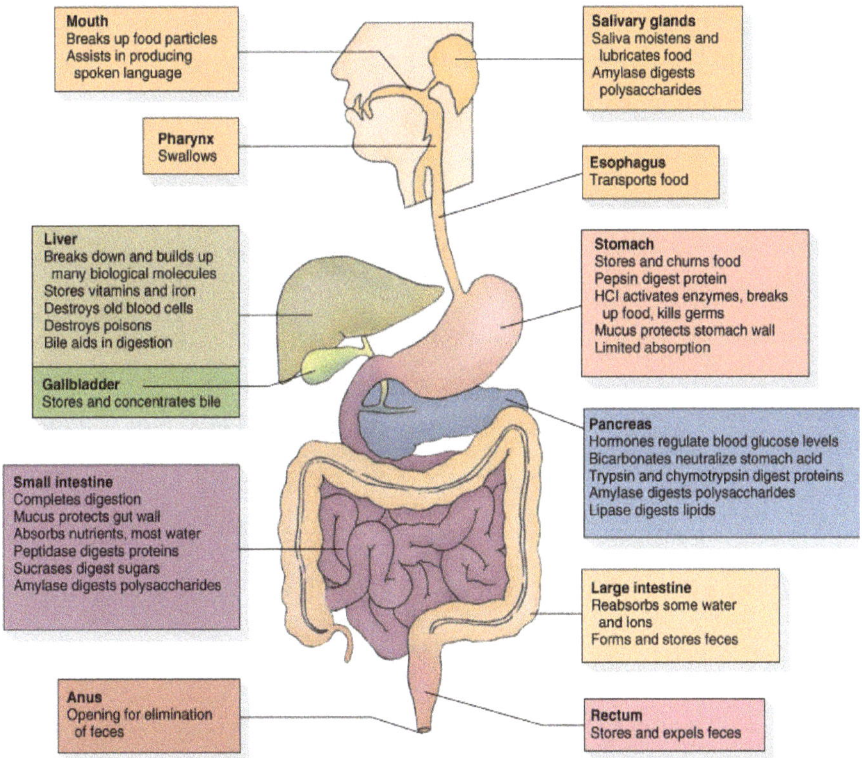
Mouth
Breaks up food particles
Assists in producing spoken language
Salivary glands
Saliva moistens and lubricates food
Amylase digests polysaccharides
Pharynx
Swallows
Esophagus
Transports food
Liver
Breaks down and builds up many biological molecules
Stores vitamins and iron
Destroys old blood cells
Destroys poisons
Bile aids in digestion
Stomach
Stores and churns food
Pepsin digest protein
HCl activates enzymes, breaks up food, kills germs
Mucus protects stomach wall
Limited absorption
Gallbladder
Stores and concentrates bile
Pancreas
Hormones regulate blood glucose levels
Bicarbonates neutralize stomach acid
Trypsin and chymotrypsin digest proteins
Amylase digests polysaccharides
Lipase digests lipids
Small intestine
Completes digestion
Mucus protects gut wall
Absorbs nutrients, most water
Peptidase digests proteins
Sucrases digest sugars
Amylase digests polysaccharides
Large intestine
Reabsorbs some water and ions
Forms and stores feces
Anus
Opening for elimination of feces
Rectum
Stores and expels feces

peptic-ulcer-disease-wikispaces.com Creative Commons License

The stomach is a churning cauldron of muscular mixing contractions, concentrated acid secretion, and potent digestive enzymes. The vagus nerve and gut hormones play a key role in the intricate balance of enzymes, acid, nutrients, and motility. When the conditions are right, the pyloric sphincter of the stomach opens to allow the acid, enzyme, and food mixture to exit. This digestive material is now called chyme as it enters the first portion of the small intestine, known as the duodenum. In Greek, this means the width equivalent to twelve fingers, which is what its small size would measure using your digits. For its small size, the duodenum plays an amazing and complex part.

The highly acid chyme would quickly damage the lining of the duodenum if it did not respond quickly with the pouring on, much like a fire extinguisher, of sodium bicarbonate. The sodium bicarbonate is produced in the duodenum itself, as well as the pancreas. The sodium bicarbonate produced in the pancreas is released through the pancreatic duct, which empties into the duodenum through the ampulla of Vater.

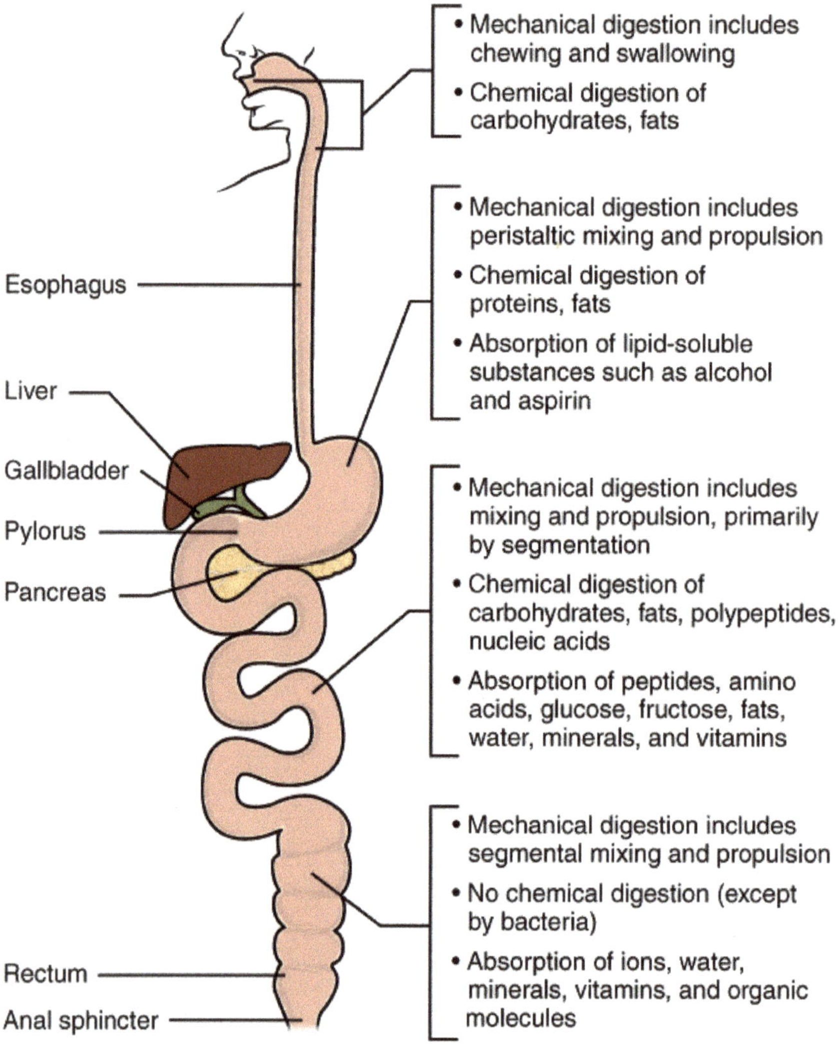
• Mechanical digestion includes chewing and swallowing
• Chemical digestion of carbohydrates, fats
• Mechanical digestion includes peristaltic mixing and propulsion
• Chemical digestion of proteins, fats
• Absorption of lipid-soluble substances such as alcohol and aspirin
Esophagus
Liver
Gallbladder
Pylorus
Pancreas
• Mechanical digestion includes mixing and propulsion, primarily by segmentation
• Chemical digestion of carbohydrates, fats, polypeptides, nucleic acids
• Absorption of peptides, amino acids, glucose, fructose, fats, water, minerals, and vitamins
• Mechanical digestion includes segmental mixing and propulsion
• No chemical digestion (except by bacteria)
• Absorption of ions, water, minerals, vitamins, and organic molecules
Rectum
Anal sphincter

Openstax College courses.candelalearning.com Creative Commons License

The fire extinguisher analogy shares another aspect of the story. Perhaps you made a fire extinguisher in a science class, or home experiment, by adding baking soda that contains sodium bicarbonate and vinegar that contains acetic acid. The active bubbling reaction that takes places is the release of carbon dioxide and water as the acid neutralizes the base. This is the same type of reaction that takes place in the duodenum, when the hydrochloric acid of the stomach meets the sodium bicarbonate released to neutralize it.

When the two react they produce water, sodium chloride commonly known as salt, and large quantities of carbon dioxide. The carbon dioxide is released as large volumes of gas that appears as bubbles arising from the reaction. The carbon dioxide is used as the active ingredient in the fire extinguisher in the science experiment since it is heavier than air, and disrupts the oxygen supply that fire requires. In the human duodenum the carbon dioxide gas generated as a side product of acid neutralization leads to bloat and distension of the gut. The body is remarkably efficient in reducing the bloat fairly quickly, in that it absorbs the carbon dioxide into the bloodstream where it travels to the lungs to be exhaled.

The bile ducts from the liver join the duct from the pancreas bringing digestive enzymes and bicarbonate that enter the duodenum through the ampulla of Vater. Within the ampulla lies the muscular sphincter of Oddi. The name sounds like a character from the story of *The Wizard of Oz*, and that would be an appropriate analogy. The coordinated release of hormones, enzymes, muscular motility, and vagus nerve input are nothing short of wizardry in action.

Major Digestive Enzymes

Enzyme	Produced In	Site of Release	pH Level
Carbohydrate Digestion:			
Salivary amylase	Salivary Glands	Mouth	Neutral
Pancreatic amylase	Pancreas	Small Intestine	Basic
Maltase	Small intestine	Small intestine	Basic
Protien Digestion:			
Pepsin	Gastric glands	Stomach	Acidic
Trypsin	Pancreas	Small intestine	Basic
Peptidases	Small Intestine	Small intestine	Basic
Nucleic Acid Digestion:			
Nuclease	Pancreas	Small intestine	Basic
Nucleosidases	Pancreas	Small intestine	Basic
Fat Digestion:			
Lipase	Pancreas	Small intestine	Basic

Subconsciously, your body can sense exactly what nutrients you have ingested. It responds by releasing the right recipe of enzymes, acid in the stomach, and bicarbonate in the duodenum, adjusting the pH as necessary. It adds just the correct amount of bile to the mix, controls the timing and volume of stomach emptying, and controls the speed of transit and intensity of mixing contractions through the length of the intestinal tract. The majority of the sensing and control feedback takes place in a small confined space the width of twelve fingers, the duodenum.

The breakdown products of the digestive process are absorbed through villi. They are the long finger like projections of the gut mucosal lining that dramatically increases the surface area for digestion and absorption. The villi are in continuous motion and are a major contributor to intestinal stirring and mixing. In spite of the relatively long length of the small intestine, its absorptive capacity would not be sufficient to maintain nutrition for an organism the size of a human without modifications to increase its surface area.

It looks like a field of waving wheat stalks, each upstanding villus is ready to use its enzymes and absorptive capacity to absorb nutrients. If you looked under the microscope you would find that each villus has thousands of even smaller villi on its surface, given the appropriate name of microvilli. All of these folds of absorptive tissue, if flattened out, would provide the equivalent absorptive capacity of a championship tennis court. This long tunnel of eagerly awaiting absorptive villi is about twenty feet long, and it is an amazingly efficient system of digestion and absorption.

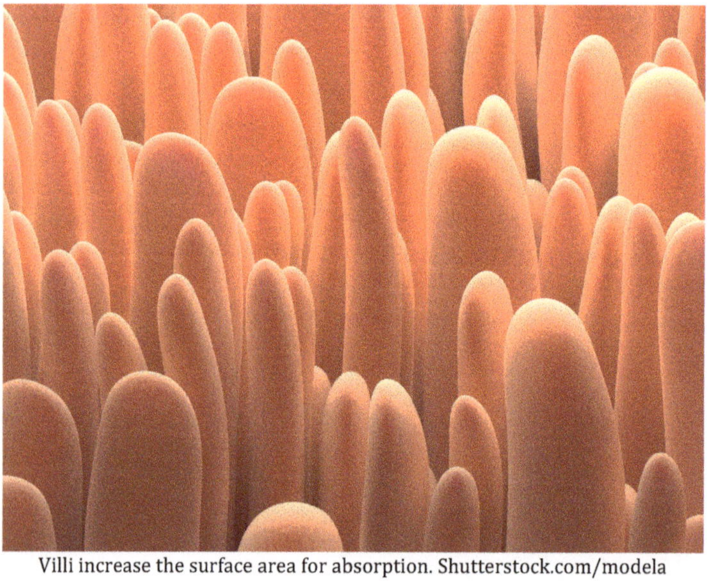

Villi increase the surface area for absorption. Shutterstock.com/modela

If injured, the ability of the small bowel to digest and absorb nutrients is compromised. A condition that temporarily damages the small intestine, such as a viral or bacterial gastroenteritis often called a stomach flu, can cause a blunting or shortening of the villi. The villus blunting will also lead to the loss of digestive enzymes that reside on the villi. A condition known as celiac disease (also known as gluten sensitive enteropathy, celiac sprue, non-tropical sprue, or sprue) is characterized by gluten induced damage to the villi resulting in blunting and impaired absorption of nutrients.

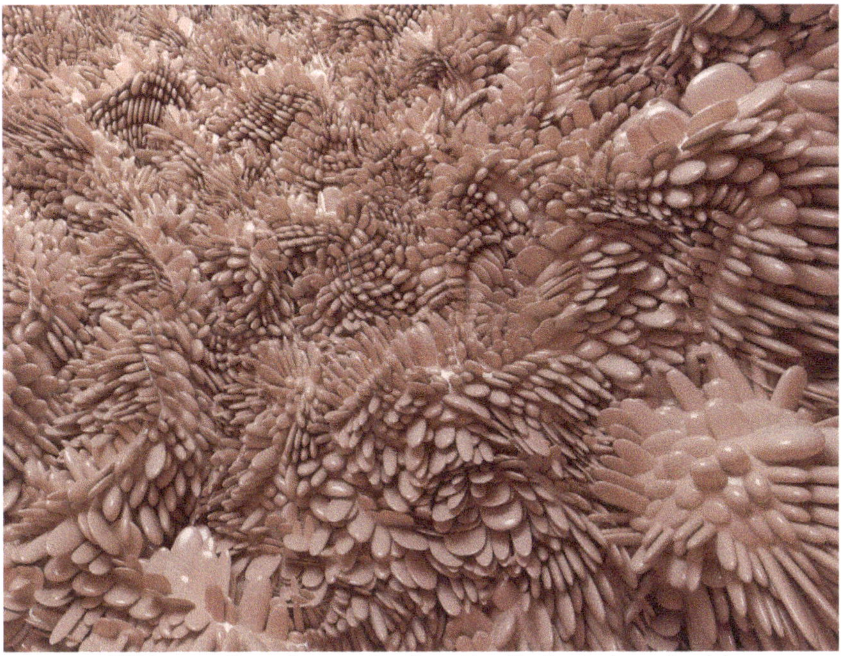

Villi increase the surface area for absorption. Shutterstock.com/modela

Without the ability to digest and absorb nutrients, the unabsorbed material can cause what is known as an osmotic diarrhea. This is one of the reasons people are often advised to avoid dairy products for a week or so after stomach flu to allow the villi and enzymes to recover. If you eat or drink lactose without waiting until the recovery is complete, you may end up with symptoms of temporary lactose intolerance such as gas and diarrhea.

When the liquid chyme leaves the jejunum and ileum of the small intestine, it goes through the ileocecal valve to enter the colon. In the cecum of the colon lies the infamous appendix, which for thousands of years mystified science as to its purpose. It looks like its function has finally, and only very recently, been identified. It stores a reservoir of intestinal bacteria, representing the healthy gut microbiome, from which the gut flora can be replenished after a bout of intestinal dysentery.

The gut microbiome is much more important than most people give it credit for. The microbes of the body far outnumber the number of human cells. In fact, if you simply go by the number of cells and not their mass, they outnumber human cells by ten to one. If you look at the proportion of genes in this unified living system, over ninety-nine percent of the genes are from microbes, and only one percent are human. In other words, you as a living system are only a fraction human, and the vast majority microbes!

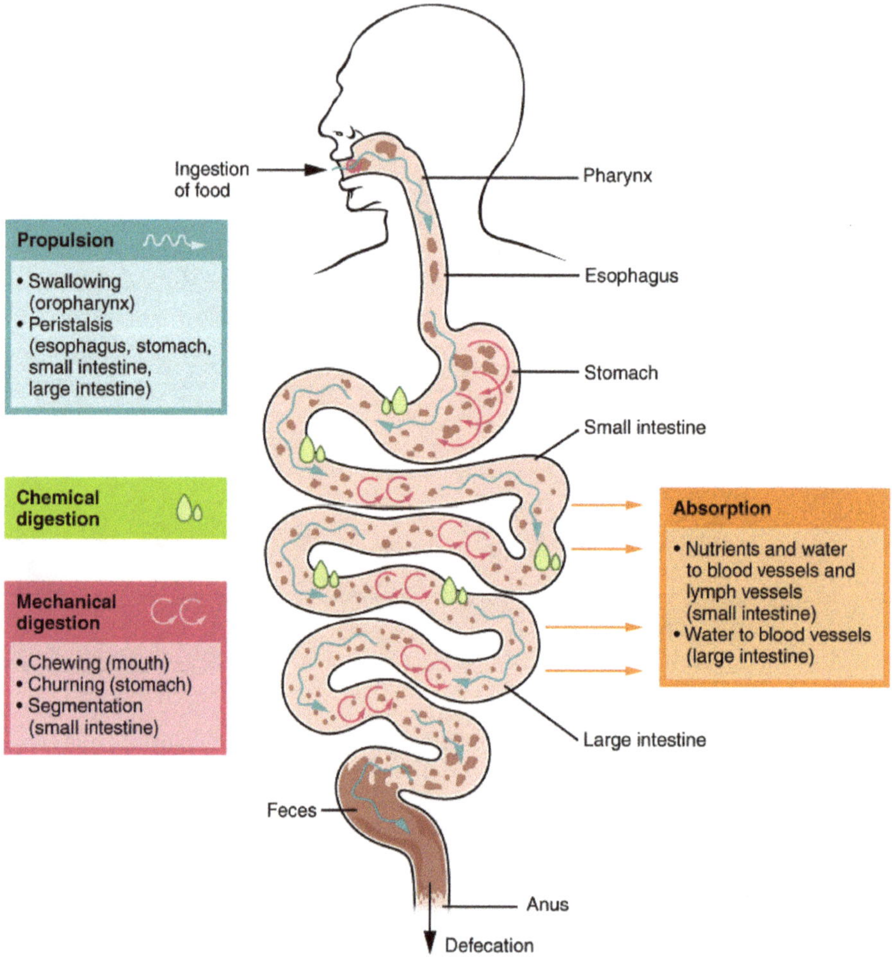
Ingestion of food
Pharynx
Esophagus
Stomach
Small intestine
Large intestine
Feces
Anus
Defecation
Propulsion
• Swallowing (oropharynx)
• Peristalsis (esophagus, stomach, small intestine, large intestine)
Chemical digestion
Mechanical digestion
• Chewing (mouth)
• Churning (stomach)
• Segmentation (small intestine)
Absorption
• Nutrients and water to blood vessels and lymph vessels (small intestine)
• Water to blood vessels (large intestine)

Openstax College philschatz.com Creative Commons License

The majority of the microbes living within and on us are commensals. This means that they are engaged with us in a symbiotic relationship from which we both benefit. They are able to process foods that would otherwise be indigestible, and convert them to absorbable nutrients and metabolites. It is not an understatement to say that they are a requirement for our health and well-being. The gut microbiome also plays a very important role in the gut-brain-microbiome-food axis, which provides for the communication of important information between its four components.

The colon, unlike the small intestine, is less involved in the digestion of foods and nutrients. It is primarily involved in the absorption of water and sodium as well as some fat-soluble vitamins such as vitamin K. The colon removes the excess moisture from the watery chyme, and the stool solidifies as it transits the gut. The ability to conserve water is very important, and without this ability the risk of dehydration would be substantially increased. The feces (also called stool, excrement, shit, and other euphemisms listed in Appendix B) are stored in the rectum and sigmoid colon awaiting the right opportunity to be eliminated through defecation.

A process or illness that impairs the colon's absorption of water will lead to more fluid in the stool and diarrhea. The loss of water and electrolytes in diarrhea may lead to dehydration, which unfortunately remains a life threatening condition in many parts of the world, especially for infants and children. If the elimination is delayed, the moisture continues to be absorbed and the stools can become harder resulting in constipation. Constipation itself aggravates the condition as the feces become harder and more difficult to pass the longer they remain in the colon. The more common treatments for constipation attempts to increase the moisture content of the feces.

The feces excreted can provide information about bowel health. For most people going about their daily activities, the passage of the feces itself is the end of the story of digestion. For other organisms, including the common housefly and dung beetle, the feces is a source of nutrition. For them the elimination of feces is just the beginning of their story of digestion, and can play an important role in the transmission of disease back to humans.

Anal Canal

The anal canal is the distal and terminal portion of the large intestine of the gastrointestinal tract, with the anus being the outlet for digestive waste. In the long tube like structure of the gastrointestinal tract, the term proximal means closest to the mouth, and distal means closest to the anus. In the intestines the term terminal means the end of the tube like structure. It is not used as the term for the end of life like the phrase terminal illness, it is more like the use of the word as in train terminal, where the travel and line ends.

The proximal portion of the anal canal begins at the superior aspect of the pelvic diaphragm, where the rectal ampulla narrows. This is at the level of the U-shaped sling formed by the puborectalis muscle. The canal is approximately one and one-half inches (three and one-half centimeters) long. The distal aspect of the anal canal ends at the anus itself, the terminal outlet of the alimentary canal.

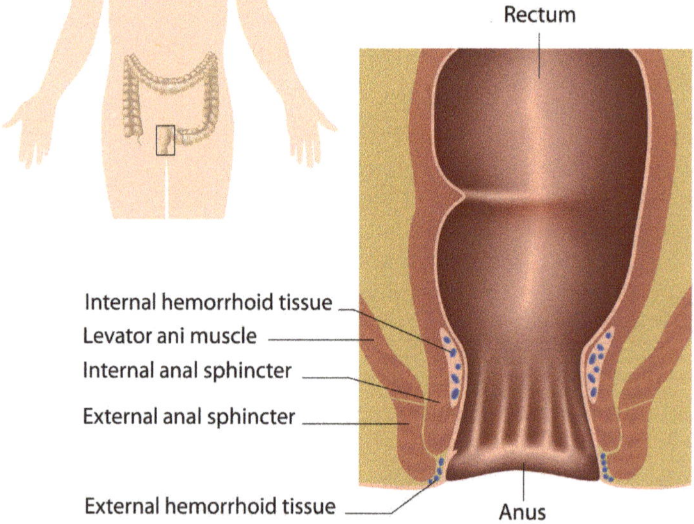
Rectum
Internal hemorrhoid tissue
Levator ani muscle
Internal anal sphincter
External anal sphincter
External hemorrhoid tissue
Anus
shutterstock.com/AlilaMedicalMedia

To fully describe anal function, a more detailed discussion of its anatomy and physiology is required. For those not needing or wanting more detail you can end your reading of this entry right here.

Fecal continence is a function of the coordinated activity of the involuntary internal and voluntary external anal sphincters. The sympathetic nervous system maintains the tone of the involuntary internal sphincter. This tone allows it to remain closed, except during filling of the rectal ampulla. The rectoanal inhibitory reflex is the involuntary internal anal sphincter relaxation in response to rectal distention. This reflex is one reason why an enema can be promptly effective in stimulating a bowel movement.

The anal sphincter tone may also be relaxed and inhibited during parasympathetic stimulation inducing contraction of the rectum. During these events, the closure must be maintained by voluntary contraction and heightened tone of the puborectalis and external anal sphincter, to prevent defecation before it is socially appropriate.

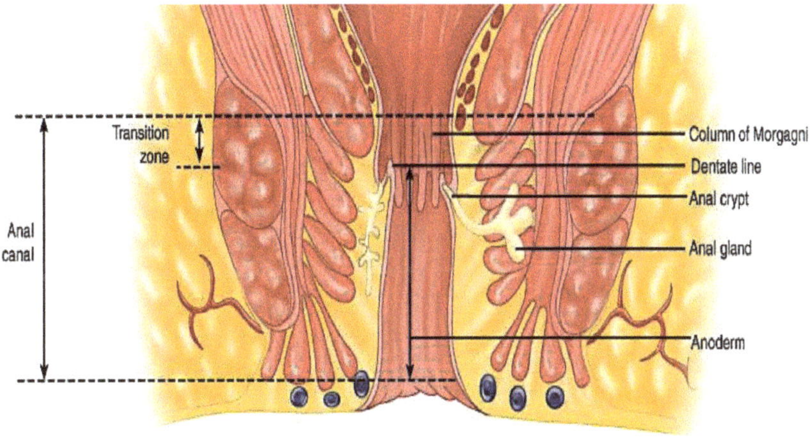
Transition zone
Anal canal
Column of Morgagni
Dentate line
Anal crypt
Anal gland
Anoderm

www.knowyourbody.net/wp- Creative Commons License

Internally the pectinate line is a visible landmark that demarcates the transition from visceral to somatic innervation and vascular supply. The canal is surrounded by superficial and deep venous plexuses, which normally have a varicose appearance. The hemorrhoidal vascular plexus contributes to the maintenance of fecal continence.

The external anal sphincter is usually under voluntary control. The sphincter is a large muscle forming a broad band across both sides of the lower two-thirds of the anal canal. The external anal sphincter is supplied through the inferior rectal nerve, which also serves the levator ani and puborectalis. They contract simultaneously to preserve continence when the internal sphincter is inhibited or relaxed, except during defecation. Internally the superior half of the anal canal has a series of longitudinal ridges called anal columns. Within these columns are the terminal vessels of the superior rectal artery and vein. The anorectal junction is demarcated by the proximal ends of the anal columns. It is at this point that the wide rectal ampulla narrows as it traverses the pelvic diaphragm.

The distal ends of the anal columns are bridged by anal valves. Proximal to the valves are small indentations called the anal sinuses. When compressed by feces the anal sinuses exude mucus, which aids in lubrication and the evacuation of feces from the anal canal. The distal limit of the anal valves forms an irregular line called the pectinate line. This line demarcates the junction of the superior and inferior portions of the anal canal.

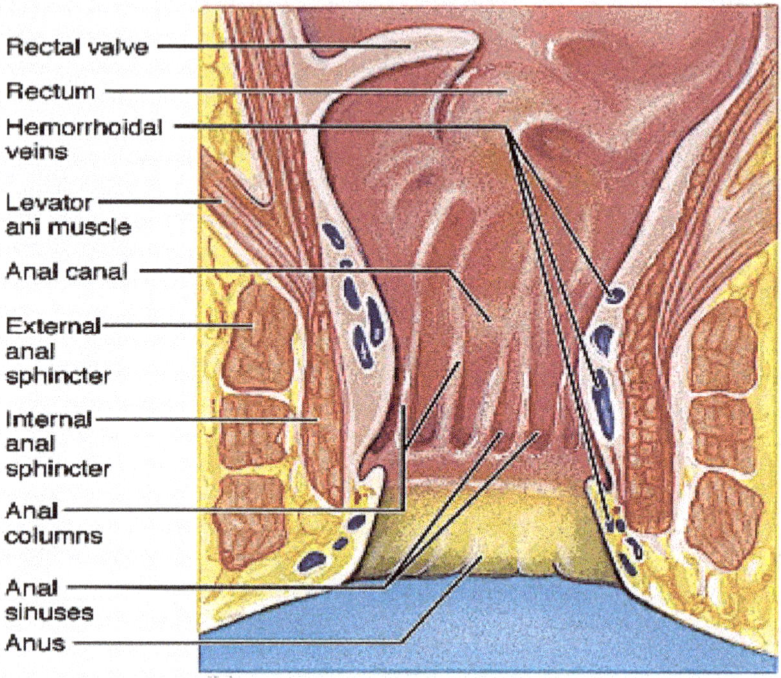
Rectal valve
Rectum
Hemorrhoidal veins
Levator ani muscle
Anal canal
External anal sphincter
Internal anal sphincter
Anal columns
Anal sinuses
Anus

Anal canal anatomy http://www.webdicine.com Creative Commons License

The anal canal proximal to the pectinate line has significant differences from the part that is distal to this landmark. The pectinate line is the anatomical landmark that separates the arterial supply, innervation, venous circulation, and lymphatic drainage of the proximal and distal portions. These differences are the result of the separate embryological origins of the proximal and distal parts of the anal canal. The proximal portion is visceral and derived from the embryonic hindgut. The distal portion is somatic and is derived from the embryonic proctodeum.

Proximal to the pectinate line, the anal canal cannot sense pain, touch or temperature. The proximal anal canal is sensitive only to stretching, which evokes sensations at both the conscious and the unconscious reflex levels. For example, distension of the rectal ampulla inhibits and relaxes the tone of the internal anal sphincter. Distal to the pectinate line, the sensory nerves of the anal canal have somatic innervation. As somatic sensory nerves they are able to sense pain, touch, and temperature. Efferent fibers of the somatic nerves cause contraction of the voluntary external anal sphincter when stimulated.

Based on the histology of cellular tissue the anal canal may be divided into three parts. The zona columnaris is the proximal portion of the anal canal and is lined by simple columnar epithelium. The distal half of the anal canal, below the pectinate line, is further divided into two zones separated by Hilton's white line. The two parts are the zona hemorrhagica lined by stratified squamous non-keratinized epithelium and the zona cutanea, lined by stratified squamous keratinized epithelium.

Anal Columns

Anal columns also known as columns of Morgagni are a number of vertical infoldings and longitudinal ridges of the mucosa and some of the underlying muscle tissue in the proximal half of the anal canal. The anal columns contain the terminal vascular branches of the superior rectal artery and vein. The distal ends of the anal columns are joined by anal valves. They are eponymously named after Giovanni Battista Morgagni (1682-1771) who also has several other anatomical structures named after him.

The anorectal junction is demarcated by the proximal ends of the anal columns. It is at this point that the wide rectal ampulla narrows as it traverses the pelvic diaphragm. The distal ends of the anal columns are bridged by anal valves. Proximal to the valves are small indentations called the anal sinuses.

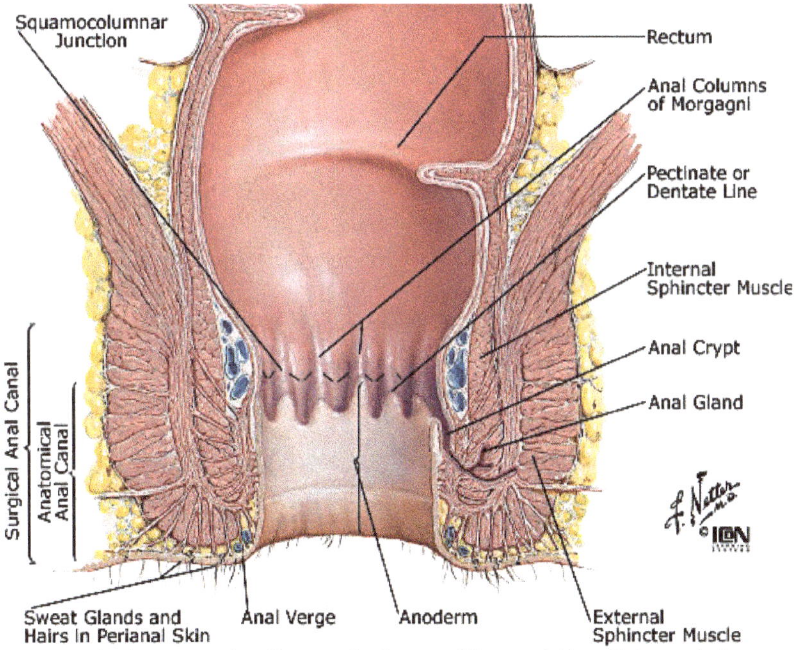
Squamocolumnar Junction
Rectum
Anal Columns of Morgagni
Pectinate or Dentate Line
Internal Sphincter Muscle
Anal Crypt
Anal Gland
Surgical Anal Canal
Anatomical Anal Canal
Sweat Glands and Hairs in Perianal Skin
Anal Verge
Anoderm
External Sphincter Muscle
Anal anatomy identifying anal columns of Morgagni. id.medicine.ucsf.edu

When compressed by feces the anal sinuses exude mucus, which aids in lubrication and the evacuation of feces from the anal canal. The distal limit of the anal valves forms an irregular line called the pectinate line. This line demarcates the junction of the superior and inferior portions of the anal canal.

Anal Expulsiveness

Anal expulsiveness describes a personality trait found in individuals who may exhibit emotional outbursts, disorganization, arrogance, rebelliousness, cruelty, and general carelessness. The term derives from the field of psychoanalysis developed by the Austrian psychiatrist Sigmund Freud (1856-1939).

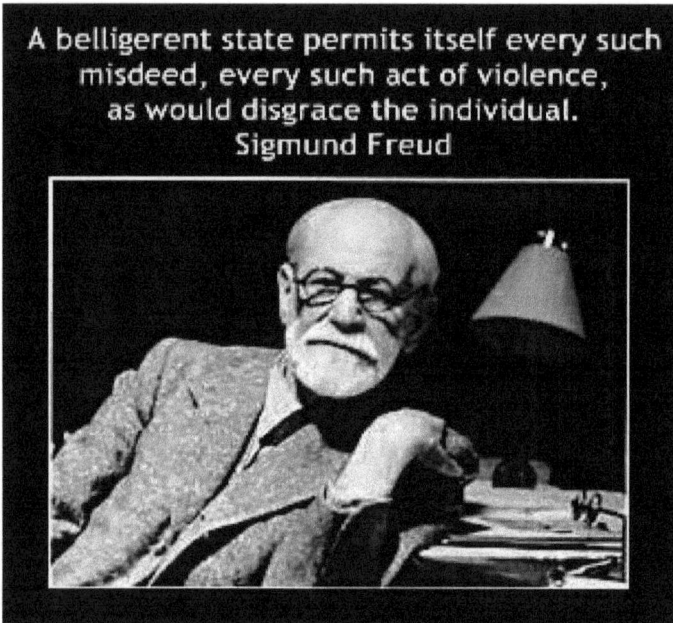
A belligerent state permits itself every such misdeed, every such act of violence, as would disgrace the individual.
Sigmund Freud

Sigmund Freud. ww1.prweb.com/Predators.png

In Freudian psychology the anal stage follows the oral stage of infant or early-childhood development. The infant's attention and focus are said to be redirected from oral stimulation to anal stimulation usually associated with the bowels but occasionally the urinary bladder. This occurs during the course of the toilet training phase and learning to control excretory functions.

For a child in this stage of development control of bowel movements allow for the expression of autonomy by withholding, refusing to comply, or soiling oneself. Conflicts with parents regarding toilet training can produce a fixation in this stage, which according to the theory can result in the development of erotic pleasure in defecation that continues through adulthood.

Anal Glands

The anal glands or sacs are sebaceous glands located in the anal canal of many mammals including dogs and cats that secrete a liquid used in the marking of territory. The anal glands are emptied passively with the passage of solid feces. With soft or loose stools the glands may not be sufficiently emptied and impaction can develop. Humans have anal glands as well, and can identify the scent of their own feces and flatus.

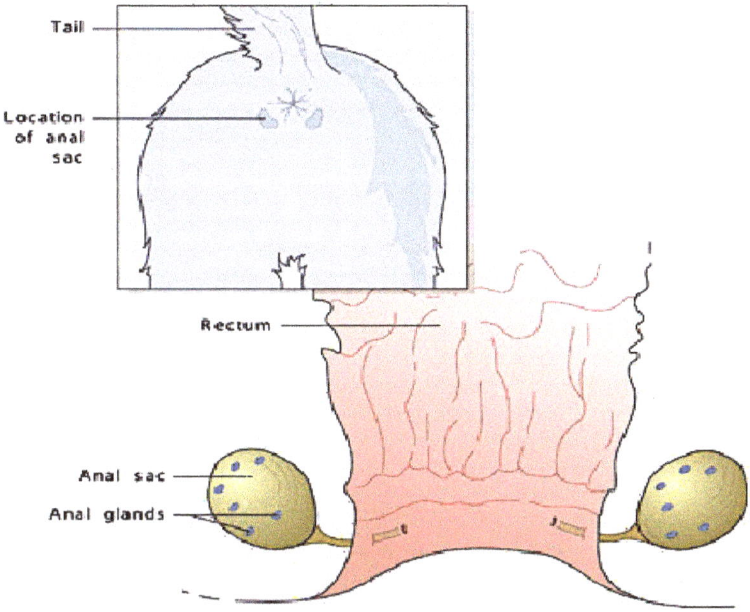
Tail
Location of anal sac
Rectum
Anal sac
Anal glands

Anal glands. www.michigananimalhospital.com

Irritation or impaction of the glands can lead to pruritus ani (anal itching), perianal pain, and abscess formation. Perirectal abscess is a very painful and potentially dangerous condition that responds to antibiotics after surgical incision and drainage. Perirectal fistula may also develop and are often associated with an inflammatory bowel condition such as Crohn disease. Perianal disease such as abscess, fistula, and fissures are best treated early for pain relief and healing.

In dogs, these glands may be referred to as 'scent glands', and butt sniffing is a means of identification of territorial markers. If the anal glands are impacted it can lead to scooting its bottom on the ground or floor, tail chasing, or licking and biting the anus. Dog groomers often perform anal sac expression for the hygiene and comfort of the animal. In cats impacted glands can cause defecation outside of the litter box. Skunks anal glands generate the foul smelling spray the utilize as a defense mechanism.

Anal Glands, Musk

Musk (Sanskrit muskies - testicle) is a class of aromatic substances used in perfumery. It is also used in Ayurveda, the traditional medical healing system developed in ancient India, where it is considered a life-saving drug in cardiac, mental, and neurological disorders. Musk was obtained from a gland of the now endangered male musk deer. By weight it is has three times the value of gold. The organic compound responsible for the musk odor is mascon. Nearly all musk used in perfumes today is synthetic.

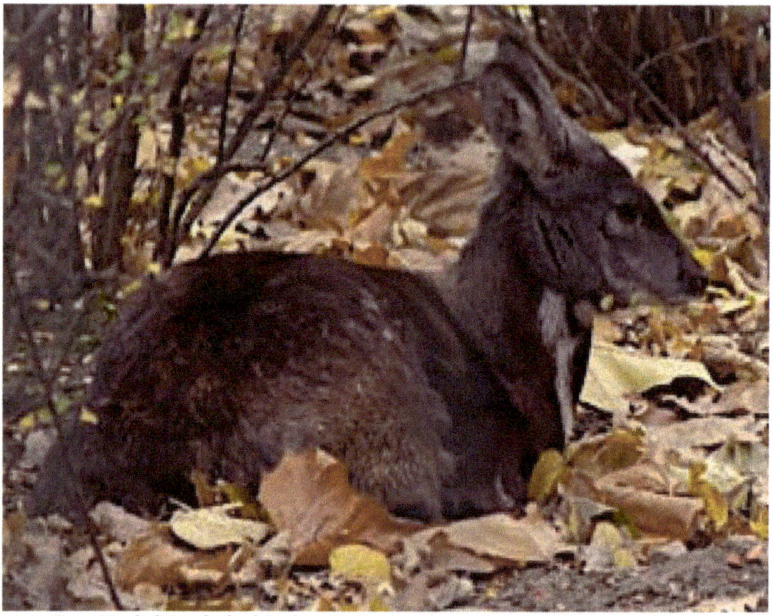

Deer Musk (Moschidae)Author: F. Spangenberg Creative Commons License

Throughout history high quality musk was stored in special containers and vessels made of gold, silver or brass. These were often placed in the royal palace for its intoxicating fragrance. Musk is produced in a special gland found in a hairy sac midway between the stomach and the genitals of the musk deer *Moschus moschiferus*. The name musk is derived from the Sanskrit term muska, which means testicle. This is actually a misnomer as the musk gland is not the testicle and the hairy sac in which it is anatomically located is not the scrotum.

The musk deer is a shy and nocturnal animal that is about three feet in length and one and a half feet tall. Hunters have historically resorted to entrapment to capture the musk deer. Its natural habitat is in the Himalaya Mountains, highlands, and forests of Tibet, as well as Siberia, and northwest China. Somewhat ironically for a product named after the testicle, the female of the musk deer species is the primary producer of black musk. This premier product is a high quality perfume additive.

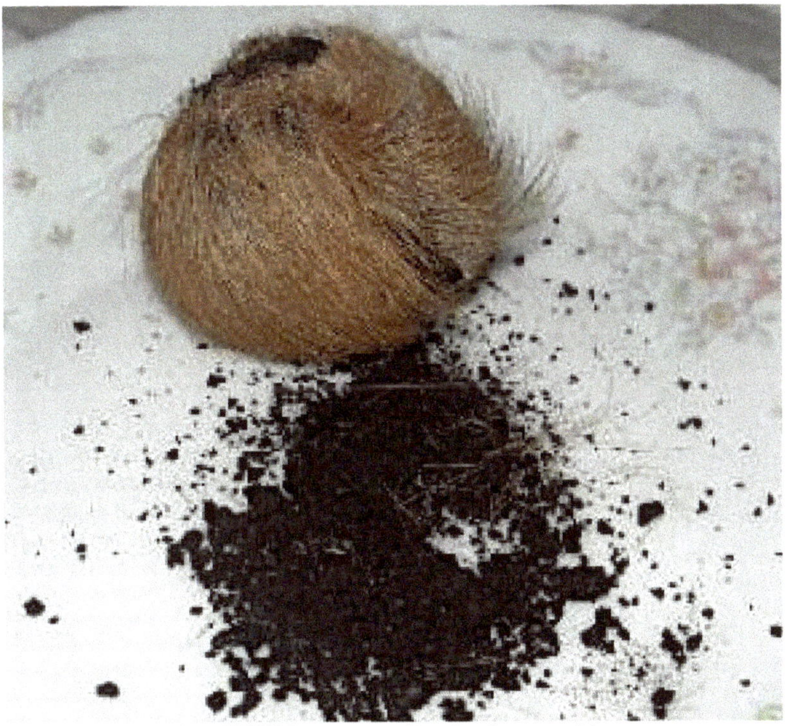

Musk sniffffffff.blogspot.com Creative Commons License

Historically, hunters would unnecessarily kill the deer for the musk sac, which is then dried under direct sunlight, or dipped in very hot oil. Musk can actually be harvested in the proper season without killing the animal. The musk deer whose life has been spared may be available for future musk harvesting. Musk comes from several countries including China, Tibet, Nepal, and Siberia in Russia.

Anal Glands, Skunk

Skunks (also called polecats) are mammals related to the ferret, which spray a liquid with a strong offensive odor from their anal glands as a defense mechanism. The skunk can aim the spray, which contains sulfur containing thiols and mercaptans, accurately over a distance of over ten feet (three meters). They are generally reluctant to release their spray, as it takes them up to two weeks to replenish the supply once dispensed.

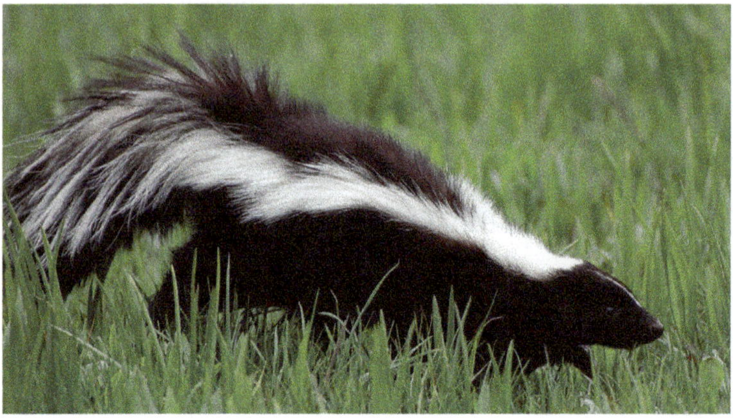

Shutterstock/JamesColeman

Anal Hygiene

Anal cleansing after defecation was historically accomplished with sticks, leaves, stones, clay, corncobs, water, or literally whatever was available at hand. The ancient Greeks used clay and stone. Romans used a water soaked sponge on a stick. Toilet paper has been used for the cleaning of the anus and urethra after elimination for well over one thousand years. The first recorded use of toilet paper was in China in the sixth century.

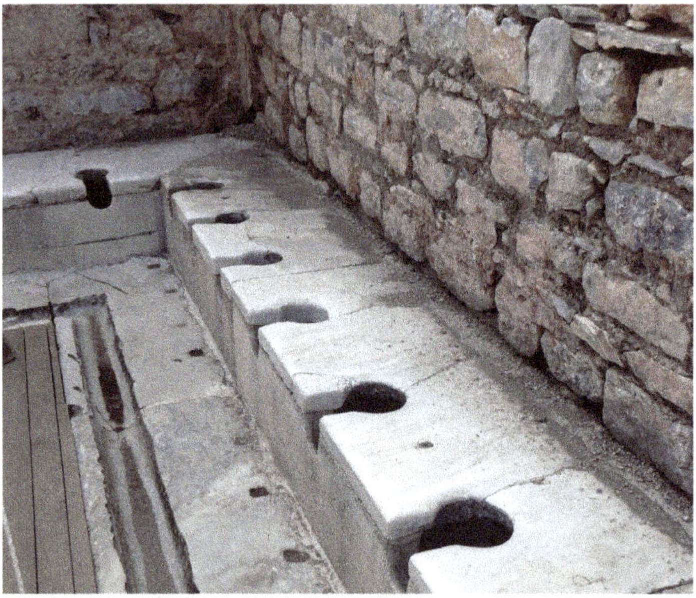

Toilets in ancient Rome had sophisticated sewer lines with running water to remove waste. Remarkably many countries around the world have more primitive systems in place today than the Romans had over two thousand years ago. shutterstock/AbelFeyman

Toilet is derived from the French word toilette meaning the act of washing, dressing, and preparing oneself. In Western society human feces waste management is usually a matter of a toilet with indoor plumbing, and a sewer or septic system. Anal cleansing after defecation was historically accomplished with sticks, leaves, stones, clay, corncobs, water, or literally whatever was available at hand. In many parts of the world only the left hand was used for wiping and cleansing after defecation. That may have contributed to the use of the right hand for social greetings and shaking hands.

The Hongwu Emperor was the first ruler of the Ming dynasty (1368-1644). Chinese imperial court documents show that fifteen thousand sheets of 'thick but soft' perfumed toilet paper were ordered in 1393. The royal family was recorded as using 720,000 sheets of toilet paper a year. The large sheets of two feet by three feet were for general use at the court, but smaller and even better quality sheets that were three inches square were designed for the exclusive use of the imperial family.

In the United States toilet paper was often simply pages torn out of the Farmer's Almanac, or the catalog of merchants such as Sears, Roebuck. & Company. They often came with a pre-punched hole in the catalog for ease of hanging by wire in the bathroom or outhouse. A humorous spinoff on the Sears Roebuck catalog was the 'Rears and Sorebutt' catalog. New York entrepreneur Joseph Gayetty invented aloe-infused sheets of Manila hemp in 1857 that he claimed prevented hemorrhoids. The product was sold in 500 sheet packages and marketed as Gayetty's Medicated Paper. The name Gayetty was imprinted on each sheet of the patented paper, and he was happy to see his name so besmirched as his fortune increased every time his customers wiped.

In 1872 John Kimberly, Charles Clark , and other investors started a paper manufacturing company in Wisconsin. In 1874 the brothers Thomas, Clarence, and E. Irvin Scott created a competing paper company and in 1890 popularized toilet paper on a roll. Scott advertised that "over 65% of middle-aged men and women suffered from some sort of rectal disease". The Scott brothers claimed that inferior toilet paper was responsible and that "harsh toilet tissue may cause serious injury". The advertisement went on to say "ScotTissue, Sani-tissue and Waldorf are famous bathroom tissues specifically processed to satisfy the three requirements doctors say toilet tissue must have to be safe: absorbency-softness-chemical purity".

In 1901 the Northern Paper Mills in Green Bay Wisconsin developed a toilet paper that was not made from hardwood pulp, but from softer pulp. They advertised it as the first toilet tissue that guaranteed you would not get wood splinters on wiping. The appeal of not getting wood splinters on wiping with toilet paper not surprisingly led to immediate market success.

Competitors soon joined in the rush to market splinter free toilet paper.

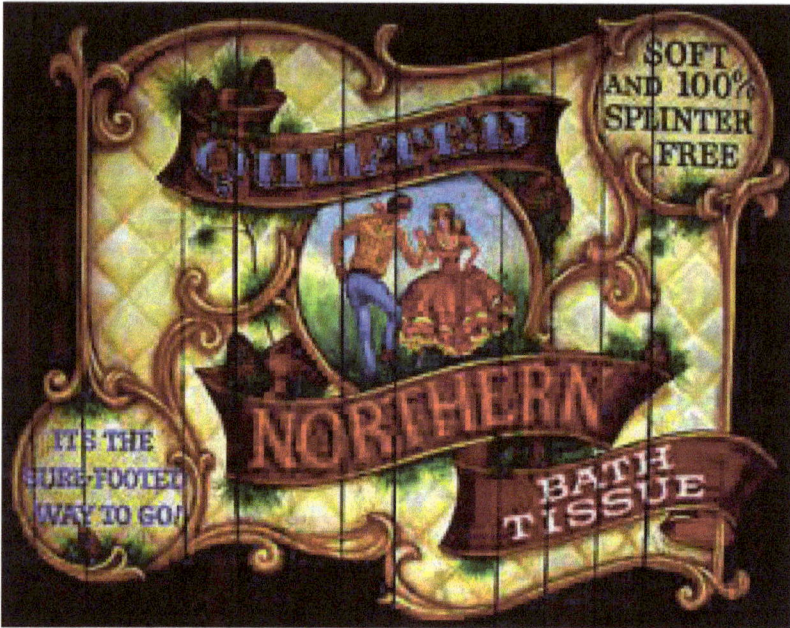
SOFT
AND 100%
SPLINTER
FREE
NORTHERN
BATH TISSUE
IT'S THE
SURE-FOOTED
WAY TO GO!

By 1925 the Scott brothers were the largest toilet paper manufacturers in the world. Acquired by Kimberly-Clark in 1995 for just under ten billion US dollars, the Scott brand name of toilet paper remains very popular. Twenty-six billion rolls of toilet paper are sold annually in the United States. Americans use an average of twenty-three and a half rolls per capita a year.

One tree produces about one hundred pounds (forty-five kilograms) of toilet paper, and global production consumes twenty-seven thousand trees daily. Perforated toilet paper for ease of tearing off sheets was patented in 1871 by New York businessman Seth Wheeler. He established the Albany Perforated Wrapping Paper Company, and toilet paper in those days was more politely referred to as wrapping paper. The patent application specified that the end of the roll of toilet paper was to be on the outside or in the 'over' position. Although the subject of ongoing debate, controversy, and arguments within a household, the official patented invention specifies 'over', and seventy percent of the public dutifully complies.

The toilet paper business in the United States is an enormous enterprise. The industry is innovative in finding ways to increase profit margins. According to the financial newspaper The Wall Street Journal in 2013 the Kimberley-Clark Corporation announced that it improved its toilet paper product by making it fifteen percent bulkier, but at the same time reduced the number of sheets by thirteen percent, a process the industry terms desheeting. Desheeting while making bulkier tissue is a money saver as Kimberly-Clark says it doesn't need additional material to make its sheets fluffier. Kimberly Clark is the largest manufacturer of toilet paper in the world with products sold in over 150 countries.

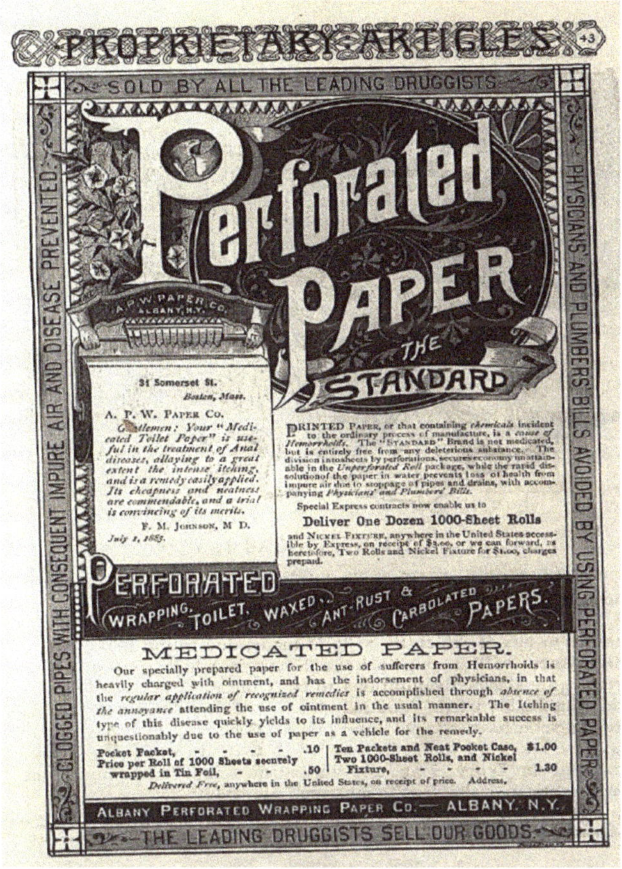
PROPRIETARY ARTICLES
43
SOLD BY ALL THE LEADING DRUGGISTS
CLOGGED PIPES WITH CONSEQUENT IMPURE AIR AND DISEASE PREVENTED.
PHYSICIANS' AND PLUMBERS' BILLS AVOIDED BY USING PERFORATED PAPER.
Perforated Paper
A. P. W. PAPER CO. ALBANY, N.Y.
THE STANDARD
31 Somerset St. Boston, Mass.
A. P. W. Paper Co.
Gentlemen: Your "Medicated Toilet Paper" is useful in the treatment of Anal diseases, allaying to a great extent the intense itching, and is a remedy easily applied. Its cheapness and neatness are commendable, and a trial is convincing of its merits.
F. M. Johnson, M. D.
July 1, 1885.
PRINTED Paper, or that containing chemicals incident to the ordinary process of manufacture, is a cause of Hemorrhoids. The "Standard" Brand is not medicated, but is entirely free from any deleterious substance. The division into sheets by perforations, secures economy unattainable in the Unperforated Roll package, while the rapid dissolution of the paper in water prevents loss of health from impure air due to stoppage of pipes and drains, with accompanying Physicians' and Plumbers' Bills.
Special Express contracts now enable us to
Deliver One Dozen 1000-Sheet Rolls
and Nickel Fixture, anywhere in the United States accessible by Express, on receipt of $3.00, or we can forward, as heretofore, Two Rolls and Nickel Fixture for $1.00, charges prepaid.
PERFORATED
WRAPPING, TOILET, WAXED, ANT-RUST & CARBOLATED PAPERS.
MEDICATED PAPER.
Our specially prepared paper for the use of sufferers from Hemorrhoids is heavily charged with ointment, and has the indorsement of physicians, in that the regular application of recognized remedies is accomplished through absence of the annoyance attending the use of ointment in the usual manner. The Itching type of this disease quickly yields to its influence, and its remarkable success is unquestionably due to the use of paper as a vehicle for the remedy.
Pocket Packet, - - - - .10
Price per Roll of 1000 Sheets securely wrapped in Tin Foil, - - .50
Ten Packets and Neat Pocket Case, $1.00
Two 1000-Sheet Rolls, and Nickel Fixture, - - - - 1.30
Delivered Free, anywhere in the United States, on receipt of price. Address,
ALBANY PERFORATED WRAPPING PAPER CO. — ALBANY, N.Y.
THE LEADING DRUGGISTS SELL OUR GOODS.

Toilet Paper was medicated, perforated, perfumed, and considered the state the art of anal hygiene in the mid-nineteenth century. Creative Commons License

According to Kimberly-Clark's research, Americans use on average forty-six sheets of toilet paper a day over five bathroom trips. Over eighty-three million rolls of toilet paper are manufactured in the United States each day. In 2012 companies sold over ten billion dollars of tissue and toilet paper, a two percent increase over the previous year. Seven billion rolls of toilet paper are sold each year in the United States. In the U.S. more than fifty miles of toilet paper are produced every second. A roll of toilet paper will last five days in the average U.S. household. The average American uses one hundred rolls of toilet paper (twenty thousand sheets) per year, and will require the processing of 384 trees during their lifetime to create the toilet paper they will use.

Most of the world has embraced the use of water cleansing for hygienic purposes wherever available. Approximately four billion people around the world do not use toilet paper. The use of only paper products for anal hygiene is counterintuitive, and is surprisingly still the procedure of choice in the United States and many Western countries. The last figures for toilet paper consumption by country were published over twenty years ago. The US led the world with 730 pounds of toilet paper consumption per resident each year. Other countries on the list with pounds of consumption per year for each resident included Finland 669, Belgium 565, Japan 526, Canada 505, Singapore 502, Taiwan 492, Switzerland 476, Denmark 471, New Zealand 468, Brazil 77, China 48, Indonesia 31, and Russia 28. Since the list was published Japan has moved into second place and China a rapidly rising third place.

Designer toiler papers are very popular. They come in various colors, but white remain the most popular followed by beige, and peach. Some come with embossed patterns, and others with writings, poetry, and images. The most exclusive designer toilet paper comes from Japan, where the Hanebisho Company creates handcrafted toilet paper that sells for nearly $20 per roll. It is created from the highest quality wood fiber pulp from Canada, and treated with the purest water fin Japan from the Nyodo River. The special drying process is constantly adjusted for humidity and temperature. The paper is then decorated by highly trained artisans and carefully wrapped and packaged in special decorative boxes. The product has been delivered to the residence of the Emperor of Japan for years.

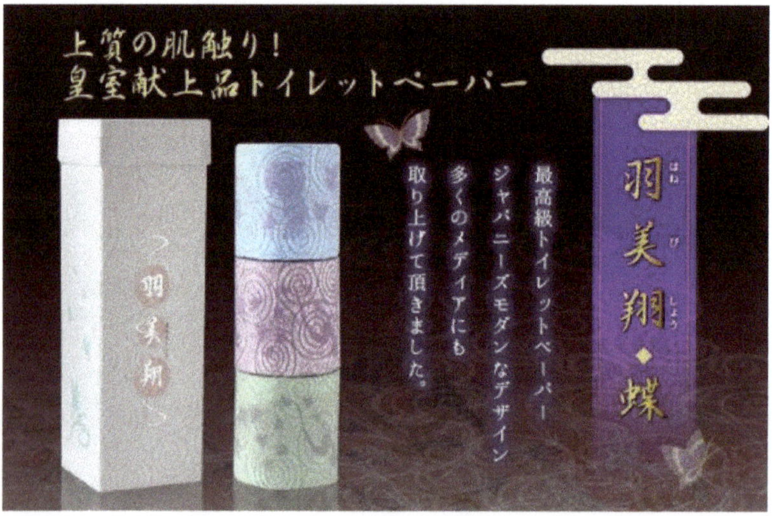
上質の肌触り！
皇室献上品トイレットペーパー
最高級トイレットペーパー
ジャパニーズモダンなデザイン
多くのメディアにも
取り上げて頂きました。
羽美翔・蝶

If you were to take toilet paper in your bare hands to wipe your pet or child's behind after a bowel movement, you would probably instantly recognize the unhygienic nature of the activity and wash your hands thoroughly. If you did not know it before now you do, toilet paper has to be at least ten sheets thick to prevent bacteria from easily transiting through the porous paper. Even double and triple folding of toilet paper allows fecal bacteria to be in direct contact with the hands. After wiping the person touches the handle to flush. It should not come as any surprise that the toilet faucet or handle has four hundred times the number of bacteria per square inch than the toilet seat.

In the United States and Western society many people wipe after a bowel movement with only porous toilet tissue paper between their fingers and fecal material. These same fingers are then often used to prepare food or pick up finger food that is often shared with others. In the United States health department codes require that restaurant and food preparation employees wash their hands after using the bathroom.

The best approach is to practice regular hand washing with an anti-microbial soap and water. The lack of hand washing after using the bathroom is commonplace, as is the lack of basic hand washing skills. The use of an ultraviolet backlight below demonstrates how the hands harbor pockets of potential sources of infection. The touching of a toilet handle and door knob on leaving the bathroom can allow the further transmission of infectious microbes.

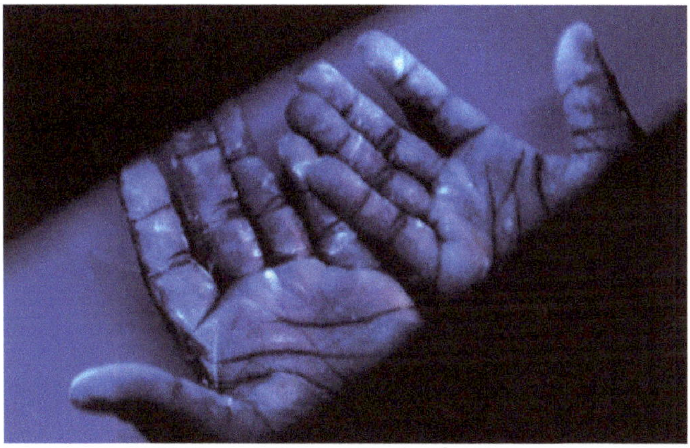

OUTFOXprevention.com. Used with Permission.

The United States Center for Disease Control publishes the following guidelines for proper hand washing. Wet the hands with clean, running water (warm or cold), turn off the tap, and apply soap. Lather the hands by rubbing them together with the soap. Lather the backs of hands, between fingers, and under the nails. Scrub the hands for at least twenty seconds. Rinse the hands well under clean, running water. Dry the hands using a clean towel or air-dry them.

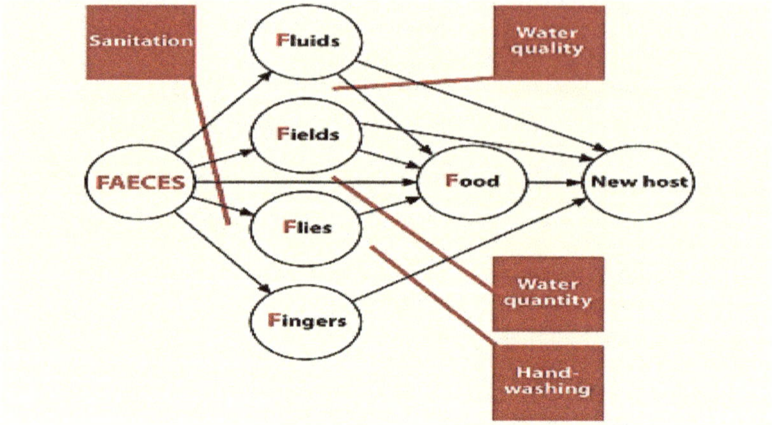
Sanitation
Fluids
Water quality
Fields
FAECES
Food
New host
Flies
Water quantity
Fingers
Hand-washing

uwcm-geog.wikispaces.com/Food+Aid Creative Commons License

The U.S. CDC advocates washing hands before, during, and after preparing food, before eating food, before and after caring for someone who is sick, before and after treating a cut or wound, after using the toilet, and after changing diapers or cleaning up a child who has used the toilet. Hand washing is also recommended after nose blowing, coughing, or sneezing, after touching an animal, animal feed, or animal waste, after handling pet food or pet treats, and after touching garbage.

Alcohol based hand sanitizers that contain at least sixty percent ethanol is also effective in reducing the transmission of contaminants and infective agents. Hopefully, the advent of high technology toilets incorporating automatic water washing features, as well as warm air blow-drying, obviating the need for toilet paper and touching the anogenital area will be more readily embraced by Western and other cultures.

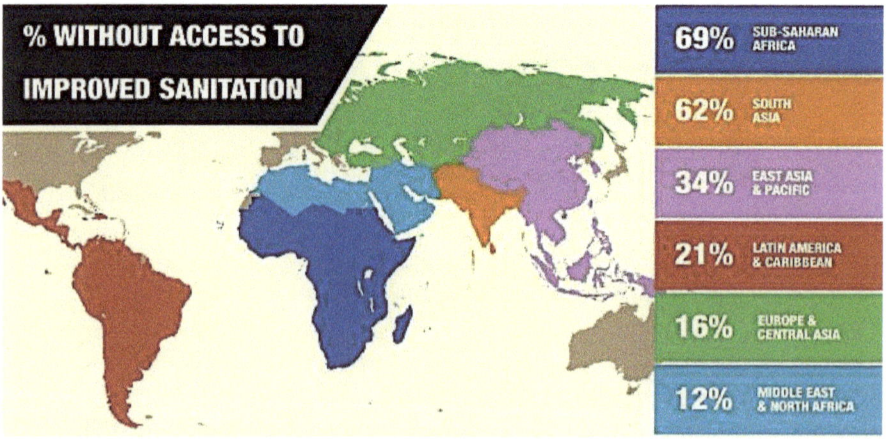
% WITHOUT ACCESS TO
IMPROVED SANITATION
69% SUB-SAHARAN AFRICA
62% SOUTH ASIA
34% EAST ASIA & PACIFIC
21% LATIN AMERICA & CARIBBEAN
16% EUROPE & CENTRAL ASIA
12% MIDDLE EAST & NORTH AFRICA

fastcompany.net Creative Commons License

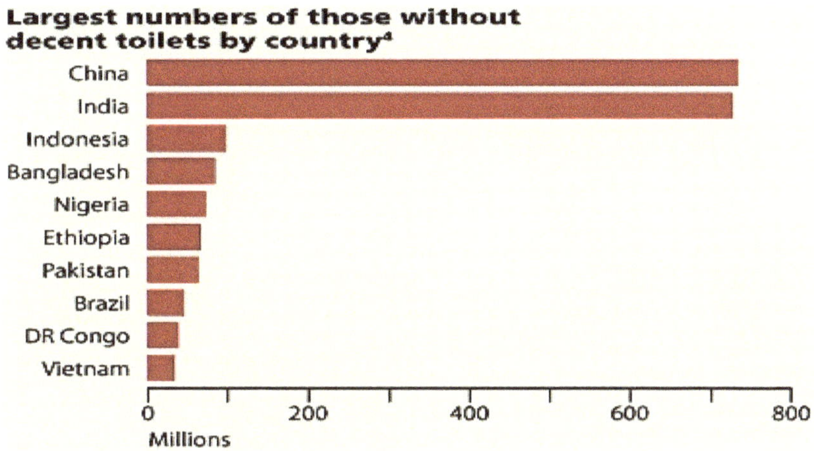
Largest numbers of those without decent toilets by country[4]
China
India
Indonesia
Bangladesh
Nigeria
Ethiopia
Pakistan
Brazil
DR Congo
Vietnam
0
200
400
600
800
Millions

uwcm-geog.wikispaces.com/Food+Aid Creative Commons License

Contrary to popular belief Thomas Crapper did not invent the indoor flush toilet. It had been developed hundreds of years before he established his manufacturing company in Victorian England. Credit for the flushing toilet is usually attributed to Sir John Harrington, a godson of Queen Elizabeth I. One rumor is that his first name is the source of the nickname 'john' for a toilet. Thomas Crapper had a successful plumbing business and the inventor Albert Giblin was an employee of his. Giblin patented a silent siphon valve and Crapper bought the patent and marketed the improved toilet from 1861-1904 at great profit and name recognition.

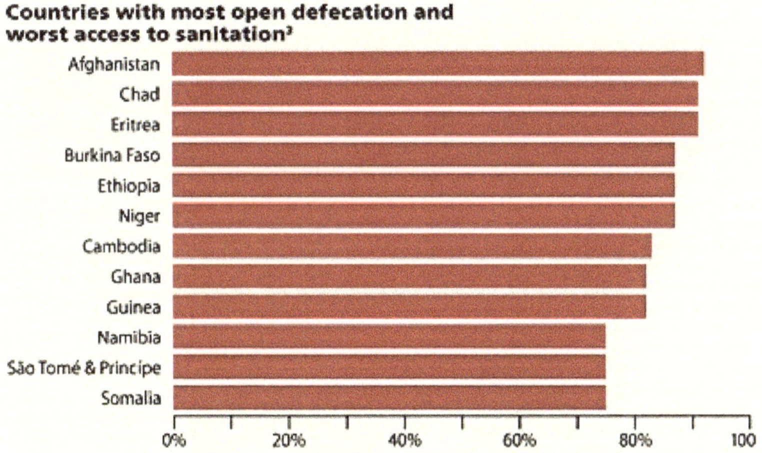
Countries with most open defecation and worst access to sanitation[3]
Afghanistan
Chad
Eritrea
Burkina Faso
Ethiopia
Niger
Cambodia
Ghana
Guinea
Namibia
São Tomé & Principe
Somalia
0%
20%
40%
60%
80%
100

uwcm-geog.wikispaces.com/Food+Aid Creative Commons License

The average person goes to the toilet 2,500 times per year, and spends a total of three years of their lifetime sitting on the toilet. For those musically inclined most toilets flush in the key of E flat. Other trivia of note, one third of Americans flush the toilet while still sitting on it, and there are 40,000 injuries a year while sitting on the toilet seat.

In France the invention of the bidet in the early eighteenth century made water cleansing popular. The word bidet means pony in French, and using the bidet required that one straddle the bowl of the bidet as if riding a pony. A bidet spray or health faucet is a hand held hose and nozzle that utilizes a water spray for perianal and genitourinary cleansing after defecation and urination. The bidet is commonplace in many countries including Spain (thirty percent), Portugal (seventy percent), Greece (eighty percent), Italy (ninety-five percent), and Japan (fifty percent). In Japan automated and high technology toilets incorporate water washing as well as air blow drying and other features. The water bidet is also very popular in the Middle East, and growing in popularity in the United States.

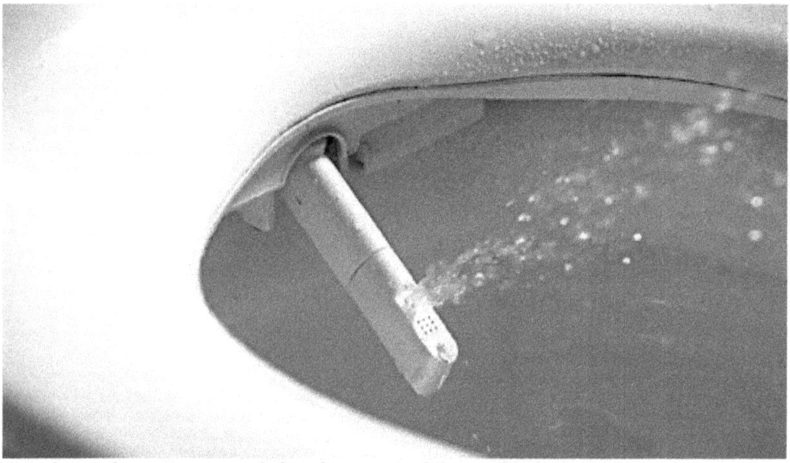

Although popular in Europe and elsewhere around the world, the United States has been very slow to adopt the preferable water based approach to anal hygiene. In addition to its increased efficacy it has environmental benefits in reducing forest product consumption and sewage disposal of paper waste products. Creative Commons License

Although popular in Europe and elsewhere around the world, the United States has been very slow to adopt the preferable water based approach to anal hygiene. In addition to its increased efficacy it has environmental benefits in reducing forest product consumption and sewage disposal of paper waste products. The reluctance of Americans to adopt the use of the bidet may be related to a misconception on the part of American and British troops during World War I. When they were first exposed to the bidet in France they assumed its purpose was purely for the washing of the genitals after sexual intercourse. The bidet incorrectly became associated as a product developed to accommodate French sexual immorality.

Although there are some very expensive models of toilets combined with bidets, the cost of an aftermarket addition of a washlet feature to a toilet is very economical. Many bidet equivalent washlets cost less than one hundred dollars, and with the savings by reduced toilet paper usage the device rapidly pays for itself. On the Indian subcontinent, in spite of the lack of bidets, over ninety-five percent of the population use water for anal cleansing. Many also use soap with water for cleansing after defecating. Use of paper is rare in this region, and hand washing after cleansing is critically important to prevent illness. In Japan the technological innovation of combining the bidet and toilet into a single product was introduced and advanced. Rapid innovations included a heated seat, automatic deodorizing, automatic lid raising and closing, directed water jets for female and male anatomy, music playing during use, vacuum fan ventilation, and warm air blow drying to obviate the need for wiping or use of toilet paper.

Genital and anal infections do not come in contact with the toilet seat in normal use. The intact skin of your buttocks is an efficient barrier against most disease organisms. Most transmission of pathogens is via the fecal to oral route is usually accomplished by way of the hands. The flush handle, sink handles, and door knob are much more likely to be a source of contamination since they are much likely to have been touched by someone whose hands had just been used to wipe their bottoms with a thin piece of toilet paper. It would be a good precaution to use toilet paper or paper towels to prevent your hands from touching the flush, faucet, and doorknobs or handles.

Most transmission of pathogens is via the fecal to oral route is usually accomplished by way of the hands. The average human stool contains three trillion microorganisms. Wiping with toilet paper nearly guarantees that the hands will come into contact with fecal microorganisms. After wiping it is not uncommon to find brown streaks on underwear because of inadequate anal hygiene. The average man's underwear contains one-tenth of a gram of feces at laundering. Another infection risk from the toilet is the splashing and aerosol formation that can occur during flushing, particularly when someone with diarrhea has used that toilet. Surprisingly one-third of Americans remain seated on the toilet when they flush, and perhaps mistakenly find the misting of their anogenital region refreshing and hygienic. If they put paper toilet seat covers down before they sit on a public toilet seat for hygienic purposes, they should definitely get off the toilet seat before they flush.

The typical toilet flush creates a mist of contaminated water droplets that can travel up to twenty feet in all directions. It includes fecal matter and pathogens that settle on any exposed surface in the flush zone, including toothbrushes, drinking cups, bath toys, handles and doorknobs. The mist can stay airborne for up to two hours and be easily inhaled. The microbial pathogens can live on surfaces for up to a week. Before you flush, lower the lid to keep the aerosolization and spread to a minimum. Worldwide there are approximately two million fatalities every year due to diarrhea. The majority of these are in children under five years of age. Simple routine hand washing with soap and water could reduce the incidence of diarrhea by approximately fifty percent, and respiratory infections by about twenty-five percent. Hand washing also reduces the incidence of skin diseases, eye infections, and intestinal worms and parasites.

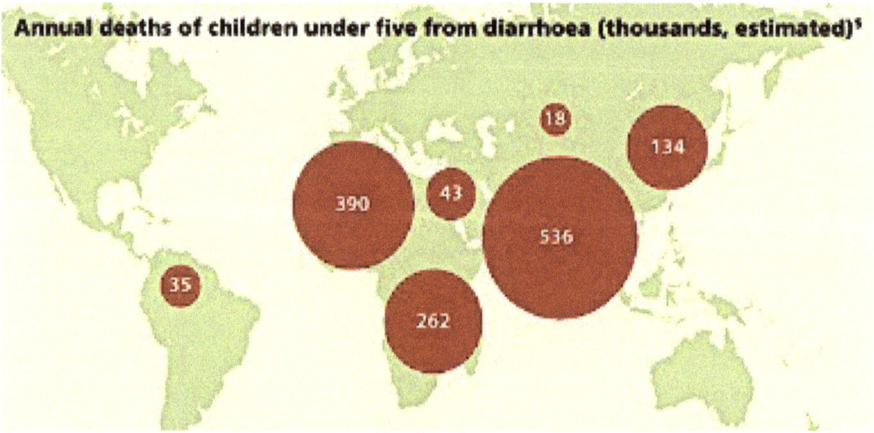
Annual deaths of children under five from diarrhoea (thousands, estimated)[5]
18
134
390
43
536
35
262

uwcm-geog.wikispaces.com/Food+Aid Creative Commons License

In most cultures and faiths food is not stored, prepared, or consumed in the vicinity of a toilet area. Both Islam and Judaism have a brief prayer of thanksgiving to be offered after the body functions of eliminating waste and the washing of hands. With the risk to health and wellness from exposure to human waste, religious customs and practices often offered practical guidance and hygiene to avoid disease. Istinja (Arabic: استنجاء), a component of Islamic hygiene practices, is the cleansing away of any residue and impurities (najasat) that remain after being passed from the urethra or anus. Istinja requires the use of water if available, and may be utilized with water alone or in combination with toilet paper. If water is not available stones, soil, or other natural material (other than bone or dung) may be utilized in the process known as 'istijmar'. The passage of intestinal gas alone does not require Istinja

Xylospongium, also known as *sponge on a stick*, is a device used to clean the perianal area after a bowel movement. It consists of a wooden stick (Greek: ξύλον, *Xylon*) with a sponge (Greek: Σπόγγος, *Spongos*) fixed at one end. In the *baths of the seven sages* in Ostia, a fresco from the 2nd century contains the Inscription *(u)taris xylosphongio* which is the first known mention of the term. Also in the early second century a papyrus letter of Claudius Terentianus to his father Claudius Tiberianus uses the term *xylospongium* in a phrase.

Shit stick is a thin stake or stick used for cleaning the perianal area after a bowel movement. It is used when water or toilet paper was not available for this purpose. The term has also been used in Chinese Buddhism and Japanese Buddhism. A well-known example is *gānshǐjué/kanshiketsu* (乾屎橛 "dry shit stick") from the Chan/Zen *gōng'àn/kōan* in which a monk asked "What is Buddha?" and Master Yunmen/Unmon answered "A dry shit stick". The presumed logic for such language was that most of the great masters of these schools did not directly state what they wished to convey. They often used a shout, or strike with a rod, or striking phrase as above to place their student in a state between comprehensibility and incomprehensibility. According to this logic it somehow promoted their development of enlightenment." Another explanation was that Zen Buddhist masters used the image of a dry shit stick to neutralize and balance of our image of a true person as sine thing other than pure or noble.
Ancient Roman latrines in Ostia Antica

Gaki zōshi 餓鬼草紙 "Scroll of Hungry Ghosts", a *gaki* condemned to shit-eating watches a child wearing *geta* and holding a *chūgi*, c. 12th century. People have used many different materials in the long history of anal cleansing, including leaves, rags, paper, water, sponges, corncobs, earthenware, pottery, and sticks. In ancient times, instruments made from bamboo, possibly in the form of spatulas ([*cèchóu*] 厠籌, [*cèbì*] 厠篦, or [*cèjiǎn*] 厠簡), may have been used with water for cleansing after a bowel movement. the assistance of water in cleaning the body after defecation.

Japanese *chūgi* from the Nara period(710-784), shown with modern toilet paper for size comparison. When monks and missionaries introduced Buddhism into China and Japan, they also brought the Indian custom of using a *śalākā, a* small stake, stick, or rod for wiping away fecal residue after a bowel movement. Translators rendered this Sanskrit word into a number of different terms based on the words of *chóu* or *chū* 籌 "small stake or stick", or *jué* or *ketsu* 橛 "short stake or stick". Such teens included the Chinese *cèchóu* 厠籌 and Japanese *chūgi* 籌木. The custom of using shit sticks became popular and had the advantages of being inexpensive, washable, and reusable.

The Chinese invented paper around the 2nd century BCE, and toilet paper no later than the 6th century CE, when Yan Zhitui noted, "Paper on which there are quotations or commentaries from the Five Classics or the names of sages, I dare not use for toilet purposes". The earliest Japanese flush toilets date from the Nara period (710–784), when a drainage system was constructed in the capital at Nara. It was designed as squat toilets built over 4 - 6 inch (10–15 cm) wide wooden conduits that users would straddle. Archaeological excavations in Nara have also found numerous *chūgi* wooden sticks that were used for fecal cleansing. Ming Dynasty Xuande Emperorplaying *touhu*, 15th century.

Chinese *chóu* and chóumù or Japanese chū 籌 or *chūgi* 籌木 (with 木 "tree; wood") and *cèchóu* 厠籌 (with 厠 "toilet") "small stake; stick" are used as the equivalent terms meaning "shit stick". The Buddhist Sanskrit term *śalāka* or *śalākā* (Pali *salākā*) is its equivalent and may be a small stake, stick, rod, or twig. In Indian Buddhist contexts, *śalākā* can also represent a stick used for purposes other than anal hygiene. particularly meant "a piece of wood or bamboo used for counting or voting". *Salaka-Grahapaka* was the wood or bamboo sticks used in counting votes in general assembly. The Jain term *salakapurusa* "illustrious or worthy person" compounds *salaka* "stick used for voting" and *purusa* "person". *Chou* 籌 originally meant "arrow used in *tóuhú* (an ancient game wth competition on the number of arrows thrown into a pot)" or "tally stick (used in counting)". *Chóu* 籌 "shit stick" was first described in writing around the 3rd century CE. The Jin dynasty (265-420) *Yulin* 語林 by Pei Qi 裴啟 has stories about the ostentatious bathrooms of wealthy merchant Shi Chong 石崇 (249-300) who mocked the politician Liu Shi 劉寔 (220-310) for not being familiar with the perfumed shit sticks offered by two female bathroom attendants.

Chinese *jué* or Japanese *ketsu* 橛 "short wooden stake; stick; peg; post" is compounded with *shi* or *shǐ* 屎 (written with 尸 "body" and 米 "rice") "shit; excrement; dung" into Japanese *shiketsu* or Chinese *shǐjué* 屎橛 "shit stick". The famous term *gānshǐjué* or *kanshiketsu* 乾屎橛 "dry shit stick", modified with *gān* or *kan*乾 "dry, dried; hollow", occurs in a famous Chan *gōng'àn* or Zen *kōan* recorded in *The Gateless Gate*. Kan-shiketsu 乾屎橛 Excrement-wiping spatula. A Zen word of abuse for a person who clings to things. Kan-shiketsu Japanese, literally a "dry shit stick"; a Zen expression designating a person who is attached to the world of appearance. Chinese *bì* 篦 "fine-tooth comb; spatula" or Japanese *hera* 篦 "spatula; scoop" is compounded into Chinese *cèbì* 厠篦 "toilet spatula" and Japanese *kusobera* 糞篦 "shit spatula" or *kusokakibera* 糞掻く篦 "shit scratching spatula". While most Japanese "shit stick" words have Sino-Japanese roots such as *chūgi* from *chóumù* 籌木 , both *kuso* 糞 "shit; crap" and *hera* 篦 "spatula; scoop" are native Japanese terms. Chinese *cèjiǎn* 厠簡 or 厕简 "toilet stick" is a synonym of *cèchóu* 厠籌 using the word *jiǎn* 簡 "bamboo and wooden slips". During the time of Queen Zhou the Elder (r. 961-964), a monk used a sharpened toilet stick to remove a tumor.

The English language has some *shit(e) stick* parallels in its lexicography parallel to these Asian language terms. The *Oxford English Dictionary* (shyte, shite, shit) quotes two early *shit-stick* examples: "a hard chuffe, a shite-sticks" (1598) and "a shite-sticks, a shite-rags, that is to say, a miserable pinch-pennie" (1659); and defines poop-stick as "a fool, ineffectual person", with the earliest usage in 1930.

Anal Hygiene, Toilet Contamination

Genital and anal infections do not come in contact with the toilet seat in normal use. The intact skin of your buttocks is an efficient barrier against most disease organisms. Most transmission of pathogens is via the fecal to oral route is usually accomplished by way of the hands. The average human stool contains three trillion microorganisms. Wiping with toilet paper nearly guarantees that the hands will come into contact with fecal microorganisms. After wiping it is not uncommon to find brown streaks on underwear because of inadequate anal hygiene.

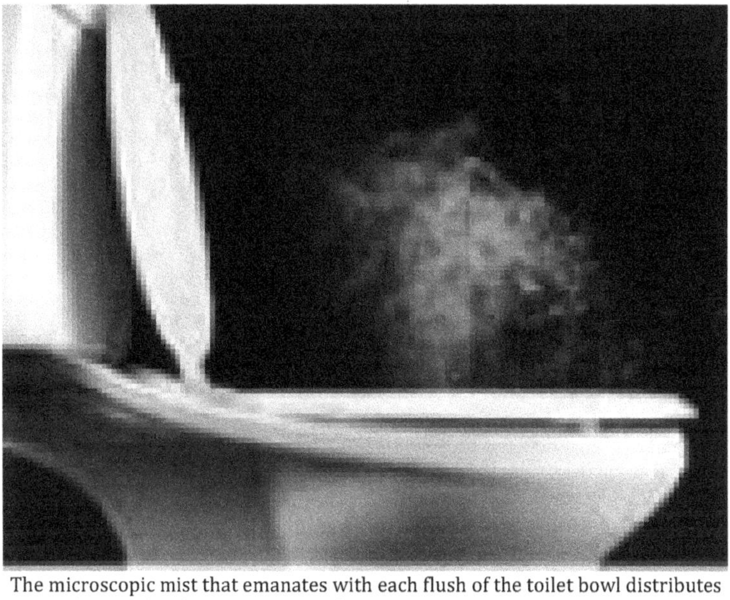

The microscopic mist that emanates with each flush of the toilet bowl distributes contaminated water droplets up to twenty feet in reach direction. Creative Commons License

The flush handle, sink handles, and door knob are much more likely to be a source of contamination since they are much likely to have been touched by someone whose hands had just been used to wipe their bottoms with a thin piece of toilet paper. It would be a good precaution to use toilet paper or paper towels to prevent your hands from touching the flush, faucet, and doorknobs or handles.

Another infection risk from the toilet is the splashing and aerosol formation that can occur during flushing, particularly when someone with diarrhea has used that toilet. Surprisingly one-third of Americans remain seated on the toilet when they flush, and perhaps mistakenly find the misting of their anogenital region refreshing and hygienic. If they put paper toilet seat covers down before they sit on a public toilet seat for hygienic purposes, they should definitely get off the toilet seat before they flush.

The typical toilet flush creates a mist of contaminated water droplets that can travel up to twenty feet in all directions. It includes fecal matter and pathogens that settle on any exposed surface in the flush zone, including toothbrushes, drinking cups, bath toys, handles and doorknobs. The mist can stay airborne for up to two hours and be easily inhaled. The microbial pathogens can live on surfaces for up to a week. Before you flush, lower the lid to keep the aerosolization and spread to a minimum.

The best approach is to practice regular hand washing with an anti-microbial soap and water. The lack of hand washing after using the bathroom is commonplace, as is the lack of basic hand washing skills. The use of an ultraviolet backlight below demonstrates how the hands harbor pockets of potential sources of infection. The touching of a toilet handle and door knob on leaving the bathroom can allow the further transmission of infectious microbes.

The United States Center for Disease Control publishes the following guidelines for proper hand washing. Wet the hands with clean, running water (warm or cold), turn off the tap, and apply soap. Lather the hands by rubbing them together with the soap. Lather the backs of hands, between fingers, and under the nails. Scrub the hands for at least twenty seconds. Rinse the hands well under clean, running water. Dry the hands using a clean towel or air-dry them.

Microbiological surveillance studies of *Escherichia coli* and other fecal bacteria have been performed in typical American household kitchens and bathrooms. The surprising finding was that toilet seats were one of the cleanest areas in the house with a very low microbe count. Faucets and refrigerator handles were more heavily contaminated. The highest concentration of microbes, more than two hundred times that of the toilet seat, were found on kitchen cutting boards. It was theorized this was from poultry, which often has fecal microbe contaminants in processing.

Public toilet seats were also surveyed and less than two percent had any *Escherichia coli* or fecal contaminants. Even this small percentage was thought to represent contamination from the water mist that is generated by flushing. The best use of the toilet seat paper protector dispensed would be to use it instead of your bare hands to touch the faucets and door handles in the bathroom. In other public places some of the highest concentrations of fecal bacteria are found on sanitary napkin dispensers, hotel TV remote control units, vending machine buttons, and drinking water fountain controls.

The following twenty-five locations were surveyed in the United States for fecal contaminants with some surprising findings. Fast food restaurants in the US serve ice that had more bacteria than the toilet water in seventy percent of locations surveyed. Public restrooms have about two million bacteria per square inch, while the average toilet seat has only fifty per square inch. The average office desk has four hundred times more bacteria than a toilet. Keyboards can have up to two hundred times more bacteria than a toilet seat. Cell phones and mobile electronic devices can have ten times more bacteria than a toilet seat, and they are frequently in close contact with the fingers, face, and mouth.

There are on average one hundred times more bacteria on restaurant menus than on restroom toilet seat. Raw meat carries a very high level of fecal bacteria, so food-chopping boards harbor more fecal contaminants than toilet seats. When the toilet is flushed the plume of toilet water with fecal contaminants often end up on toothbrushes left exposed. With two hundred thousand bacteria per square inch, carpets are four thousand times dirtier than a toilet seat. Humans shed one and one-half million skin cells every hour that helps feed the bacteria carpeting the carpets.

Most refrigerators test positive for the fecal contaminant *Escherichia coli* because thorough cleaning and disinfecting is an infrequent undertaking. Reusable shopping bags have more fecal matter than underwear and are rarely washed. In many households the television remote control is one of the most contaminated items handled. Hands are one of the dirtiest parts of the body, and they are frequently used to grasp and hold doorknobs, which are a reservoir of contaminants. Light switches can have up to two hundred and seventeen bacteria per square inch.

The kitchen sink is usually dirtier than the bathroom and is often overlooked when cleaning. The bathtub, although thought of as a place to get clean, typically harbors nearly twenty thousand bacteria per square inch around the drain. Dead skins cells, dust mites, fungal spores, pollens, and other body secretions build up on the pillow, the place the head usually rests at night. After ten years a mattress will nearly double in weight thanks to the number of dust mites and dust mite feces that it has collected. The inside rim of a pet bowl alone contains over two thousand bacteria per square inch.

Currency bank notes can harbor up to two hundred thousand bacteria. It's a good idea to wash the hands after directly handling cash and currency. It brings new meaning to those having lots of money being known as 'filthy rich'. Draperies collect pet fur, mold, dander, debris, dust mites, and dust mite feces. The warm, dark, and moist insides of showerheads are popular breeding grounds for bacteria. Handbags contain cell phone, money, hairbrush, lipstick, cosmetics, and other items teeming with contaminants. Handbags are rarely cleaned and are a notorious source of potential contaminants. The kitchen sponge is nearly always the most heavily contaminated item in the house. With ten million bacteria per square inch the kitchen sponge is nearly a quarter of a million times dirtier than a toilet seat. The toilet seat is usually very clean, and the reason is really pretty simple, it gets cleaned often.

Worldwide there are approximately two million fatalities every year due to diarrhea. The majority of these are in children under five years of age. Simple routine hand washing with soap and water could reduce the incidence of diarrhea by approximately fifty percent, and respiratory infections by about twenty-five percent. Hand washing also reduces the incidence of skin diseases, eye infections, and intestinal worms and parasites.

In most cultures and faiths food is not stored, prepared, or consumed in the vicinity of a toilet area. Both Islam and Judaism have a brief prayer of thanksgiving to be offered after the body functions of eliminating waste and the washing of hands. With the risk to health and wellness from exposure to human waste, religious customs and practices often offered practical guidance and hygiene to avoid disease.

Analingus

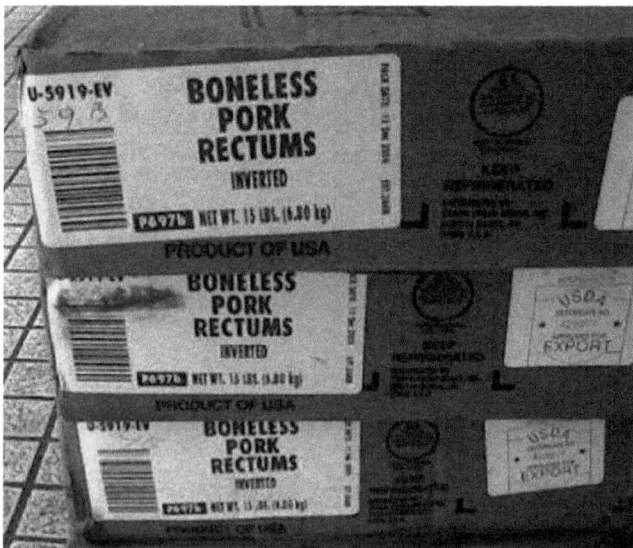
U-5919-EV
BONELESS
PORK
RECTUMS
INVERTED
PRODUCT OF USA
BONELESS
PORK
RECTUMS
EXPORT
BONELESS
PORK
RECTUMS

Although not the intended use for the word analingus, eating these delicacies may well qualify for the definition. fbcdn-sphotos-c-a.akamaihd.net Creative Commons License

Analingus (Latin *anus* + *-lingus* tongue) is a form of sexual practice that results in anal-oral contact. It is widely considered a taboo act in many cultures and parts of the world. It encourages the transmission of disease spread by the fecal-oral route and the recognition of its spread of disease may have contributed to its wide cultural recognition as a taboo practice.

Diseases which may be transmitted by anal-oral contact facilitated by analingus include shigellosis, hepatitis A, hepatitis B, hepatitis C, hepatitis E, poliomyelitis, human papillomavirus (HPV), herpes simplex virus, intestinal parasites, chlamydia, gastroenteritis, conjunctivitis, gonorrhea and other sexually transmitted infections. There is also a suggested correlation between throat cancer and exposure to the human papillomavirus that may be transmitted by analingus.

Anal Reflex

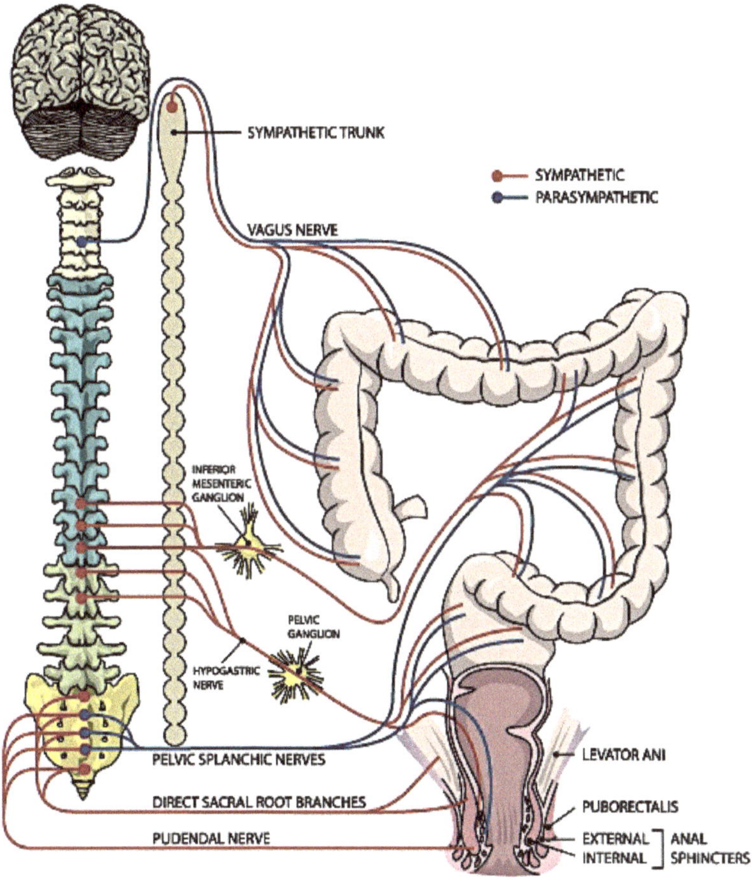
SYMPATHETIC TRUNK
SYMPATHETIC
PARASYMPATHETIC
VAGUS NERVE
INFERIOR MESENTERIC GANGLION
PELVIC GANGLION
HYPOGASTRIC NERVE
PELVIC SPLANCHNIC NERVES
DIRECT SACRAL ROOT BRANCHES
PUDENDAL NERVE
LEVATOR ANI
PUBORECTALIS
EXTERNAL
INTERNAL
ANAL SPHINCTERS

rjh.goingeast.ca/wp-content/SCI4/NeurogenicBowel Creative Commons License

The anal reflex is also known as the anal wink, perineal reflex, and anocutaneous reflex. The anal reflex is the contraction of the muscles of external anal sphincter upon stimulation of the skin around the anus. The stimulation of the perianal skin is detected by the pressure receptors known as nociceptors. The sensory stimulation is transmitted via the pudendal nerve. This reflexive response is integrated by the spinal cord sacral segments S2 through S4. Reflex anal dilation is a reflex in which the anus dilates to a diameter greater than two centimeters. The reflex response occurs with the parting of the buttocks or anal stimulation.

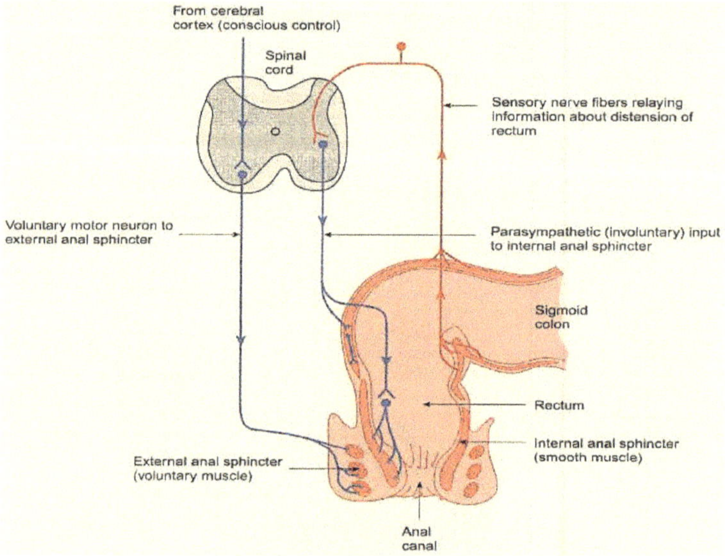
From cerebral cortex (conscious control)
Spinal cord
Sensory nerve fibers relaying information about distension of rectum
Voluntary motor neuron to external anal sphincter
Parasympathetic (involuntary) input to internal anal sphincter
Sigmoid colon
Rectum
Internal anal sphincter (smooth muscle)
External anal sphincter (voluntary muscle)
Anal canal

zavantag.com/tw_files Creative Commons License

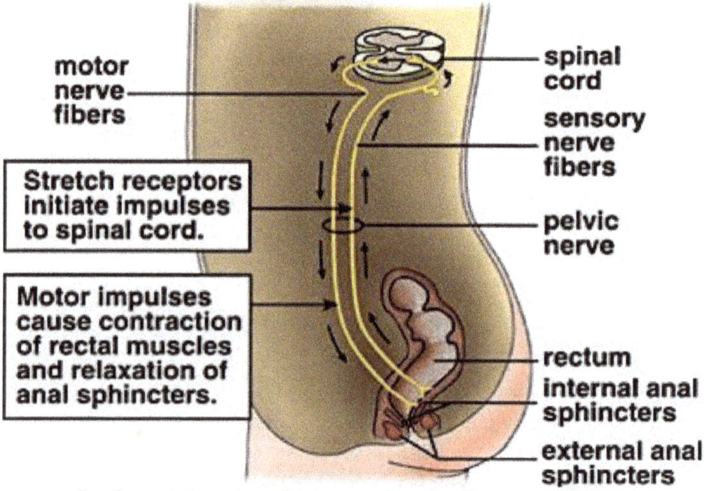
motor nerve fibers
Stretch receptors initiate impulses to spinal cord.
Motor impulses cause contraction of rectal muscles and relaxation of anal sphincters.
spinal cord
sensory nerve fibers
pelvic nerve
rectum
internal anal sphincters
external anal sphincters

hamber.vsb.bc.ca/mambo/images Creative Commons License

Anal Retentive

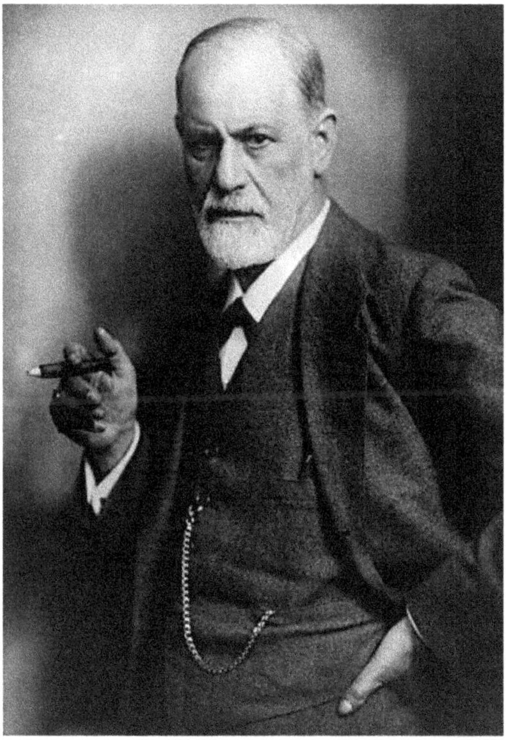

Sigmund Freud, founder of psychoanalysis Author Max Halberstadt Public Domain

Anal retentive, often abbreviated to 'anal' when describing personality traits, is an adjective used to describe a person who pays excess attention to detail. The term derives from psychoanalysis developed by the Austrian psychiatrist Sigmund Freud. In Freudian psychology the anal stage follows the oral stage of infant or early-childhood development. The infant's attention and focus are said to be redirected from oral stimulation to anal stimulation usually associated with the bowels, but occasionally the urinary bladder. This occurs during the course of toilet training phase and learning to control excretory functions.

Freud theorized that children who were in conflict with parents or others during the period of toilet training became fixated on bowel control. They developed 'anal' personality traits associated with toilet training including orderliness, stubbornness, and a compulsion for control. The term 'anal-retentive' remains in common usage, especially as a pejorative criticism. Freud's theories of causation and psychoanalysis in general have fallen out of favor. Those who reject that they have any anal-retentive characteristics are often jokingly said to have 'anal expulsive' personality types.

Anal Sex (see Anal Stimulation)

Anal Sphincter, External

The external anal sphincter is a striated muscle under voluntary control. The sphincter is a large muscle forming a broad band across both sides of the lower two-thirds of the anal canal. The external anal sphincter is supplied through the inferior rectal nerve branches from spinal nerves S4 which also serves the levator ani and puborectalis. They contract simultaneously to preserve continence when the internal sphincter is inhibited or relaxed, except during defecation.

Anatomically, the external anal sphincter is attached to the perineal body anteriorly, and to the coccyx via the anococcygeal ligament body posteriorly. The sphincter blends together with the puborectalis muscle in its proximal aspect. The sphincter has three distinct zones comprising subcutaneous, superficial, and deep parts.

When under contraction the external anal sphincter can double the pressure generated to maintain closure of the anal canal. The rectoanal inhibitory reflex is an involuntary internal anal sphincter relaxation in response to rectal distention. This allows the bowel's sampling of some of the rectal contents, which then enter into the anal canal. Here it is brought into contact with specialized sensory mucosa to detect consistency.

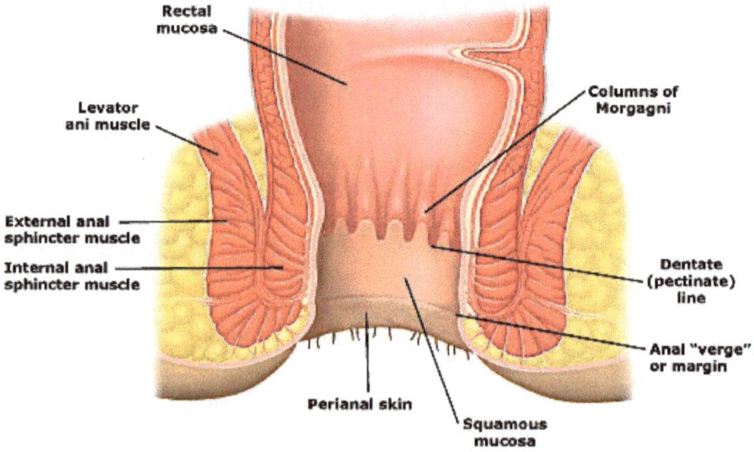
Rectal mucosa
Levator ani muscle
Columns of Morgagni
External anal sphincter muscle
Internal anal sphincter muscle
Dentate (pectinate) line
Anal "verge" or margin
Perianal skin
Squamous mucosa

Anal sphincter anatomy. www.aboutcancer.com Creative Commons License

The external anal sphincter plays only a secondary yet important role compared to the internal anal sphincter in maintaining fecal continence. When the internal anal sphincter relaxes, it is only the voluntary contraction of the external anal sphincter that is maintaining continence and preventing a bowel movement at an inopportune time.

The rectoanal excitatory reflex is initially a semi-voluntary contraction of the external anal sphincter and puborectalis muscle. This reflex returns the normal tonality of the sphincter following the rectoanal inhibitory reflex.

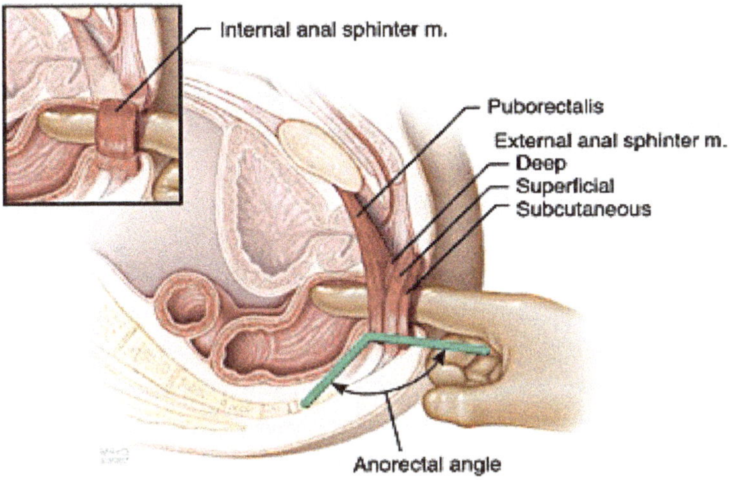
Internal anal sphinter m.
Puborectalis
External anal sphinter m.
Deep
Superficial
Subcutaneous
Anorectal angle

www.nature.com/ajg

Anal Sphincter, Internal

The internal anal sphincter is a circular muscular ring that surrounds about one to one-and-one-half inches (two-and-one-half up to four centimeters) of the length of the anal canal just proximal to the external anal sphincter. The activity of the internal anal sphincter is entirely involuntary.

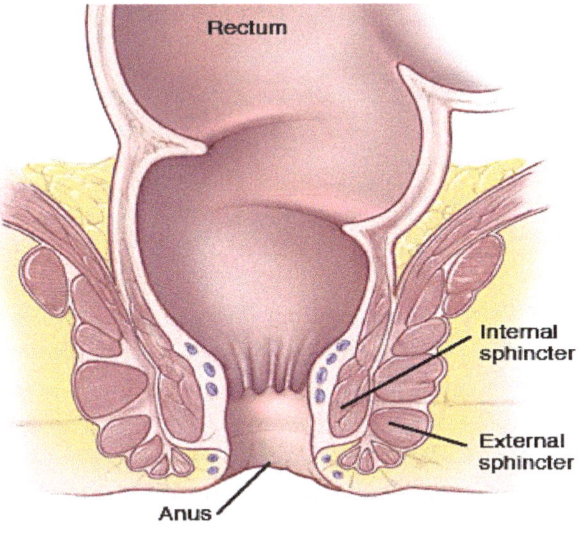
Rectum
Internal sphincter
External sphincter
Anus

www.sparrow.org/Health Library Creative Commons License

The sphincter is in continuous contraction to prevent the passage of feces and intestinal gas. Parasympathetic stimulation causes the sphincter to relax allowing the passage of material. The internal anal sphincter contributes approximately sixty percent of the tonal pressure of the anal canal and is very important for bowel continence, especially for liquid and gas.

The contraction tone is stimulated and maintained by the sympathetic fibers of the autonomic nervous system from the superior rectal and hypogastric plexuses. Contraction of the internal anal sphincter is inhibited by parasympathetic fiber stimulation. This occurs on both an intrinsic basis in relation to peristalsis, as well as an extrinsic basis via fibers passing through the splanchnic nerves of the pelvis.

This sphincter remains nearly continuously contracted to prevent leakage of fluid or intestinal gas. The internal anal sphincter is inhibited and relaxes temporarily in response to the stretching of the rectal ampulla by feces or gas. When involuntary internal anal sphincter relaxation occurs, voluntary contraction of the external anal sphincter and puborectalis muscle forming the anorectal angle are required to prevent defecation or the passage of flatus.

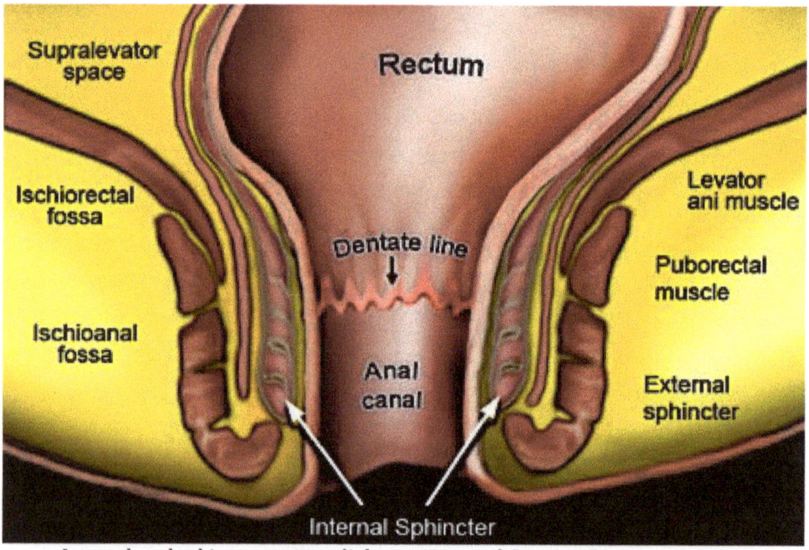
Supralevator space
Rectum
Ischiorectal fossa
Levator ani muscle
Dentate line
Puborectal muscle
Ischioanal fossa
Anal canal
External sphincter
Internal Sphincter
Internal anal sphincter www.radiologyassistant.nl Creative Commons License

When the rectum fills and the rectal walls are distended, the defecation cycle may be triggered. This begins with the rectoanal inhibitory reflex, which inhibits the contraction, thus relaxing the internal anal sphincter. A small amount of rectal contents descends into the anal canal where special receptors of the mucosa determine whether the material in the rectum is gas, liquid or solid. The rectal ampulla relaxes after initial distension when peristalsis subsides.

The internal anal sphincter tone returns to its normal baseline until the next peristalsis, or until a significant level of distension occurs. Once this occurs, the inhibition of the internal anal sphincter is continuous until distension is relieved by defecation or passage of flatus. Only the continued contraction and tone of the external anal sphincter maintains continence at this point. Disorders of the internal anal sphincter and external anal sphincter may lead to various degrees of fecal incontinence to liquids, solids, or mucus discharge.

Anal Stimulation

In both males and females, the anus actively participates in the involuntary muscular contractions of orgasm just as they are manifested in the genitalia. During orgasm in the human male the anal sphincter experiences rapid rhythmic contractions of the anal sphincter, lasting ten to fifteen seconds on average. These occur simultaneously with the orgasmic contractions of the penis and prostate. A woman's orgasm lasting twenty seconds on average consists of a series of muscular contractions of the anus in addition to the pelvic muscles, vagina, and uterus.

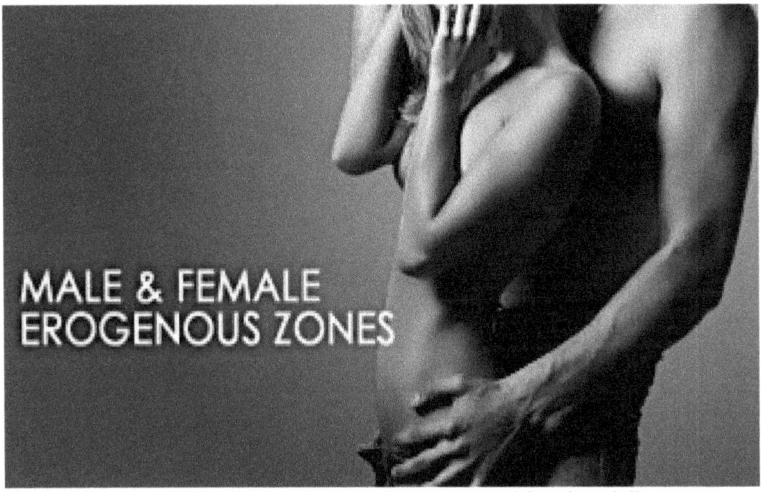
MALE & FEMALE
EROGENOUS ZONES

Anal stimulation involves an erogenous zone in males and females of all orientations.
www.romancehelpguide.com

In both sexes, stimulation of the sensory region of the anus may be pleasurable. Sexual penetration of the anus may provide concomitant prostate stimulation in the male, which may also be pleasurable. For women, anal penetration may provide local as well as indirect stimulation of the clitoral nerve endings that extend along the labia minora to the anus and by the shared sensory pudendal nerves. Contractions of the anal sphincter during orgasm may be perceived as more intense if the anal canal is physically occupied and the sphincter muscles thereby stretched to a degree.

While the responses may be pleasurable in some, in others they can be uncomfortable or painful. Supplemental lubrication, hygiene, sensitivity, and common sense are required as the anus can be injured in such activities. The hygienic preparations and precautions include avoiding introduction of any anal contamination into the vagina or urinary bladder as infections can result. Regular engagement in anal penetrative activities can affect the sphincter tone and ability to maintain anal competence to withhold the passage of gas and non-gas contents.

Anal Valves

Anal columns, also known as columns of Morgagni, are a number of vertical infoldings and longitudinal ridges of the mucosa and some of the underlying muscle tissue in the proximal half of the anal canal. The anal columns contain the terminal vascular branches of the superior rectal artery and vein. The distal ends of the anal columns are joined by anal valves. They are eponymously named after Giovanni Battista Morgagni (1682-1771) who also has several other anatomical structures named after him.

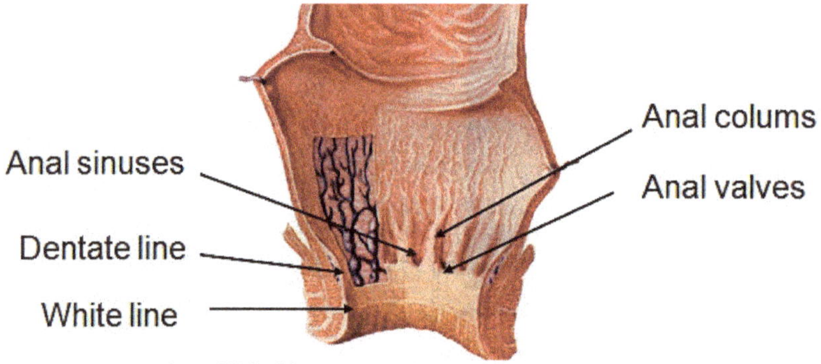
Anal colums
Anal sinuses
Anal valves
Dentate line
White line

http://3.bp.blogspot.com Creative Commons License

The anorectal junction is demarcated by the proximal ends of the anal columns. It is at this point that the wide rectal ampulla narrows as it traverses the pelvic diaphragm. The distal ends of the anal columns are bridged by anal valves. Proximal to the valves are small indentations called the anal sinuses. When compressed by feces the anal sinuses exude mucus, which aids in lubrication and the evacuation of feces from the anal canal. The distal limit of the anal valves forms an irregular line called the pectinate line. This line demarcates the junction of the superior and inferior portions of the anal canal.

Anal Wink

The anal wink, also known as the anal reflex, perineal reflex, or anocutaneous reflex, is the involuntary contraction of the external anal sphincter upon stimulation of the perianal and perineal skin. The stimulus is sensed by the nociceptors in the perineal and perianal skin. The reflex is transmitted via the pudendal nerve, which is innervated by the spinal cord sacral segments S2 through S4. Reflex anal dilation is a reflex in which the anus dilates to a diameter greater than two centimeters. The reflex response occurs with the parting of the buttocks or anal stimulation.

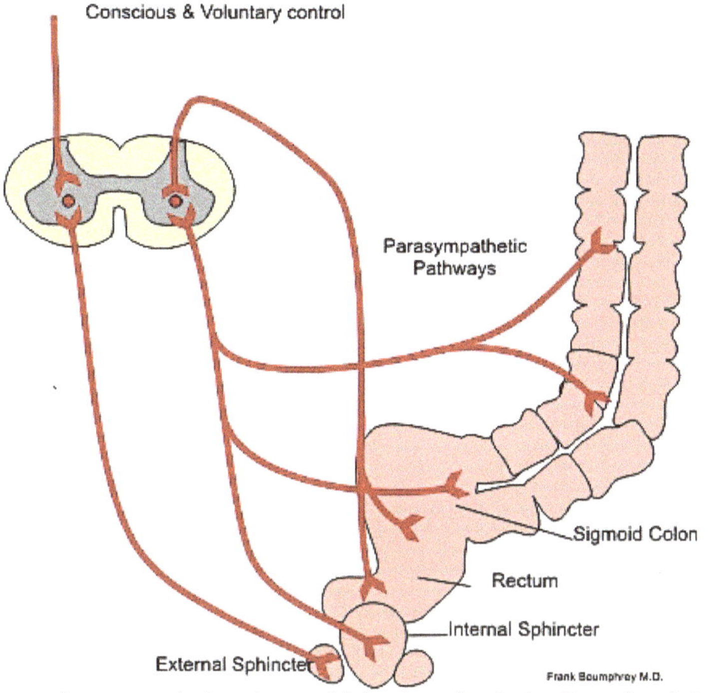
Conscious & Voluntary control
Parasympathetic Pathways
Sigmoid Colon
Rectum
Internal Sphincter
External Sphincter
Frank Boumphrey M.D.

Voluntary and parasympathetic pathways of defecation reflex Author Boumphreyfr Creative Commons License

Anoscopy

Anoscopy, proctoscopy, rectoscopy, and sigmoidoscopy are all procedures to inspect the anus, rectum, and sigmoid colon depending on the length of the instrument. Historically these instruments were always rigid tube like devices that were sometimes referred to euphemistically as the 'silver stallion'. Anoscopy using a rigid instrument does offer a better view of the anal canal because it distends the sphincter and may allow otherwise unseen anal fissures and other pathology to be visualized. Most physicians and patients prefer the more comfortable flexible instruments.

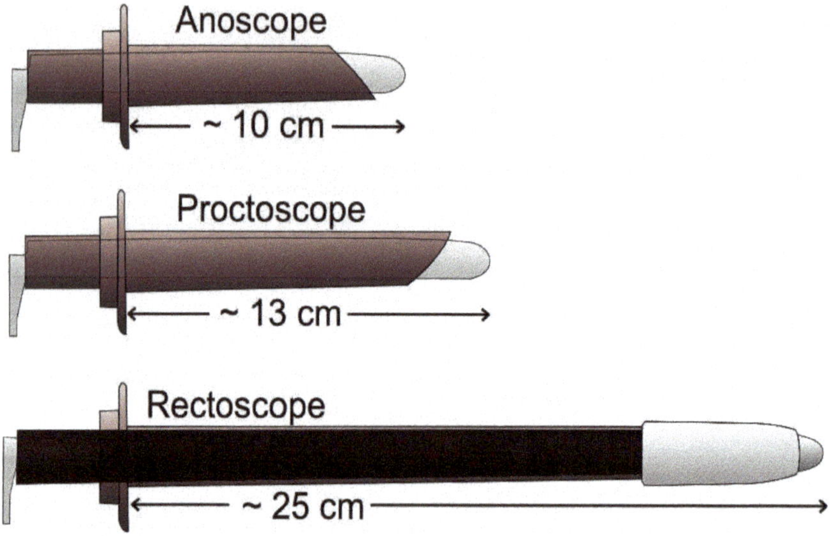
Anoscope
~ 10 cm
Proctoscope
~ 13 cm
Rectoscope
~ 25 cm

An anoscope, a proctoscope and a rectoscope, with approximate lengths.
Source: Gima International Catalogue Author Mikael Häggström Creative Commons License

Aroma, Feces

Olfaction, also known as olfactics, is the scientific term for the sense of smell. Olfaction occurs when odorant molecules bind to specific sites known as the olfactory receptors. The olfactory receptors are specialized sensory cells in the nasal cavity of vertebrates. Invertebrates, such as insects, typically house their olfactory sense organ on their antennae. In the snake the olfactants are acquired by the tongue, which taking advantage of its forked anatomy deposits them on the olfactory cells on the respective sides of the nasal cavity.

The difference in concentration of the olfactants on each side of the nasal cavity allows the receptors to discriminate and localize the source of the scent, much like binocular vision allows depth perception. Because humans and other animals have two nostrils, each with separate inputs to the brain, it is possible for them to have perceptual rivalry in the olfactory sense akin to binocular vision.

Many vertebrates, including most mammals and reptiles, have two distinct olfactory systems. The main olfactory system identifies general odorants while the accessory olfactory system is used mainly to detect pheromones. For air-breathing animals the main olfactory system detects volatile aerosolized chemicals, and the accessory olfactory system detects chemicals usually in the fluid phase. Olfaction, along with taste, is a form of chemoreception. Although taste and smell are separate sensory systems in land animals, water-dwelling organisms often have one chemical sense.

Odors are also commonly called scents, and these terms can refer to both pleasant and unpleasant stimuli. The terms fragrance and aroma are used primarily by the food and cosmetic industry to describe a pleasant odor, often referred to as a perfume or bouquet. In contrast malodor, stench, reek, and stink are used specifically to describe unpleasant odor. The sense of smell gives rise to the perception of odors, mediated by the olfactory nerve. The olfactory receptor (OR) cells are neurons present in the olfactory epithelium, a small patch of tissue in back of the nasal cavity.

There are millions of olfactory receptor neurons, each neuron has hair like projections known as cilia. The cilia have receptor proteins that are in direct contact with air and bind directly with the odorant chemicals and molecules initiating a neuron mediated electric signal. Volatile small molecule odorants, non-volatile proteins, and non-volatile hydrocarbons may all produce olfactory responses and sensations. Much like some animal species are able to visualize ultraviolet or infrared beyond the spectrum visible to humans a number can smell carbon dioxide and other odorants that are not detectable and thus considered odorless based on human sensitivity.

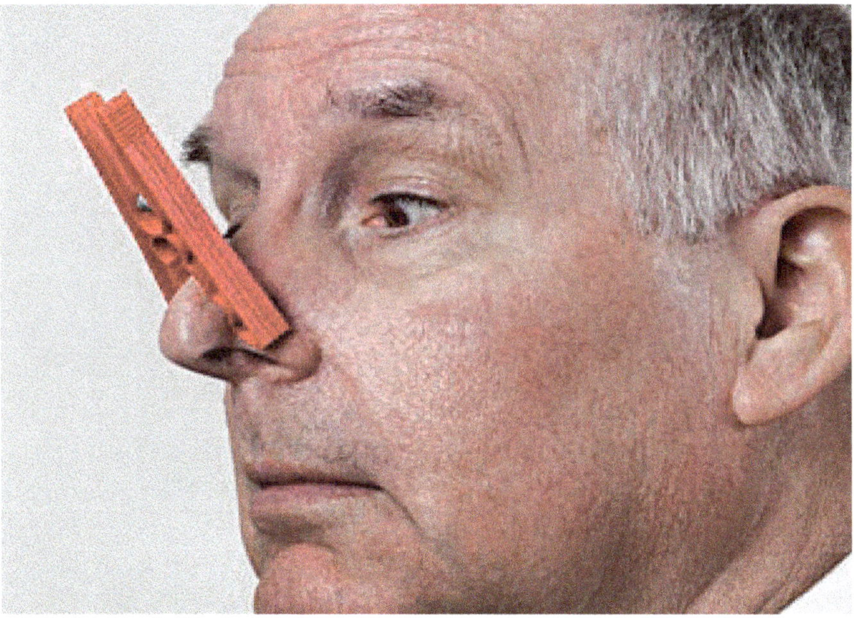

www.theguardian.com

Olfaction, taste, and trigeminal receptors with a property known as chemesthesis together contribute to flavor. The human tongues us able to distinguish five distinct qualities of taste, salt, sweet, acidic, bitter, and umami. The nose and olfactory sense of smell has a much greater sense of discrimination can distinguish among hundreds of substances, even in extremely minute quantities. The olfactory sense of smell takes place during inhalation, while the olfactory contribution to flavor occurs during exhalation. The olfactory system is unique among the human senses in that the neural pathway bypasses the thalamus and provides neural input directly to the forebrain. In human females the sense of olfaction is strongest around the time of ovulation, significantly stronger than during other phases of the menstrual cycle and stronger than the sense in males. The association of heightened olfactory sensitivity in association with ovulation has raised speculation about pheromone activity in humans but it has yet to be scientifically confirmed.

Scent hounds as a group can smell one- to ten-million times more acutely than a human, and bloodhounds , which have the keenest sense of smell of any dogs, have noses ten- to one-hundred-million times more sensitive than a human's. They were bred for the specific purpose of tracking humans, and can detect a scent trail a few days old. The second-most-sensitive nose is possessed by the Basset Hound, which was bred to track and hunt rabbits and other small animals. The silvertip grizzly bear found in parts of North America, have a sense of smell seven times stronger than that of the bloodhound. This keen sense of smell is essential for its skill in locating food underground. Bears can detect the scent of food from up to 18 miles away.

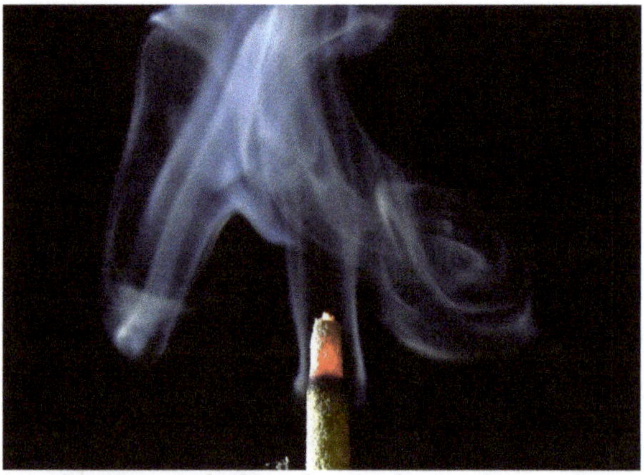

Most odorants are in the form of vapors. Creative Common License.

Olfaction, the sense of smell, is a form of chemo-perception that in humans occurs when odorant molecules bind to olfactory receptors. It is the oldest and most sensitive of the senses. Cloning of olfactory receptor proteins and identifying that odor molecules that bind to specific receptors led to the 2004 Nobel Prize award to Linda B. Buck and Richard Axel.

Feces and farts have a characteristic aroma that most find people find unattractive or offensive. Females have greater olfactory sensitivity than males, particularly at the time of ovulation. More than pheromones are involved and females can detect by olfaction potential mates that have a genetic diversity that would be beneficial for their offspring. Odor information is retained in long-term memory and the olfactory system is anatomically associated with the limbic system, a region of the brain associated with emotion. It has been long recognized that odors can trigger memories and emotions from remote times.

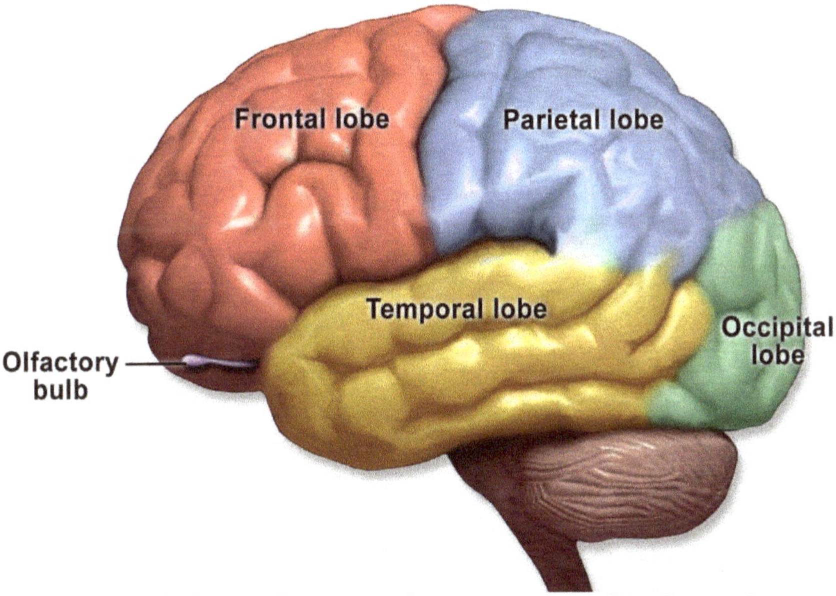
Frontal lobe
Parietal lobe
Temporal lobe
Occipital lobe
Olfactory bulb

Blausen.com staff. "Blausen gallery 2014". *Wikiversity Journal of Medicine*. Creative Commons License

The olfactory nerve is a cranial nerve and its neuronal endings known as dendrites extend to the olfactory bulb of the upper aspect of the nasal passages. They are the only nerve endings that have elongated non-motile cilia that are directly exposed to the external environment. The life span of an olfactory neuron is between thirty and forty days, the shortest life span of all nerve cells. The stem cells in the olfactory epithelium are the source of the new replacement olfactory neurons.

An odorant is a chemical or molecule that stimulates a receptor when in contact with the cilia. An odorant is a volatile chemical or molecule, which has become a vapor as it has exceeded its boiling point. It binds to and stimulates a receptor on the olfactory cilia. Each cilia has approximately one million receptors and may transmit complex signals depending on the receptors activated. When the receptor is stimulated the information is transmitted via the axons of the olfactory nerve directly to various centers of the brain including the cortex and limbic system.

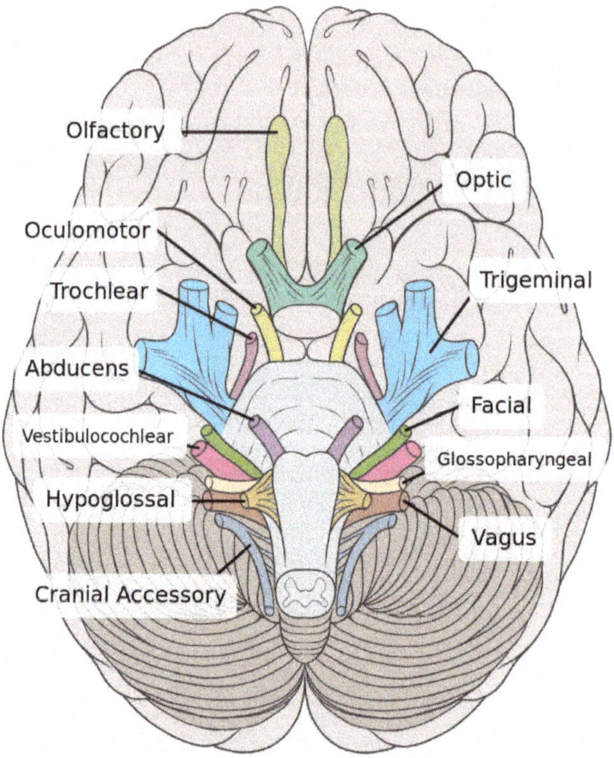
Olfactory
Optic
Oculomotor
Trigeminal
Trochlear
Abducens
Facial
Vestibulocochlear
Glossopharyngeal
Hypoglossal
Vagus
Cranial Accessory

Olfactory nerve (one of the twelve cranial nerves) and bulb at base of the human brain. Peter J. Lynch, medical illustrator, Creative Commons License.

The sense of olfaction is the most sensitive of all human senses. The nose can identify the single scented molecule hiding amongst two billion unscented ones. To use a visual analogy, paint one single square sheet of a toilet paper roll the color red. Now wrap that unlimited length roll of toilet paper around the twenty-five thousand mile long equator of the planet earth, and go around a second time, a third, a fourth, and a full fifth time. Your nose can instantaneously identify the single red square of a one-hundred-and-twenty-five thousand mile roll of toilet paper. Are you impressed with the human sense of smell? Just like wealth and beauty there is always another who has more to keep us from being number one.

Human's olfactory epithelium occupies less than ten percent of the surface area of a dog's olfactory epithelium. As if that were not enough, they also have one hundred times more receptors per square centimeter. Bloodhounds have olfactory receptors up to one hundred million times the sensitivities of humans and are trained to track a human trail several days old. North American grizzly bears have the keenest sense of smell known, seven times greater than the bloodhound.

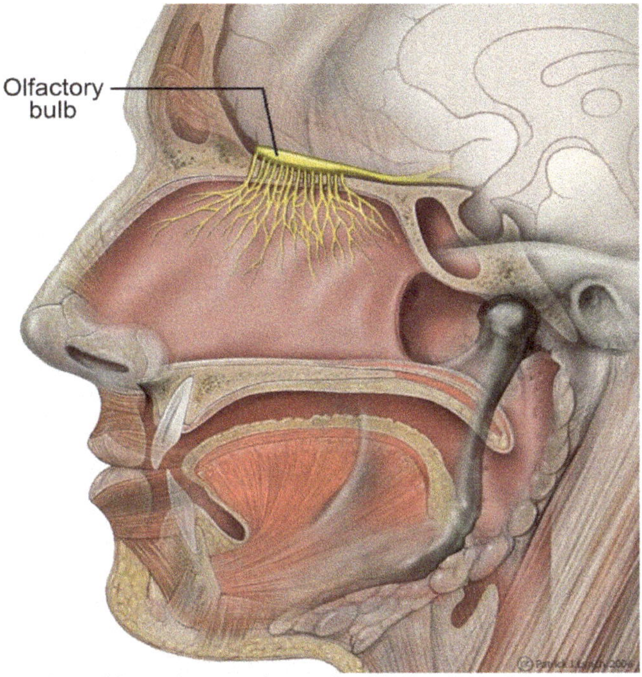
Olfactory bulb

Olfactory nerve (one of the twelve cranial nerves) and bulb at base of the human brain. Peter J. Lynch, medical illustrator, Creative Commons License.

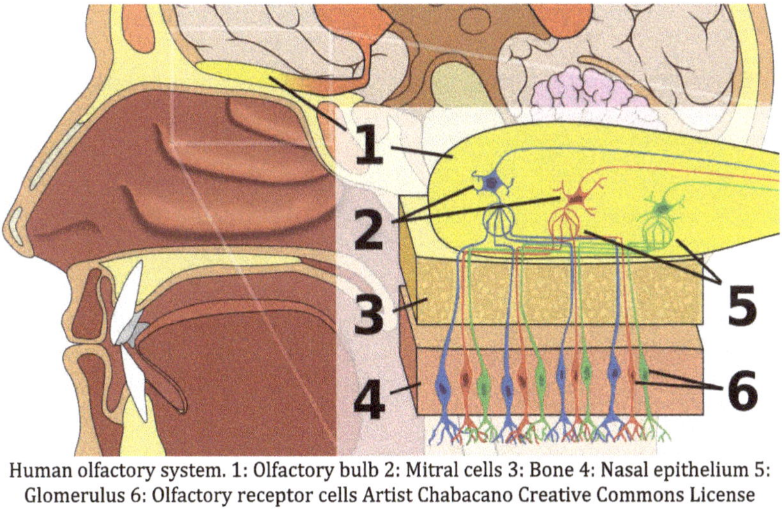
1
2
3
4
5
6

Human olfactory system. 1: Olfactory bulb 2: Mitral cells 3: Bone 4: Nasal epithelium 5: Glomerulus 6: Olfactory receptor cells Artist Chabacano Creative Commons License

Salmon utilize their keen sense of smell in ocean waters to locate the stream from which they were hatchlings years earlier to return to spawn. A mosquito smelling the 'odorless' carbon dioxide that mammals exhale to locate their next blood meal illustrates the olfactory sensitivity of the receptors located on their antennae. The aromas generated by feces and by farts are normally considered unattractive or offensive. There is a surprising percentage of the normal population, predominantly males, who profess enjoyment and pleasure with the olfactory stimulation generated by their own farts, but not those of others. Perhaps being the author and creator of their 'distinct' talents gives rise to pride of ownership.

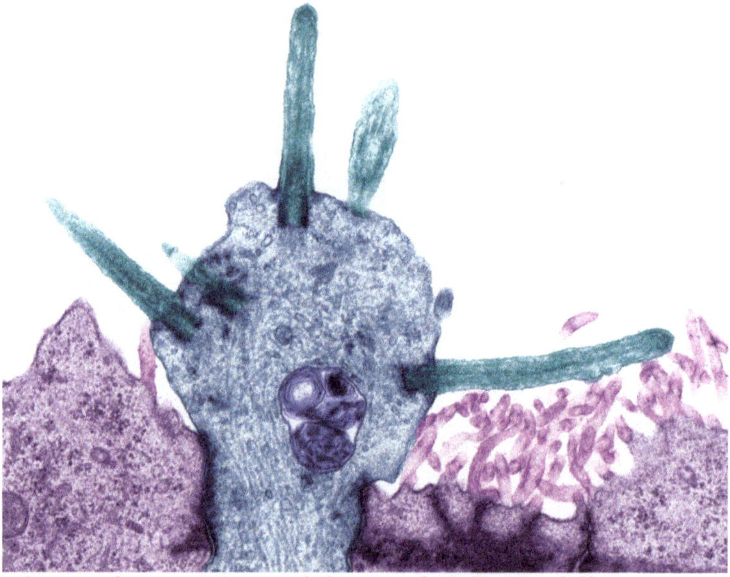

Scanning electron microscopy of cilia arising from dendrite of olfactory nerve.

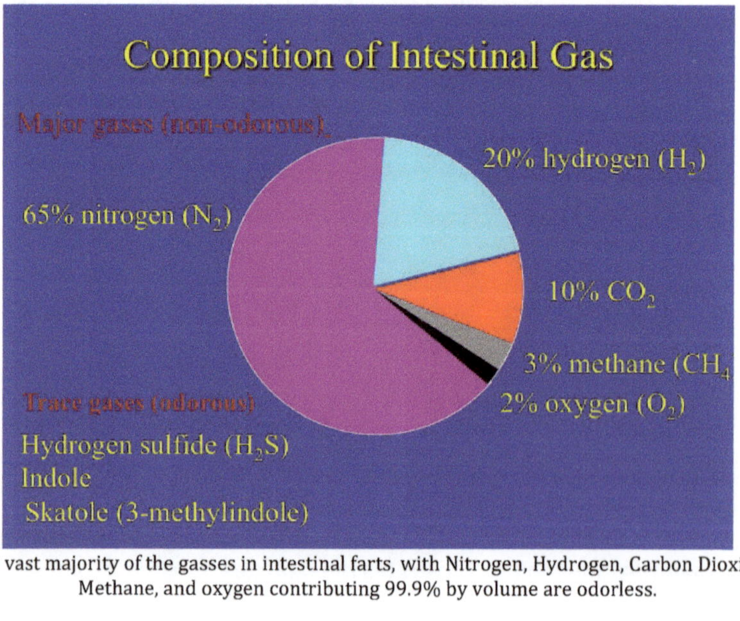
Composition of Intestinal Gas
Major gases (non-odorous)
20% hydrogen (H_2)
65% nitrogen (N_2)
10% CO_2
3% methane (CH_4
2% oxygen (O_2)
Trace gases (odorous)
Hydrogen sulfide (H_2S)
Indole
Skatole (3-methylindole)

The vast majority of the gasses in intestinal farts, with Nitrogen, Hydrogen, Carbon Dioxide, Methane, and oxygen contributing 99.9% by volume are odorless.

Indole

Indole is an organic compound known as an aromatic heterocyclic because it consists of a six-membered benzene ring fused to a five-membered nitrogen-containing pyrrole ring. Indole is often used as a component of fragrances and is used in the production of a number of pharmaceutical products. The amino acid tryptophan is the precursor of the neurotransmitter serotonin and is an example of an indole derivative.

Tryptophan is one of the twenty-two amino acids, and is also considered an essential amino acid. Essential amino acids are those amino acids that cannot be synthesized by humans, and therefore must be obtained through the diet. Because of its importance as an essential amino acid, tryptophan is a common constituent of most protein foods and supplements. A diet rich in tryptophan can contribute to the fecal aroma of intestinal gas. Indole occurs naturally in human feces and contributes to the characteristic fecal odor. Surprisingly, at very low concentrations it has a flowery smell and is a constituent of many perfumes. The name indole is a portmanteau created from the words indigo and oleum. Indole was first isolated by the dye industry in treatment of the deep blue indigo dye with oleum.

Indole is widely distributed in the natural environment and can be produced by a variety of bacteria as a degradation product of the amino acid tryptophan. tryptophan is an indole derivative and the precursor of the hormone melatonin, the neurotransmitter serotonin, and the plant hormone auxin. Indole serves as an intercellular signal molecule,

indole regulates various aspects of bacterial physiology, including spore formation, plasmid stability, resistance to drugs, biofilm formation, and virulence. It takes several million jasmine blossoms to make one pound of natural jasmine oil, which is two-point-five percent indole. It is priced over one thousand times as much as synthetic jasmine, which takes advantage of the commercial production of indole.

Skatole

Skatole (from the Greek το σχατος = feces), or methylindole, is a mildly toxic organic compound belonging to the indole family. It is the primary source of the odor of feces and is produced from the breakdown of the important amino acid tryptophan, the precursor of the neurotransmitter serotonin. Surprisingly, in low concentrations skatole has a very pleasant flowery smell and is found in orange blossoms, jasmine, and other flowers and essential oils. It is used as a fragrance in many perfumes.

Skatole is attractive to males of various species of bees, who gather the chemical to synthesize pheromones. It is also an attractant to gravid (pregnant) mosquitos. The U. S. military has used skatole as a non-lethal malodorant weapon. The German physician Ludwig Brieger, who also identified cadaverine and putrescence, discovered skatole in 1877. His neighbors were probably not pleased with the smell coming from his laboratory as the names he gave his discoveries were derived from their source material.

Skatole also plays a major role in the aroma of pork obtained from mature male pigs (boars). After puberty, under the influence of the male hormone androstenone, the gut microbiome of the male pig generates skatole. This odorant is deposited in the fat and muscle giving it an offensive smell and taste known as taint. Because it cannot be sold at market, male pigs are typically castrated at a young age or slaughtered before puberty. The male of the human species, under similar hormonal influence is also a larger producer of skatole contributing to the enhanced offensive potency of male farts after puberty.

Of particular interest to some scientists is that androstenone, and its effect on skatole, appear to have a pheromone like effect on the human female. Much like color-blindness, there appear to be some odors that cannot be smelled by all people. Initial studies suggested that about thirty percent of human females could not sense androstenone. Further studies revealed that the majority of the non-scenters could be trained to identify it, yet there remained a small proportion of less than five percent who could not perceive the scent. The ability to sense androstenone was found to be genetic and the gene responsible was identified.

The sense of smell in the human female is intimately tied to the menstrual cycle. The height of olfactory sensitivity peaks at the time of ovulation. The androstenone and skatole scents are perceived to be less offensive or more attractive at the time of ovulation. The androstenone skatole connection also explains why the feces and flatus of males are considered more powerful or offensive than that of females. Diet also plays a role in that the ingestion of more meat and fat also leads to more skatole production than a diet with higher fiber content. This is partly due to the diet containing more tryptophan, the amino acid precursor of skatole, as well as the diet induced change in the microbiome. Androstenone also occurs naturally in some plants, including celery, parsnip, and truffle. The celery has long had a reputation as an aphrodisiac dating from Greek and Roman times.

Thiol, Sulfhydryl, Mercaptans

The sulfur hydrogen functional group may also be referred to as a thiol group or a sulfhydryl group. Thiols are also referred to as mercaptans. The term mercaptan (Latin mercurium captans 'capturing mercury') is used because the thiolate group bonds so strongly with mercury compounds.

Hydrogen sulfide is known for its characteristic odor of smelling like rotten eggs. Surprisingly women tend to produce more hydrogen sulfide then men. Diet certainly plays a role as cruciferous vegetables such as broccoli, cabbage, cauliflower, and Brussels sprouts are common offenders. Dried fruits such as apricots are often treated with sulfur products that create odiferous gasses. Red meat, beer, garlic, and aromatic spices are other significant contributors. The offensive smell of sulfur products led to religions ascribing an association between the devil and sulfur.

Hydrogen sulfide is a toxic substance in high concentrations yet very valuable and beneficial on a cellular level when present in minute quantities. The human nose is exceptionally sensitive to this toxin and can identify it in minute concentrations, such as in a fart. When present in very high concentrations the olfactory cells are overwhelmed and can no longer sense it. This has led to a sever hazard for farmers and workers in animal waste manure pits and sewage treatment facilities. A worker collapses on exposure to the high concentration of hydrogen sulfide and fellow workers coming to their aid are likewise stricken because there was no olfactory warning. With a toxic potency equivalent to cyanide workers in such hazardous occupations are urged to use self-contained breathing apparatus to avoid exposure.

Volatile thiols have distinctive and strong garlic like odor. The spray of skunks consists mainly of thiols and derivatives. These compounds are detected by the human nose at concentrations as low as ten parts per billion. Human sweat contains methyl-sulfanylhexan (MSH), found in higher concentrations in females, and has a fruity onion-like odor. Not all thiols have unpleasant odors. The aroma of roasted coffee is due to thiols as is the characteristic scent of grapefruit. Dimethyl sulfide has an aroma that is often described as sweet. Natural gas distributors were required by law to add odorants such as thiols to odorless natural after a tragic school explosion in New London, Texas, in 1937.

Most natural odorant additives used today contain mixtures of mercaptans and sulfides. T-butyl mercaptan is often utilized as the main odorant constituent. The characteristic and pungently offensive odor of animal flesh decay is caused by putrescence and cadaverine. Putrescence and cadaverine are the breakdown products of the amino acids ornithine and lysine, respectively. Cadaverine and putrescence were also used as odorant additives for natural before improved odorants became commercially available.

<u>Methanethiol</u>

Methanethiol (methyl mercaptan) is a flammable, colorless with a powerful smell like rotten cabbage or decomposing vegetables. It is a natural substance found in certain foods such as some nuts and cheese, and is released from decaying organic matter. Methanethiol is also a byproduct produced by the metabolism of asparagus. The change in the odor of urine may be apparent within thirty minutes of eating asparagus. It is one of the main chemicals responsible for bad breath and the smell of feces and flatus.

Natural gas and propane are colorless and odorless, and an undetected leak can lead to tragic consequences. To serve as an odorous marker that a leak is occurring small amount of methyl mercaptan or ethyl mercaptan may be added as an odorant. The addition of an odorant is often required by law to prevent the danger of natural leaks going undetected

Fatty Acids

A fatty acid is a saturated or unsaturated carboxylic acid with a long aliphatic tail or chain. Fatty acids with carbon–carbon double bonds are known as unsaturated, and those without as saturated. Fatty acids are derived from triglycerides or phospholipids, and when unattached to other molecules are described as "free". Fatty acids are an important cellular fuel and yield large quantities of ATP when metabolized. Many cell types can use either glucose or fatty acids for this purpose. Heart and skeletal muscle prefer fatty acids although most cells can use glucose interchangeably. The brain has the ability to use fatty acids, glucose, or ketone bodies as a fuel.

Fatty acids that must be obtained via the diet because humans cannot synthesize them are called essential fatty acids. Fatty acid chains are categorized by their length. Short-chain fatty acids (SCFA) have aliphatic tails of fewer than six carbons. Medium-chain fatty acids (MCFA) have tails of six to twelve carbons and can form medium-chain triglycerides. Long-chain fatty acids (LCFA) have tails of thirteen to twenty-one carbons, while very long chain fatty acids (VLCFA) are longer than twenty-two carbons.

Short- and medium-chain fatty acids are absorbed by the intestines directly into the blood stream and travel via the portal vein for further processing in the liver. Long-chain fatty acids are absorbed into the cells of the intestinal villi and converted into a triglyceride. The triglycerides formed are coated with cholesterol and a protein coat in a compound known as a chylomicron. These enter lymphatic capillaries called lacteals and are transported via the thoracic duct of the lymphatic system, eventually entering the circulatory system via the left subclavian vein. The chylomicrons can transport the triglycerides to tissues where they are stored or metabolized.

Fatty acids absorbed in the blood circulation may be processed in the liver and subsequently circulate as very low-density lipoproteins (VLDL), low-density lipoproteins (LDL), and high-density lipoproteins. Fatty acids serve as a fuel for the mitochondria where they produce ATP through beta-oxidation for muscular contraction and general metabolism.

When released from adipocytes, fatty acids exist in the blood as free fatty acids. It is believed that fatty acids in the skin of mammals, in conjunction with lactic acid and pyruvic acid, creates a distinctive aroma. Animals with a keen sense of smell appear to be able to identify individuals based on their unique aromatic profile.

Aromatic Amino Acids

Aromatic amino acids are amino acids that include an aromatic ring. Examples include phenylalanine, tryptophan, histidine, and tyrosine. Phenylalanine, histidine, and tryptophan are essential amino acids in that animals cannot synthesize them and they must be obtained from the diet. Tyrosine is semi-essential in that it can be synthesized but only if phenylalanine is ingested. The disorder phenylketonuria occurs when there is an absence of the enzyme phenylalanine hydroxylase, which is required for tyrosine synthesis.

All plants and microorganisms synthesize their aromatic amino acids, unlike animals, which obtain them through their diet. Animals have lost these energy-intensive metabolic pathways, since they obtain aromatic amino acids through their diet. Herbicides and antibiotics inhibiting enzymes involved in aromatic acid synthesis are toxic to plants and microorganisms dependent on this pathway, but not to animals that do not utilize these enzymes.

Volatile Organic Compounds

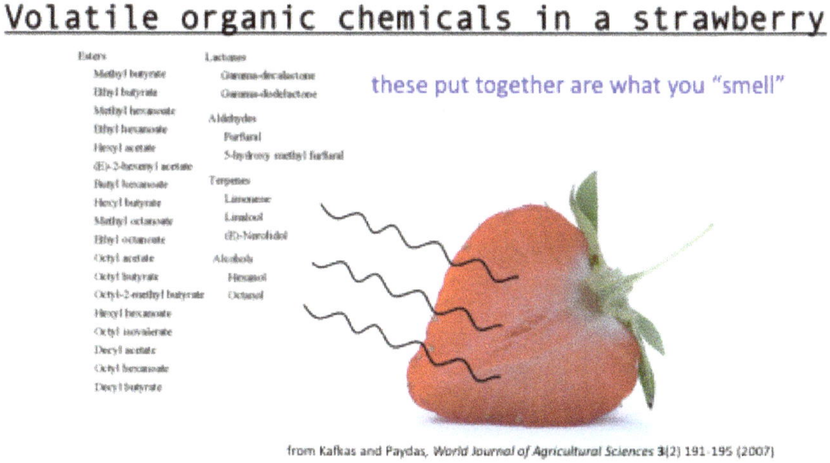
Volatile organic chemicals in a strawberry
these put together are what you "smell"
from Kafkas and Paydas, World Journal of Agricultural Sciences 3(2) 191-195 (2007)
clearscience.tumblr.com/post/610596286/a-list-of-the-volatile-organic-compounds

The term volatile refers to the ability of a substance to evaporate or readily vaporize at room temperature. Most instances of vaporization refer to evaporation where a liquid becomes a gas, such as liquid water boiling into gaseous steam and water vapor. Some solids vaporize from the solid state directly without entering an intermediate liquid phase, a process is known as sublimation. One example would be dry ice, frozen carbon dioxide, which leaves the solid state and is immediately transformed into a gas.

Vaporization also has another form that is not evaporation, but is the scattering or diffusing of molecules or particles through the air. The particles have so little mass that they can remain airborne for extended periods of time, and become airborne again upon being disturbed or moved even by a gentle gust of air. This is frequently noticed when a bright beam of light enters a darkened room and the dust particles circulating in the air become visible.

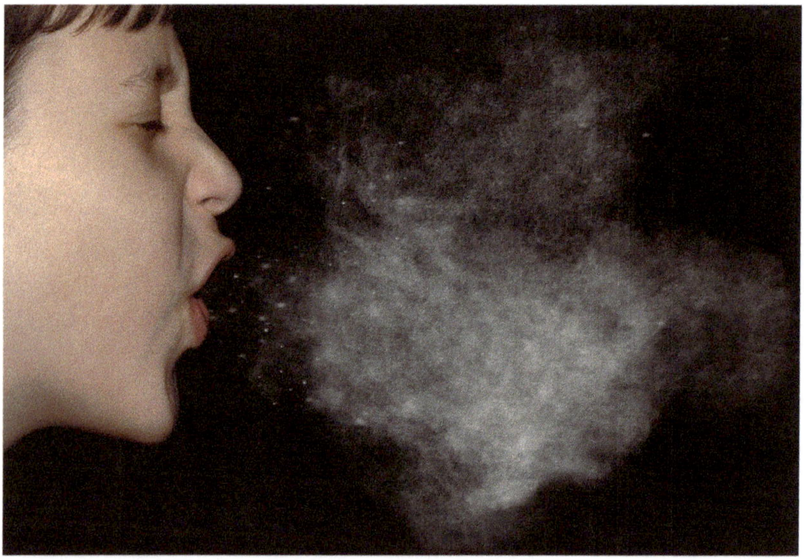

Mold, spores, pollens, viruses, bacteria, fecal matter of mites, volatile organic compounds and others can circulate and spread through large open spaces. Allergies, acquiring viral or bacterial infections from the sneeze or cough of others even hours earlier, occur because of this aerosolization. The ability to detect the aroma of certain compounds, and volatile organic compounds are the result of this form of vaporization as well as they can vaporize at room temperatures.

A list of the volatile organic compounds found in strawberries includes approximately two dozen chemicals including methyl butyrate, octyl acetate, hexanol, and others. Since these compounds are volatile they may vaporize and if they reach your olfactory receptors you may detect them and identify them as coming from a strawberry.

Therapeutic Options

Many individuals have issues with unpleasant fecal odors, and unfortunately it is not as easily remedied as flushing or walking away. The fecal aroma generated by the gut microbiome that smells in defecated feces is the identical aroma that may be discharged with intestinal gas, fecal incontinence, fistula, ostomies, diarrhea, inflammatory bowel disease, after gastric bypass surgery, and a host of other conditions. The numbers of individuals affected is in the millions in the United States alone. Unfortunately, the majority of the general public remains uninformed and impose a social stigma on a medical condition over which they have limited or no control.

Fortunately there are a number of effective therapeutic options available, but too many sufferers are not aware of or have access to them. They range from external appliances and clothing, to external and internal deodorants and suppressants. Of course there are also tongue-in-cheek suggestions, such as getting a dog to blame as the source of the fart odor. The Merck Manual a few years back suggested working on perfecting one's glare, just glare at someone else as if they were the source.

More direct references to farts have been employed in the advertising campaign of air-freshener company Poo-Pourri. Although the advertising campaign received a nomination as one of the worst ads by a national newspaper, it was a major hit on social media with over thirty million views. For a holiday themed advertisement Santa Claus is farting on the toilet while an attractive model sings a parody of a seasonal tune.

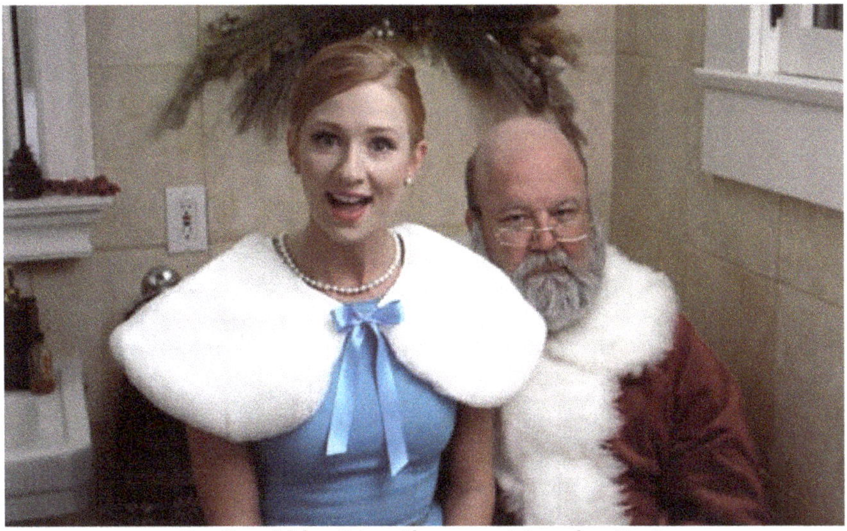

Poo-Pourri Advertising video www.ninjamarkweting.it

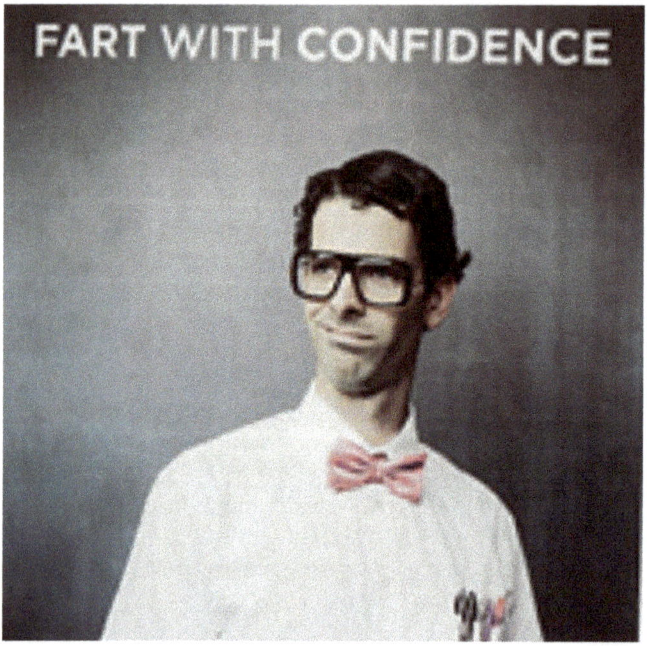
FART WITH CONFIDENCE

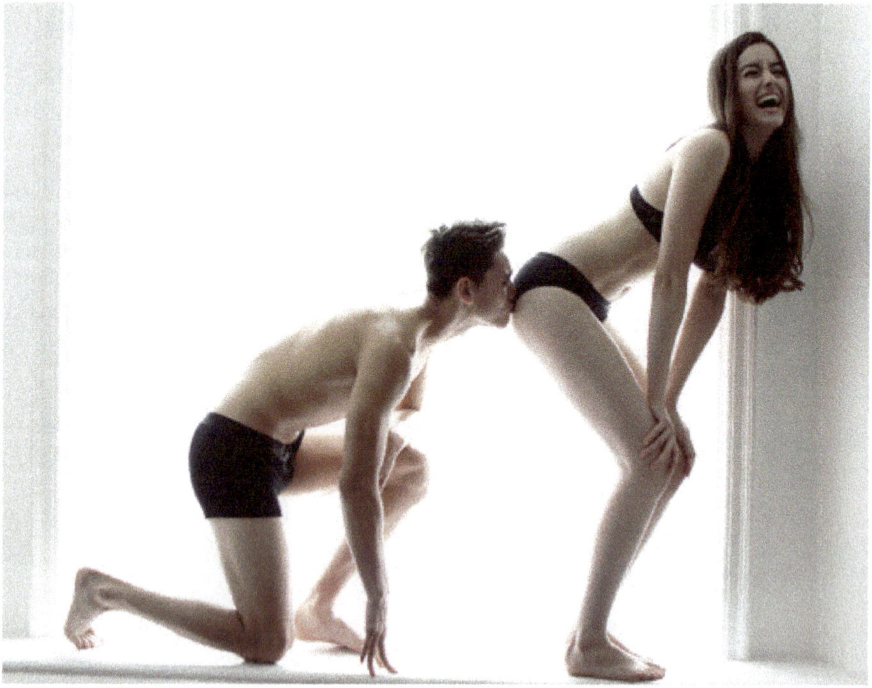

Shreddies advertising campaign for activated charcoal odor adsorbing underwear
myshreddies.com/store/gifts/

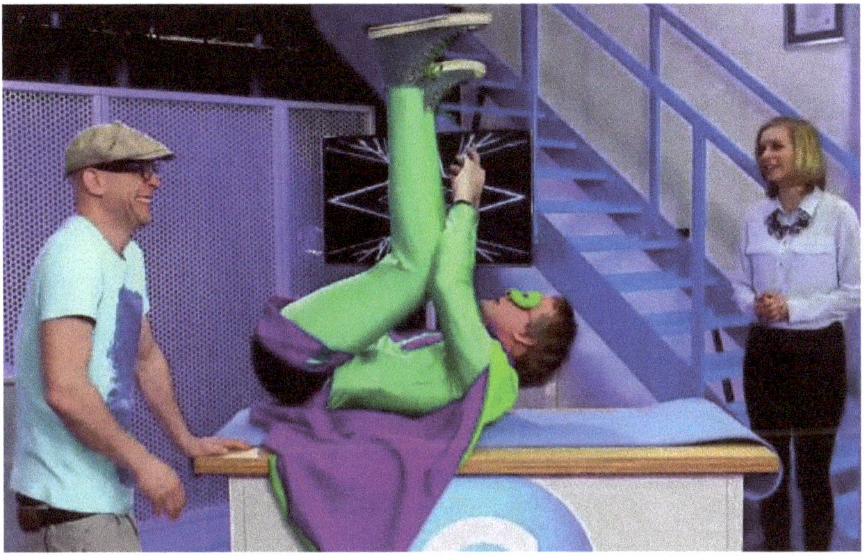

Mr. Methane demonstrating effectiveness of activated charcoal in a pair of Shreddies on *The Gadget Show* myshreddies.com/media/?a=1

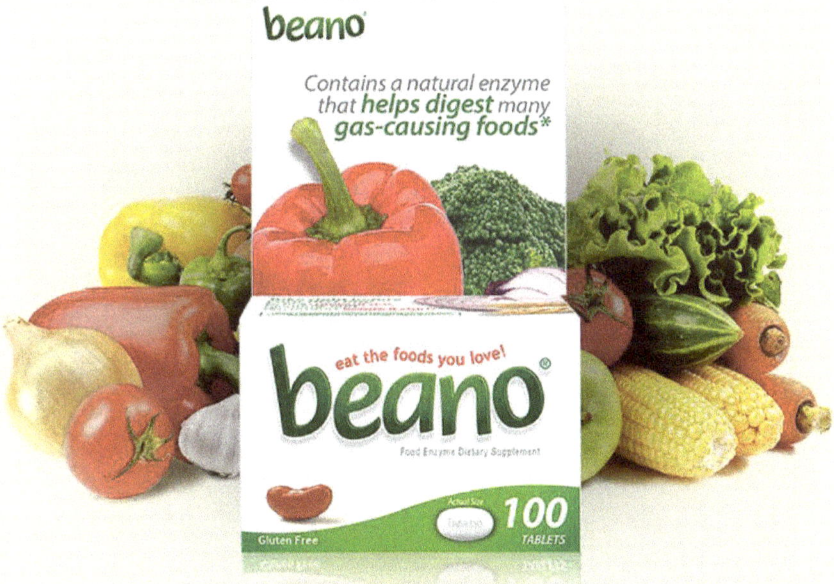
beano
Contains a natural enzyme that helps digest many gas-causing foods*
eat the foods you love!
beano
100
TABLETS
Gluten Free

Beano was one of the first products to advertise a product designed to reduce intestinal gas. Its ad first appeared in Vegetarian Times

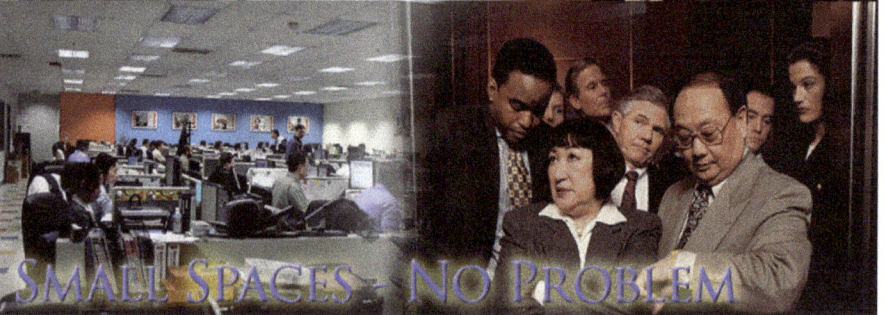

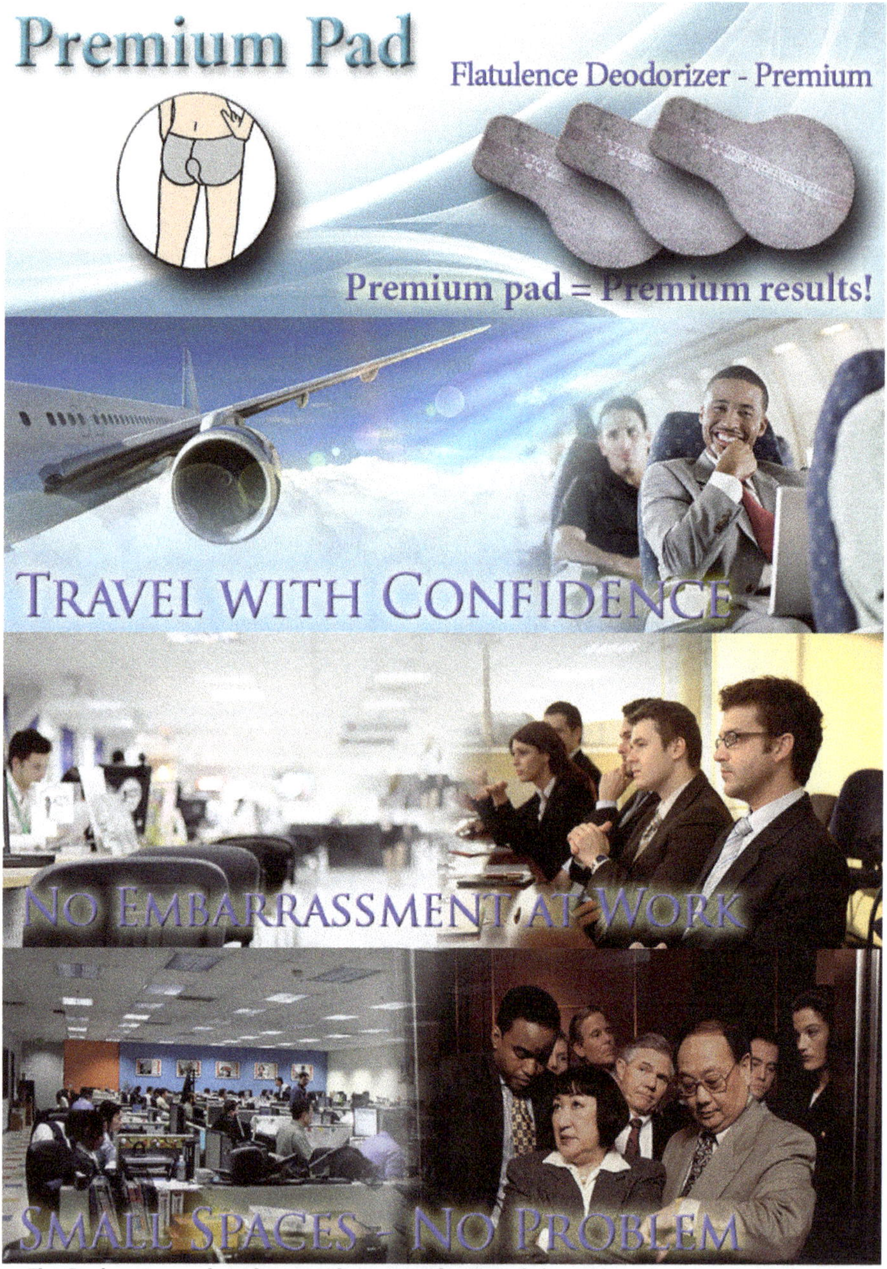
Premium Pad
Flatulence Deodorizer - Premium
Premium pad = Premium results!
TRAVEL WITH CONFIDENCE
NO EMBARRASSMENT AT WORK
SMALL SPACES - NO PROBLEM

Flat-D advertises and markets a wide variety of activated charcoal products to adsorb the aroma of flatus and other body odors. www.flat-d.com

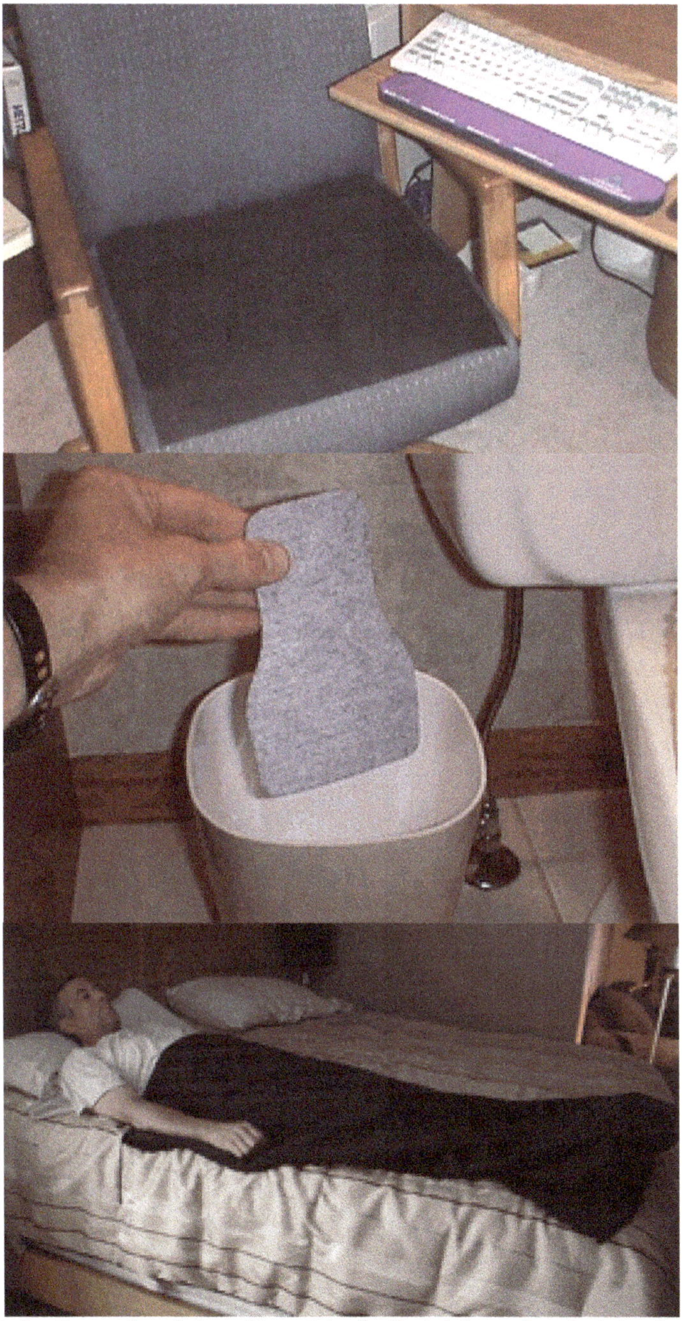

Flat-D advertises and markets a wide variety of activated charcoal products to adsorb the aroma of flatus and other body odors. Activated charcoal seat cushions, liners for underwear and clothing, and sleeping sack are amongst the numerous products they offer. www.flat-d.com

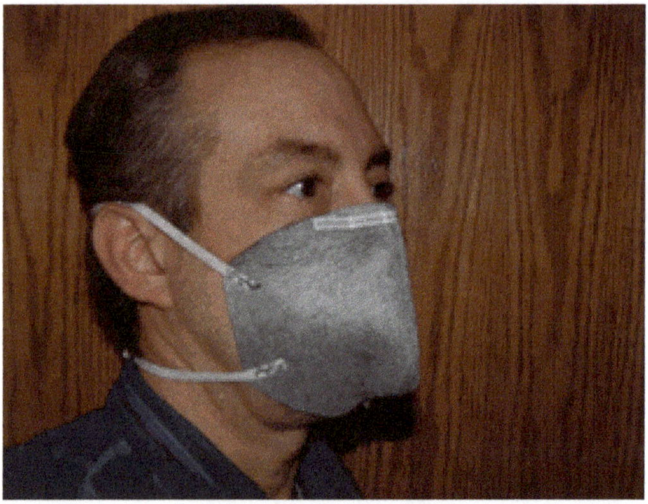

Flat-D offers another approach to protecting the individual from offensive odors, by wearing an activated charcoal facemask covering the mouth and nose. www.flat-d.com

Surprisingly where it can provide relief and comfort to many sufferers, some media outlets refuse to place advertisements for products dealing with flatulence and ostomy odors. Deodorants, feminine hygiene douches, tampons, sanitary napkins for menstruation, diapers for adults with incontinence, erectile dysfunction prescriptions, etcetera have been seen by the public and the country still stands. Devrom, an effective internal deodorant that suppresses fecal odor was not allowed to place their advertisement in Reader's Digest or AARP (Association for the Advancement of Retired People) because it contained the word stool and smelt flatulence. Somehow the publications did not see the irony in that their policy did not pass the smell test.

Devrom is an over the counter preparation of bismuth subgallate and has been marketed for over fifty years as an internal deodorant. Bismuth does have antibacterial properties it may change the microbiome by reducing the organisms that contribute to offensive flatulence. Another bismuth product that has been popular in the marketplace is Pepto-Bismol, which is a bismuth subsalicylate. Bismuth subsalicylate is related to aspirin (salicylic acid) and does not appear to provide as significant relief from the unpleasant odors as has been reported with Devrom.

It has been particularly popular for individuals who have undergone gastric bypass surgery, inflammatory bowel disease, as well as those with ostomies, and others. With advances in surgery, and the ability to preserve sphincters or create artificial sphincters, ostomies are seen less frequently. This is where the intestinal discharge exits the body through an artificial opening, the ostomy, created at surgery. Because the bowel is diverted from the colon less moisture is absorbed, and the feces may be semi-formed or liquid.

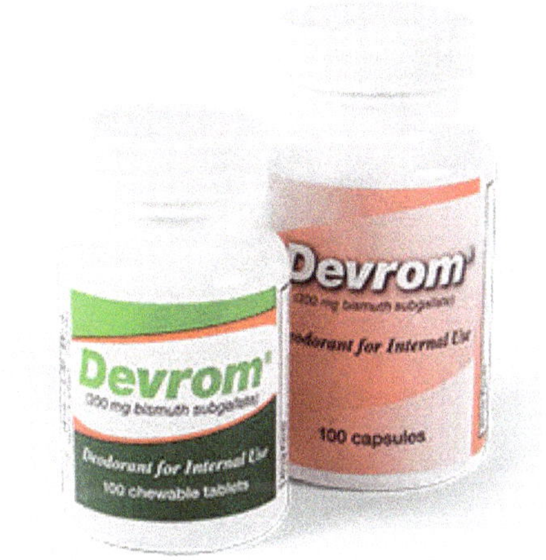
Devrom
Devrom
100 capsules

The more liquid form allows for the more rapid vaporization of volatile organic compounds and gasses that give rise to the feculent odor. In spite of being in otherwise excellent health, many individuals with these issues find themselves socially restricted in their activities because of concern about embarrassment or offending others. Safe and effective products are available, but many individuals are unaware and suffer unnecessarily because of the lack of information and understanding.

Bismuth is a chemical element, number eighty-three on the periodic table, which has a long history of being used in preparations designed to treat gastrointestinal complaints. It is a heavy metal with a low level of toxicity. Its various compound have also been used historically to treat syphilis and the severe diarrhea from cholera. Bismuthinite is a mineral consisting of bismuth sulfide (Bi_2S_3) and is an important ore for bismuth.

The mechanism of action is unknown and may be related to its known antimicrobial activity, perhaps inhibiting the microbes that generate some of the more offensive gasses that are usually contain sulfur as well as aromatic and volatile organic compounds. Bismuth also reacts directly with sulfur generating bismuth sulfide, a dark black insoluble compound. This can cause darkening or blackening of the tongue if sulfur is found in high concentrations in the saliva. It will also cause blackening of the stool as it binds with the sulfur that would otherwise give rise to hydrogen sulfide and other offensive sulfur gasses. The dark black color of the stool may be mistaken for melena, a sign of internal bleeding that results from the digestive process on blood cells and hemoglobin. The black coloration is not a health concern and is temporary clearing with cessation of bismuth intake.

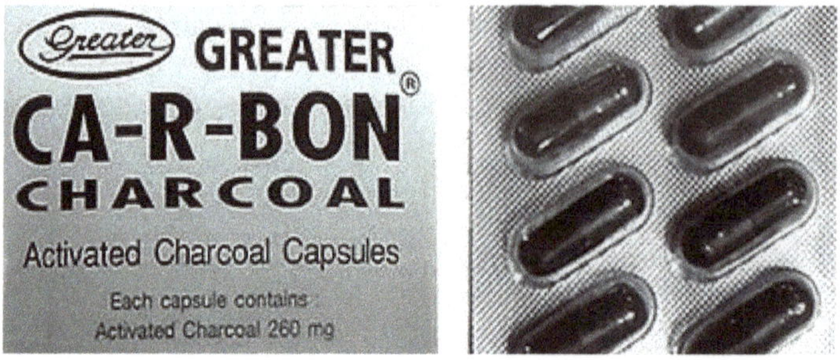
Greater
GREATER
CA-R-BON
CHARCOAL
Activated Charcoal Capsules
Each capsule contains
Activated Charcoal 260 mg
Capsules of activated charcoal are commonly used as a treatment for intestinal gas.

Activated carbon is used to treat oral poisonings by binding to and preventing the poison from being absorbed by the gastrointestinal tract. Charcoal biscuits were marketed in the early 19th century as an antidote to flatulence, and are still marketed today for diarrhea, indigestion, flatulence, and as a pet care product. Orally ingested charcoal pills are of limited effectiveness in reducing intestinal gas. This may be because the adsorptive capacity of the activated charcoal is usually fully utilized before it finally gets to the colon where its gas adsorbing properties are needed. Fortunately, bismuth products do provide a significant advantage by binding to the sulfur compounds and eliminating them without producing offensive gas.

Asshole

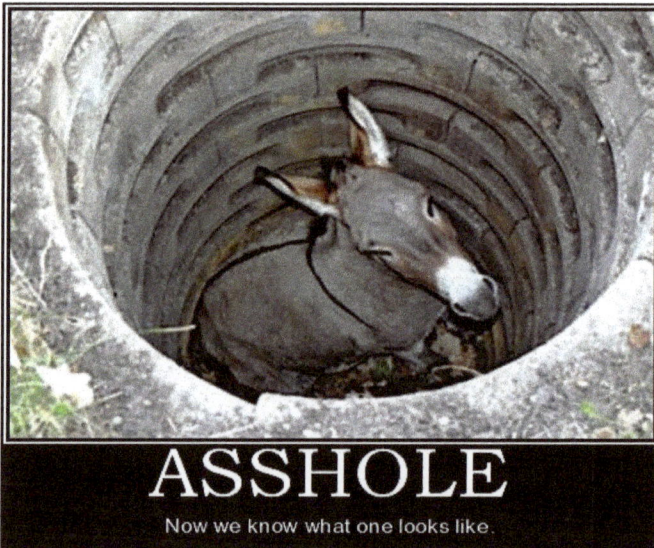
ASSHOLE
Now we know what one looks like.
www.ceremonyheals.com/wp

The word asshole is an Americanized variant of the British English word arsehole a common (vulgar is a description of a word used by common people in a given language) term to describe the anus. It is often utilized as a derogatory term to describe a person who behaves in an offensive manner. The word arse in old English derives from the Germanic root 'arsaz' which can be tracked back to its original Proto-Indo-European root 'ors' meaning the buttocks or backside. The English word ass (especially when used outside of the US and Canada) refers to a donkey derived from its zoological name *Equus asinus.* It may also be utilized as a term of contempt for a person with deficiencies of social graces or boorish behavior.

Assume

To assume (Latin assmere to take) is the act of taking something for granted or accepted as true without proof. In medicine, as in many other fields where accuracy is paramount, the traditional teaching is to never assume anything. The word's real meaning is often described within the word itself as if one assumes anything from another person the result would be to make an: "ASS (out of) U and ME"!

Autointoxication

Autointoxication is an outdated and disproved theory that any fecal residue in the colon can lead to toxic consequences from their absorption. In the early twentieth century adherents underwent regular colon irrigations and high enemas. Other approaches were to increase the amount of fiber and roughage in the diet to speed the passage of fecal material through the bowel in the shortest amount of time. The entry on enemas highlights some of the more popular remedies of the day, including the Battle Creek Sanitarium under the direction of Dr. John Harvey Kellogg.

Ayurveda

The word agni is Sanskrit term for 'fire'. Sanskrit is in the Indo-European family of languages as is Latin, English, Greek and others. The Sanskrit word 'agni' is the equivalent of the Latin 'ignis', which is the root of the English word ignite often used as descriptive action to start a fire. Agni is a central concept in Ayurveda, as it represents the fire energy equivalent produced by the metabolic process of digestion. It allows the breakdown, absorption, and assimilation of food nutrients while eliminating waste and toxins, known as the Ayurveda term 'ama', from the body. The accumulation of ama results in the slow but progressive deterioration of the body which ultimately leads to ill health and disease.

Agni also refers more broadly to our ability to process and digest all aspects of life, including food, experiences, memories, and sensory impressions. It transforms the physical matter of food into the useable forms of energy the cells of the body require. *Jathar-agni* determines the production of hydrochloric acid in the stomach, while *Bhuta-agni* determines the production of bile in the liver. *Kloma-agni* determines the production of the pancreatic enzymes, while *Jatru-agni* regulates the thyroid gland. *Dhatu-agni* is the agni at the level of tissue and cellular metabolism. The Ayurvedic concept of agni beliefs continues to an even subtler level of *Indrya-agni,* described as the door of perception, which transforms external information into internal knowledge. In Ayurveda a stronger agni allows for a stronger and clearer body and mind. The nature and quality of the various *agnis* depend on the individual's blend of the three doshas: vata, pitta, and kapha. In individuals with a predominance of the vata and kapha doshas the agni tends to be weak resulting in a digestive system that is cold, irregular, and sluggish. This is believed to contribute to signs and symptoms of constipation, malabsorption, and excess intestinal gas. In pittas the fires of agni is excessive and can result in heartburn, acid reflux, colitis, and other burning symptoms.

Culinary herbs and spices are used in Ayurveda to enhance the level of agni between and during meals. The meals should be balanced and provide a sampling of each of the tastes, sweet, sour, astringent, bitter, salty, and pungent. One popular Ayurvedic practice is to consume a small piece of fresh ginger with a few drops of lemon juice prior to eating a meal. This allows a slow and progressive awakening of the fire of digestive Agni. Other aromatic spices that aid in digestion include black pepper, cayenne pepper, cardamon, and liquorice. They are believed to aid in the cooking and predigestion of foods. The spices also stimulate the secretions of saliva and digestive enzymes which reduces the work load of the Agni and results in less fatigue after eating. By assisting digestion the Herb's and spices reduce gas and ama. When digestion is incomplete, fermentation takes place and it is this process which produces gas and ama which can contribute to gastrointestinal signs and symptoms. Fennel is a common herb offered in Indian restaurants as a carminative. The seeds are chewed, the juice swallowed, and the pulp spit out. It relaxes the lower esophageal sphincter to allow swallowed air to be released and may reduce gas, discomfort, and fatigue. Hing is also used in Ayurveda cooking to assist weak agni and digestion. It is a resinous sap from the asafetida plant and, when combined with other aromatic and carminative herbs in the Ayurveduc remedy hingavashtak, it is believed to promote the deeper assimilation of nutrients.

Ojas is the Ayurveduc term for the vital nectar of life. To achieve optimal health it is important to eliminate ama and focus on the production of Ojas, the Sanskrit term meaning 'vigor'. Ojas is the pure and subtle essence that has been extracted from food that has been completely and properly digested. It circulates throughout the body tissues and heart, sustaining the physical body, providing clarity to the mind, and nurturing emotional balance. A diet of pure easily digested foods, described in Ayurveda as 'Sattvic', promotes the creation and flow of Ojas. Sattvic foods include organic milk, almonds, honey, sesame, rice, and fruits.

Some foods are difficult if not impossible for the body to convert into ojas, including meat, poultry, fish, oily foods, cheese, processed food, and items with an excess of sour or salty tastes. Freshly prepared meals produce more Ojas than foods that has been canned, frozen, or reheated. Alcohol and tobacco use reduce and eliminate ojas. Signs of Ojas includ: You feel rested upon awakening, Your skin has a healthy glow, Your tongue is clear and pink, Your body feels light, regardless of the number on the scale, You feel centered throughout the day, Your digestion is strong without bloating, You feel energized & enthusiastic, Your mind is clear, Your body has a pleasant smell, You rarely get sick. Signs of Ama include: Bad breath, Coated tongue, Dull appetite, Delicate digestion, Sluggish or irritable elimination, Generalized pain, Fatigue, Depression, Susceptibility to infections, Difficulty manifesting intentions.

Oma's is the essence of the processing of all signals our body receives, not just the foods we eat. Much as important as the quality and character of the foods, is the quality of our experience and environment. If we are in a stressful or uncomfortable environment creating ojas cannot take place because we are experiencing what are basically indigestible emotions that are distributing distressed chemical messages throughout our cells and organs. To create a nurturing atmosphere for meals it is important to pay attention to all of the senses — taste, sound, sight, touch, and smell. Here are a few suggestions to enhance the production if ojas

- Eat in a comfortable environment and atmosphere
- Do not eat when you are upset.
- Sit down comfortably to enjoy your meal.
- Do not multitask while you are eating, do not eat while reading, watching television, or while on a computer or mobile device.
- Only eat when you are hungry.
- Dine at a moderate pace. Chew your food well and with enjoyment of the taste, texture, and aroma. Don't gulp down your food or eat too slowly.
- Moderate the quantity of raw foods, which are harder to digest than cooked ones.
- Include all six tastes (sweet, sour, astringent, bitter, salty, and pungent) with each meal.
- Drink water to maintain adequate hydration
- Use spices and herbs that assist the digestive process
- Enjoy pure Sattvic foods they are easily digestible, including organic milk, almonds, honey, sesame, rice, and fruits.

Barium Enema

Barium studies are not performed as often today, but they can provide valuable diagnostic information. A number of years ago I had a patient who was scheduled to have a barium enema to examine the colon, to be followed a few days later by a barium swallow to examine the esophagus. In about twenty percent of patients undergoing barium enema, the contrast material passes through the ileocecal valve and into the small bowel. This can be useful in providing additional diagnostic information about the distal small bowel, such as the presence of inflammatory bowel disease. In this individual, it entered the small intestine but before the radiologist could reduce the pressure of the barium flow it refluxed all the way into his stomach and esophagus and the patient vomited up the barium. With disgust, the patient told the radiologist to cancel the barium swallow. When asked why, the patient told him he would never be able to drink the barium because it tasted like shit!

Bashful Bowel

Parcopresis (shy bowel, bashful bowel) is a condition of psychogenic fecal retention characterized by the inability to defecate unless in an area that offers a certain level of privacy. The degree of the condition is extremely variable as some individuals find that they can only defecate in the privacy of their own bathroom at home, and others can defecate comfortably anywhere just not in the outdoors even if no one is in the area. The fear may be one of being observed in the actual act of defecation, or just being observed in the vicinity where such acts take place.

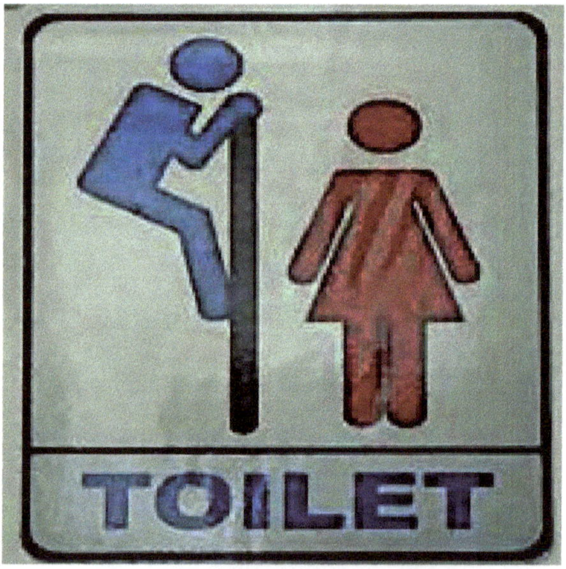
TOILET

www.websophist.com/MenWmn_ToiletB.

It is in the category of conditions known as 'toilet phobia' that refers to any anxiety disorder involving toilets. This includes the fear of contamination, fear of using a public bathroom, specific object phobias such as black toilet seat phobia, inability to use squat type toilets or an outhouse, paruresis (shy bladder, bashful bladder), etcetera. Continued voluntary suppression of the urge to defecate can lead to constipation as the stool within the rectum and bowel becomes progressively harder with continued water absorption by the colon and rectal mucosa.

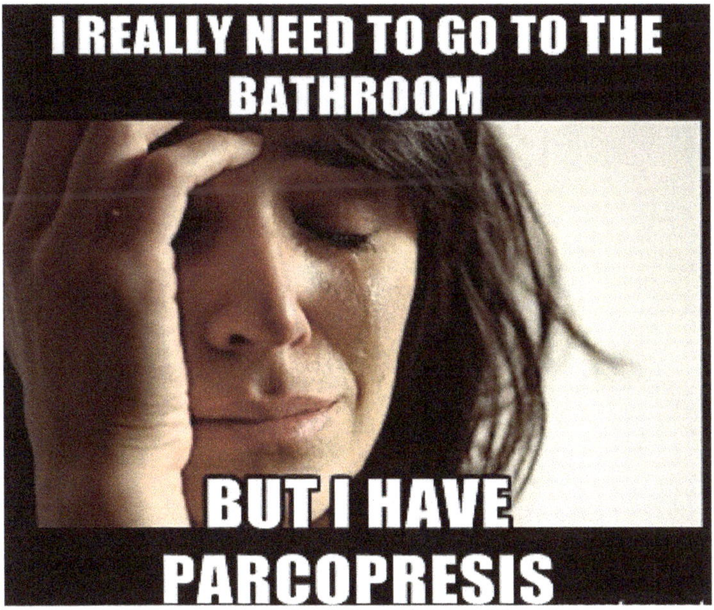
I REALLY NEED TO GO TO THE BATHROOM
BUT I HAVE PARCOPRESIS
memegenerator.net/instance

Bidet (see Anal Hygiene)

Anal cleansing after defecation was historically accomplished with sticks, leaves, stones, clay, corncobs, water, or literally whatever was available at hand. The ancient Greeks used clay and stone. Roman's used a water soaked sponge on a stick. The first recorded use of toilet paper was in China in the sixth century. In France the invention of the bidet in the 1710's made water cleansing popular.

A bidet spray or health faucet is a hand held hose and nozzle that delivers a spray of water to assist in cleansing after defecation and urination. The bidet is commonplace in many countries including Spain (30%), Portugal (70%), Greece (80%) and Italy (95%), Japan (50%.) It is also very popular in the Middle East, and growing in popularity in the United States.

Although there are some very expensive models of toilets combined with bidets, the cost of an aftermarket addition of a washlet feature to a toilet is very economical. Many bidet equivalent washlets cost less than one hundred dollars, and with the savings by reduced toilet paper usage the device rapidly pays for itself.

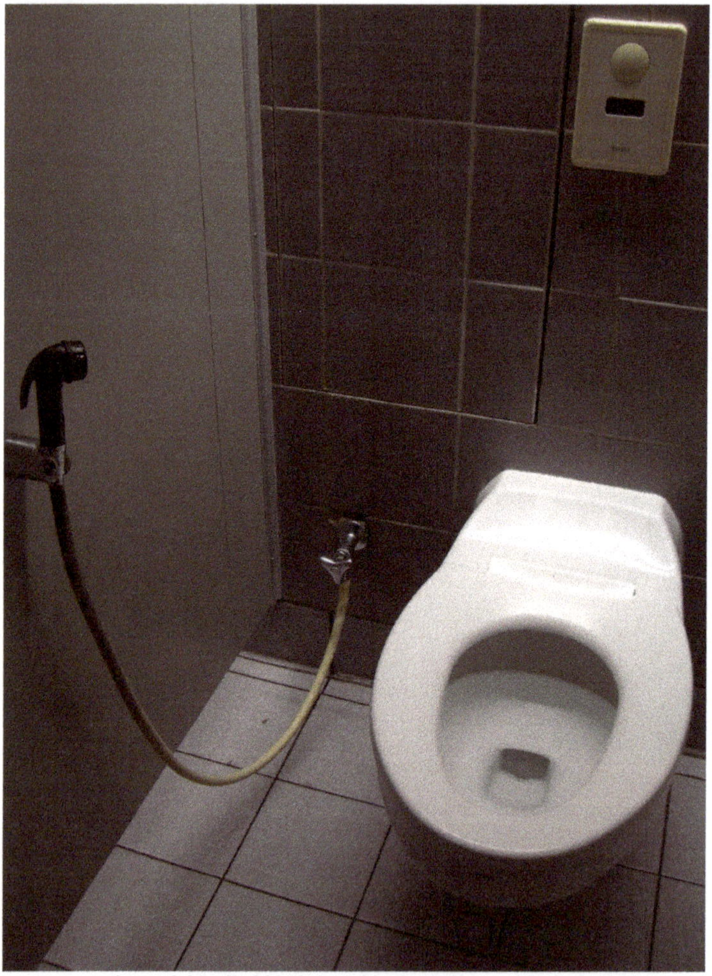

Dubai airport toilet with handheld bidet washlet hose Akaitori flic.kr/p/Rr9ny Creative Commons License

On the Indian subcontinent in spite of a lack of bidets over 95% of the population use water with or without soap for cleansing after defecating. Use of paper is rare in this region and hand washing after cleansing is critically important. It is surprising that it is not more universally popular as it adds another dimension of hygiene and provides an attractive and more hygienic approach than using one's hands and dry paper for anogenital cleansing.

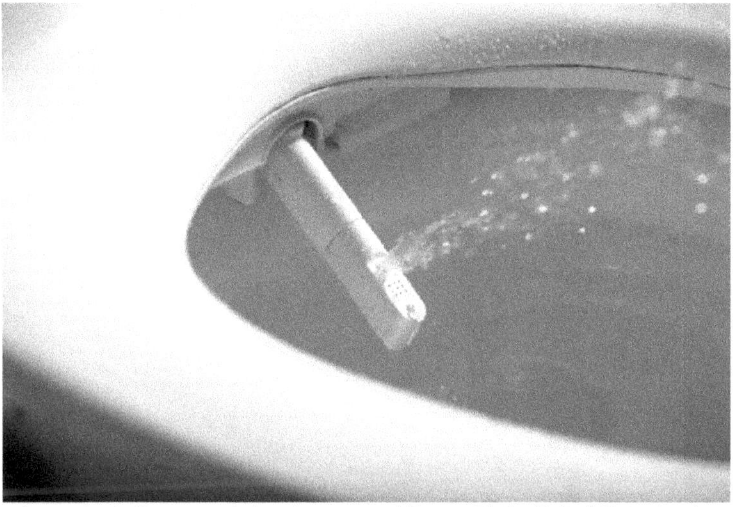

Although popular in Europe and elsewhere around the world, the United States has been very slow to adopt the preferable water based approach to anal hygiene. In addition to its increased efficacy it has environmental benefits in reducing forest product consumption and sewage disposal of paper waste products. Creative Commons License

Most transmission of pathogens is via the fecal to oral route is usually accomplished by way of the hands. The average human stool contains three trillion microorganisms. Wiping with toilet paper nearly guarantees that the hands will come into contact with fecal microorganisms. After wiping it is not uncommon to find brown streaks on underwear because of inadequate anal hygiene.

Bismuth

Bismuth is a chemical element, number eighty-three on the periodic table, which has a long history of being used in preparations designed to treat gastrointestinal complaints. It is a heavy metal with a low level of toxicity. Its various compound have also been used historically to treat syphilis and the severe diarrhea from cholera. Bismuthinite is a mineral consisting of bismuth sulfide (Bi_2S_3) and is an important ore for bismuth.

Bismuth subgallate, with a chemical formula $C_7H_5BiO_6$, is the active ingredient in Devrom, an over the counter product described as an internal deodorizer. The term 'sub' refers to the high oxygen content in the molecule and the presence of bismuth oxygen compounds. It is used to reduce the fecal odor arising from flatulence and fecal incontinence. Those with gastric bypass bariatric surgery, inflammatory bowel disease, irritable bowel syndrome, and ostomy appliances commonly use it. It has also been used to treat *Helicobacter pylori* infection and is in wound therapy.

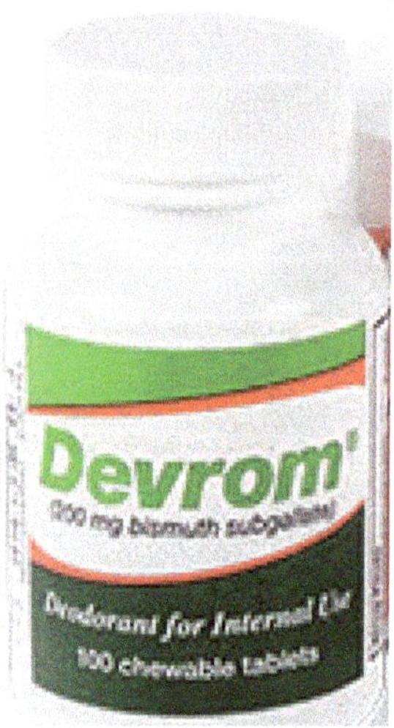
Devrom

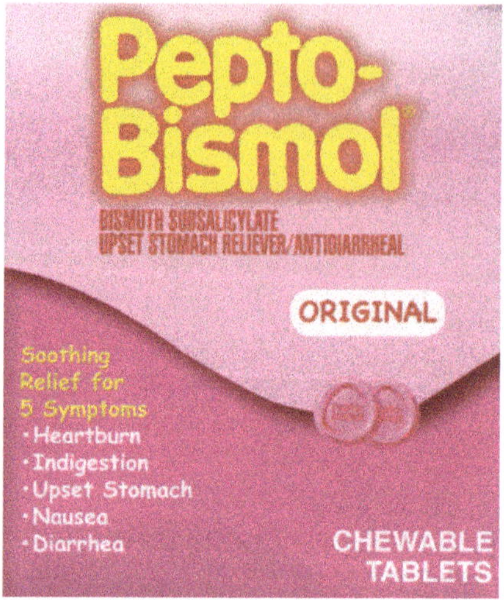
Pepto-Bismol
BISMUTH SUBSALICYLATE
UPSET STOMACH RELIEVER/ANTIDIARRHEAL
ORIGINAL
Soothing Relief for 5 Symptoms
·Heartburn
·Indigestion
·Upset Stomach
·Nausea
·Diarrhea
CHEWABLE TABLETS

The mechanism of action is unknown and may be related to its known antimicrobial activity, perhaps inhibiting the microbes that generate some of the more offensive gasses that are usually contain sulfur as well as aromatic and volatile organic compounds. Bismuth also reacts directly with sulfur generating bismuth sulfide, a dark black insoluble compound.

This can cause darkening or blackening of the tongue if sulfur is found in high concentrations in the saliva. It will also cause blackening of the stool as it binds with the sulfur that would otherwise give rise to hydrogen sulfide and other offensive sulfur gasses. The dark black color of the stool may be mistaken for melena, a sign of internal bleeding that results from the digestive process on blood cells and hemoglobin. The black coloration is not a health concern and is temporary clearing with cessation of bismuth intake.

Bismuth subsalicylate has a bismuth oxide core structure with salicylate ions attached to its surface. It is used as an antidiarrheal and is the active ingredient in Pepto-Bismol, as well as the U.S. version of Kaopectate since it was reformulated in 2004. It is a popular remedy for indigestion, nausea, heartburn, and as a preventative for traveler's diarrhea. It is also used to treat some other gastro-intestinal diseases and infections including the microorganism *Helicobacter pylori*, which is associated with peptic ulcer disease and stomach cancer.

The antimicrobial property may be as a result of an oligodynamic effect, where toxic small doses of heavy metal ions are toxic to microbes. Another antimicrobial effect may arise from the release of salicylic acid as the compound is of the compound is hydrolyzed. It is believed the salicylic acid acts as an antimicrobial for toxigenic *Escherichia coli,* an important cause of traveler's diarrhea.

As a derivative of salicylic acid, bismuth subsalicylate also displays anti-inflammatory properties as well as some adverse effects of salicylates. Because salicylate levels can accumulate and lead to toxicity any use beyond a few weeks length is discouraged. Children should not take bismuth subsalicylate while suffering from a viral infection between of the associated risk of acquiring Reye's syndrome and liver failure. Nursing mothers should not use bismuth subsalicylate as it is excreted in breast milk and may pose a risk of Reye's syndrome in nursing children.

Blue Ice Fall

Blue ice is the term given to the frozen bathroom overflow that is occasionally released from an airplane flying at high altitude. It is a mixture of human waste and the blue disinfectant deodorant utilized in the aircraft sewage holding tank. Several dozen incidents have been reported, including those that have resulted in the destruction of property and human injury. The size and speed of the frozen falling objects can lead to fatalities on the ground. Most of the reported blue ice falls have occurred on the landing approach to airports, as the frozen material begins to thaw and becomes dislodged with the aircraft descent to warmer temperatures.

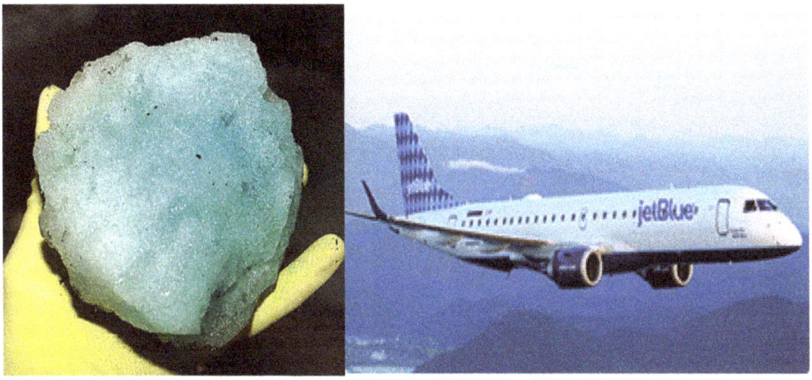
jetBlue

tierra.rediris.es Creative Commons License

If the material has thawed sufficiently it may assume a consistency more in line with the commonly experienced, and less dangerous, bird droppings. Droppings delivered from heights may also be experienced by those under a tree with a depositing bird or animal in a higher branch. It was also experienced in historical times when night stools were emptied out of windows of higher storied buildings to the streets below. Theoretically, once can also expect the infrequent release of human waste from other flying modalities that do not have human waste receptacles such as hot air balloons, skydivers, hang gliders, helicopters, dirigibles, etc.

Bowel (see Digestion)

Bowel is one of several alternative words used to describe the tubular gastrointestinal tract distal to the stomach. Other words used include gut, alimentary tract or canal, large and small intestine, digestive tract.

Bowel Flora (see Gut Flora, Microbiome)

Bowel Management

Bowel management is a practical approach to manage fecal incontinence or constipation. The definition of fecal incontinence is the inability to voluntarily hold feces in the rectum. This can lead to significant disruption in social activities and reduction in the quality of life. Bowel management is the purposeful clearing of colonic contents on a schedule that prevents uncontrolled bowel movements. Daily enemas, laxatives, and a controlled diet may be components of a bowel management regimen. Bowel management programs are usually necessary when dealing with neurogenic bowel dysfunction.

For those dependent on a daily enema as part of the regimen a creative approach has been the development of an operation to convert the appendix to an access port for the administration of fluid into the colon. Called a continent appendicostomy or Malone procedure, a catheter to administer the enema fluid is inserted into a small orifice usually located near the belly button. This allows full control of the enema process to the individual to maintain independence.

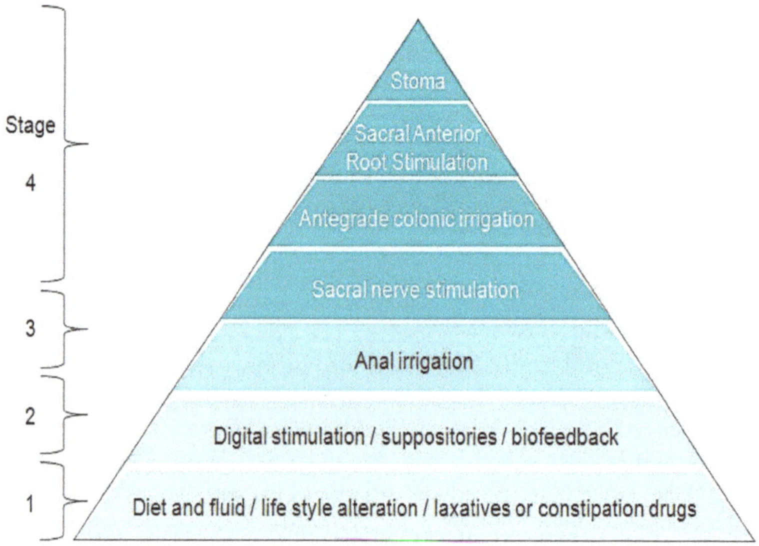
Stage
4
3
2
1
Stoma
Sacral Anterior Root Stimulation
Antegrade colonic irrigation
Sacral nerve stimulation
Anal irrigation
Digital stimulation / suppositories / biofeedback
Diet and fluid / life style alteration / laxatives or constipation drugs

my-bowel.co.uk/wp Creative Commons License

Bowel Movement

Defecation, a bowel movement or often named for its abbreviated initials BM, is the elimination of fecal waste material from the digestive tract via the anus. The stimulus to defecate is the distention of the rectum or sigmoid colon with feces. This reflex can be triggered by manual stimulation of the rectal wall stretch receptors. Voluntary control of defecation is part of the toilet training process and is typically mastered during childhood. This control can be lost again with neurological, psychological or senescent changes. The involuntary release of feces is known as fecal incontinence, often called encopresis in children.

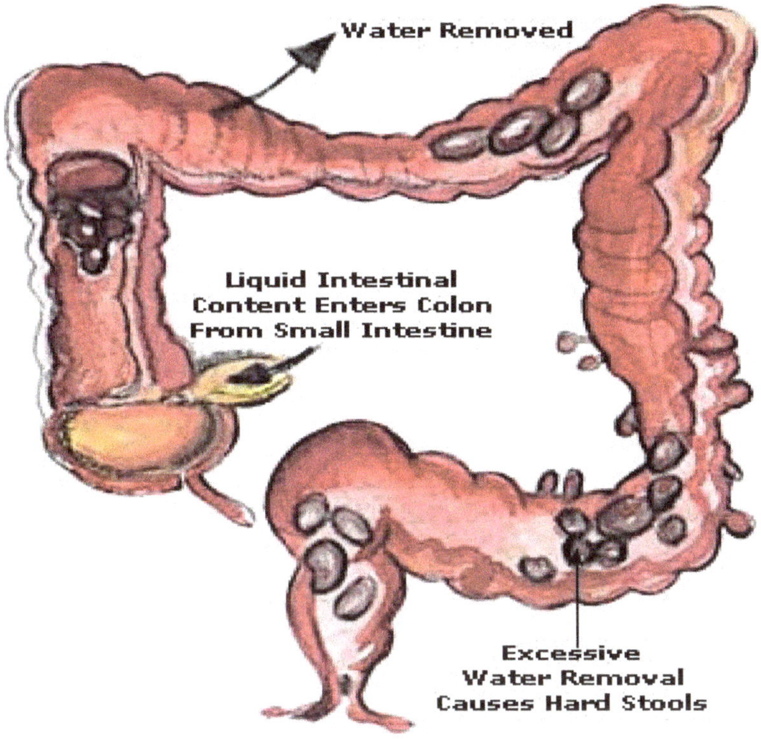
Water Removed
Liquid Intestinal Content Enters Colon From Small Intestine
Excessive Water Removal Causes Hard Stools

Creative Commons License

Defecation is a complex reflex coordination of neuromuscular activity that relaxes the puborectalis muscle straightening the normally ninety-degree anorectal angle and initiates the relaxation of the internal anal sphincters. There is a strong urge to defecate but the external anal sphincter contracts to prevent defecation until voluntarily released to initiate the process. Colonic contractions, along with increased intra-abdominal pressure by performance of the Valsalva maneuver (attempting to exhale against a closed epiglottis), then push the fecal material out of the rectum via the anus.

The frequency range of normal bowel movements is variable and can range from two bowel movements per day to once per week, often dependent on diet. The squatting position is most conducive to defecation. Using Western style sitting toilets, as opposed to squat toilets found in non-Western locales, can be problematic especially if the feet cannot reach the ground, as in young children. An elevated footrest to allow the thighs and legs to be flexed can greatly assist in the ease of elimination for both children and adults.

The puborectalis sling forming the anorectal angle is responsible for gross continence of solid stool. The internal anal sphincter is an involuntary muscle that contributes about fifty-five percent of the resting anal pressure. Together with the hemorrhoid vascular cushions, the internal anal sphincter maintains continence of flatus and liquid during rest.

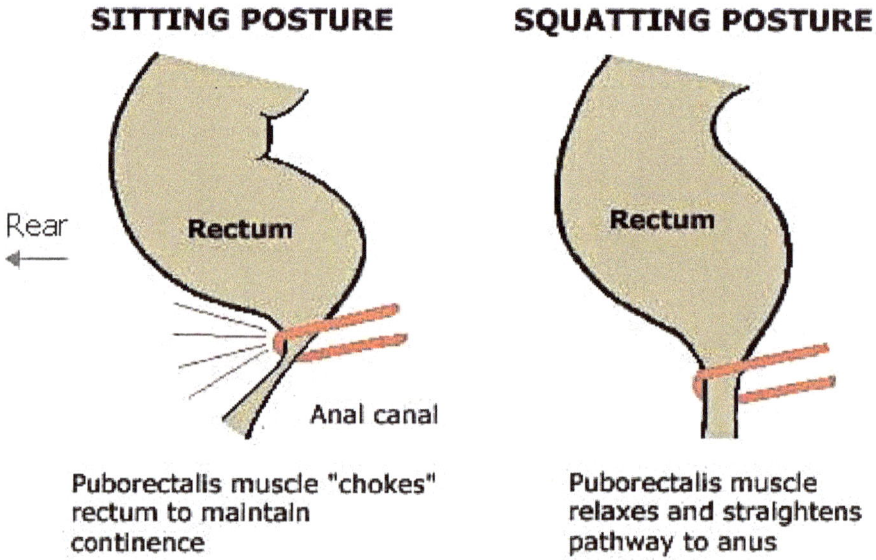
SITTING POSTURE
SQUATTING POSTURE
Rear
Rectum
Rectum
Anal canal
Puborectalis muscle "chokes" rectum to maintain continence
Puborectalis muscle relaxes and straightens pathway to anus

www.jcrows.com Creative Commons License

The external anal sphincter is a voluntary muscle, doubling the pressure in the anal canal during contraction. The rectoanal inhibitory reflex is an involuntary internal anal sphincter relaxation in response to rectal distention. This allows a sampling of some of the rectal contents to descend into the anal canal. Here it is brought into contact with specialized sensory mucosa to detect consistency. The rectoanal excitatory reflex is an initial semi-voluntary contraction of the external anal sphincter and puborectalis, which returns tone following the rectoanal inhibitory reflex.

Other factors include the specialized anti-peristaltic function of the last part of the sigmoid colon, the sensory ability of the lining of the rectum and the anal canal to detect the consistency and quantity when of stool present, and the normal rectoanal reflexes and defecation cycle that completes evacuation.

Humans can defecate in a number of different postures. The two most common are the squatting posture and the sitting posture. The squatting posture is used for squat toilets and is also commonly used for defecation in the absence of toilets or other devices. It is commonly used in non-Western cultures. The sitting defecation posture is used in Western toilets with either a leaning forward posture or a ninety-degree sitting upright posture. The posture chosen appears to be largely a cultural decision although there is evidence that the squatting posture is more efficacious and induces the least bodily strain.

The sitting position can cause the defecating human being to repeat the Valsalva maneuver many times and with great force. This can lead to diverticulosis, hemorrhoids, hernias and cardiovascular stress and defecation syncope. For those with underlying cardiac disease the additional stress induced by defecating in the sitting position as opposed to the more natural squatting position may be surprisingly life threatening The magnitude of straining during defecation is at least three times greater than with the squatting posture.

Difficulty with the seated position is particularly true if the feet cannot reach the floor, as is commonly seen when small children are placed on adult height toilets. The adults may become frustrated that it is taking the child so long to defecate, not realizing that without being able to brace their feet and apply resistance that are unable to generate the intra-abdominal pressure needed to promote defecation.

The affectionate term 'potty' is often used with children especially during toilet training. The term potty is also used to describe the child-size chamber pot type toilets that are at the appropriate height with a child-size seat. When a child sits on an adult-size toilet seat there is a genuine fear of falling in, which can inhibit having a bowel movement.

Regular adult toilets, which have an opening that is normally too large and frightening for a child, may be used if a child seat adapter is provided. To remind you that their fear is not unjustified American adults suffer 40,000 toilet related injuries per year. Falling off a toilet directly contributed to the death of King George II of Great Britain. Because the height of the adult toilet does not allow their feet to touch the ground, a foot stool can be a great help. This gives their feet a place to rest and to assume the squatting posture. This eases the initiation of a bowel movement and can accelerate toilet training.

Bowel Sounds

Bowel sounds, also known as abdominal sounds, if audible at a distance are known by the onomatopoeia borborygmi. Onomatopoeia is a word created to imitate the sound it is meant to describe. Bowel sounds may also have a bubbling, gurgling, rushing fluid sound and is generated by the peristaltic movement of the contents along the gastrointestinal tract.

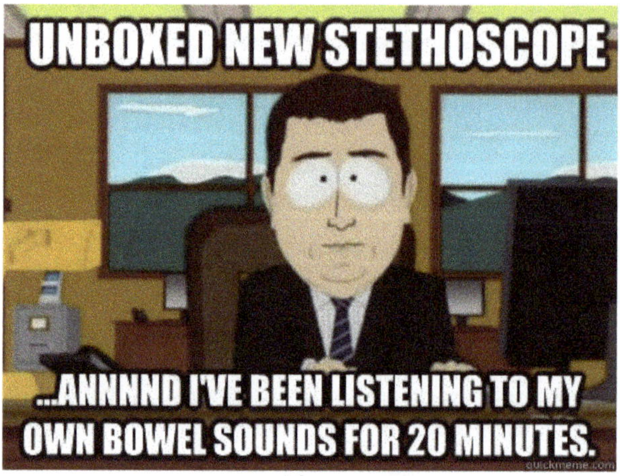
UNBOXED NEW STETHOSCOPE
...ANNNND I'VE BEEN LISTENING TO MY OWN BOWEL SOUNDS FOR 20 MINUTES.

www.quickmeme.com

These sounds are usually audible only by placing the listening ear on the abdominal wall or with the aid of a stethoscope. The presence of bowel sounds indicates that peristaltic activity is occurring. Changes in the bowel sounds, such as hyperactivity or absence may be indicative of a gastrointestinal disorder such as bowel obstruction or ileus.

Bristol Stool Scale

The Bristol stool scale (or chart), developed by Dr. Ken Heaton at the University of Bristol, classifies human feces into seven stool types based on appearance and consistency.

Type 1: Separate hard lumps, like nuts (hard to pass)
Type 2: Sausage-shaped, but lumpy
Type 3: Like a sausage but with cracks on its surface
Type 4: Like a sausage or snake, smooth and soft
Type 5: Soft blobs with clear-cut edges (passed easily)
Type 6: Fluffy pieces with ragged edges, a mushy stool
Type 7: Watery, no solid pieces. Entirely liquid

The transition from constipation at Type 1 to diarrhea as Type 7 is indicative of stool moisture content and its effect on morphology.

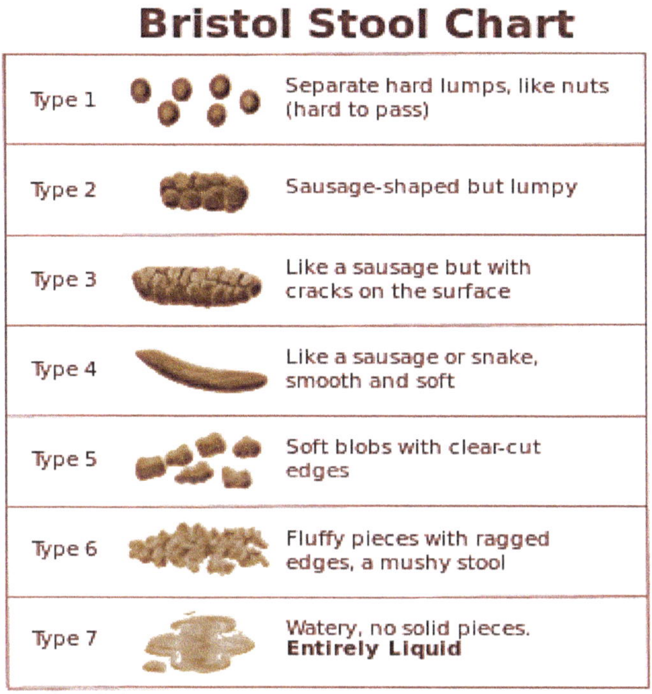
Bristol Stool Chart
Type 1
Separate hard lumps, like nuts (hard to pass)
Type 2
Sausage-shaped but lumpy
Type 3
Like a sausage but with cracks on the surface
Type 4
Like a sausage or snake, smooth and soft
Type 5
Soft blobs with clear-cut edges
Type 6
Fluffy pieces with ragged edges, a mushy stool
Type 7
Watery, no solid pieces.
Entirely Liquid

Bristol Stool Chart 2011 Author Kyle Thompson Creative Commons License

Bullshit (see Manure)

Bullshit, also known as bullcrap is a common English slang profanity meaning 'nonsense' and often shortened to the euphemism bull or the initials BS. 'Bull' meaning nonsense, dates from the 17th century and may have been derived from the Old French word *boul* meaning fraud or deceit. The term 'bullshit' has been used as early as 1915 in American slang, and came into popular usage during World War II. The celebrated poet T. S. Eliot wrote an unpublished poem as a ballad in the early 1900's entitled *The Triumph of Bullshit*.

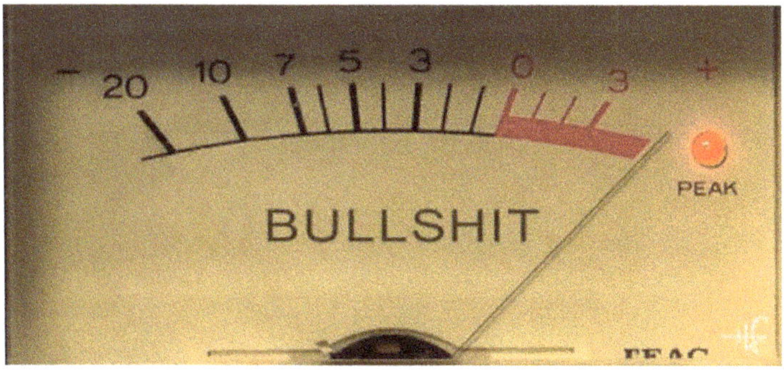
20
10
7
5
3
0
3
+
PEAK
BULLSHIT

thehoopla.com.au/bullshit-meter-hits-red-zone

Bullshit is a common rebuke to actions that are perceived to be false, misleading, or deceptive. Bullshit does not necessarily have to be an untruthful fabrication. It can also be an attempt to impress others that one has a greater mastery of a subject, often by excessive verbosity implying knowledge when in actuality it is merely filler without substance.

Harry Frankfurt, Professor of Philosophy at Princeton University, wrote the treatise *On Bullshit* proposing that bullshit is related to but distinct from lying. Frankfurt believes the liar knows the truth and deliberately misleads. The bullshitter does not care about the truth and is only seeking to impress.

From *On Bullshit* by Dr. Harry Frankfurt (written in 1986, and published in 2005): "It is impossible for someone to lie unless he thinks he knows the truth. Producing bullshit requires no such conviction. A person who lies is thereby responding to the truth, and he is to that extent respectful of it. When an honest man speaks, he says only what he believes to be true; and for the liar, it is correspondingly indispensable that he considers his statements to be false.

For the bullshitter, however, all these bets are off: he is neither on the side of the true nor on the side of the false. His eye is not on the facts at all, as the eyes of the honest man and of the liar are, except insofar as they may be pertinent to his interest in getting away with what he says. He does not care whether the things he says describe reality correctly. He just picks them out, or makes them up, to suit his purpose."

Cathartic

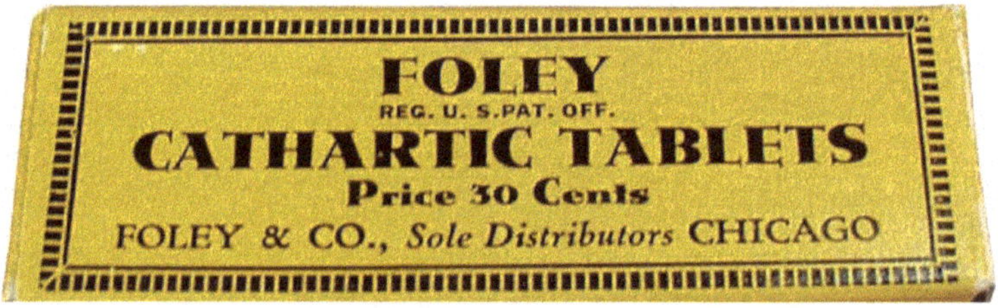
FOLEY
REG. U. S. PAT. OFF.
CATHARTIC TABLETS
Price 30 Cents
FOLEY & CO., Sole Distributors CHICAGO

The term catharsis is derived from the Greek κάθαρσις *katharsis* meaning purification or cleansing. It is a term used in literature, psychology, sociology, and a number of fields other than medicine. In physiology and medicine it is used to describe the accelerated release of material from the genitourinary or digestive systems. A cathartic is a product that accelerates this process, especially a purgative that stimulates the prompt evacuation of the bowels. A laxative is the term used for a product that eases the passage of fecal material, such as a lubricant. Some products have both cathartics and laxative properties.

Chamber Pot

A chamber pot (French: pot de chambre) is a pit like receptacle for receiving human waste. It was usually kept in the same chambers and under the sleeping bed and since the sixteenth century often enclosed in a stool with a lid.

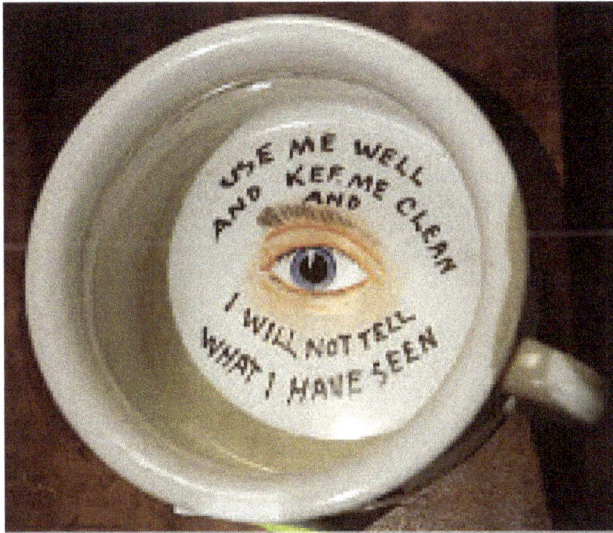
USE ME WELL
AND KEEP ME CLEAN
AND
I WILL NOT TELL
WHAT I HAVE SEEN

ginirifkin.blogspot.com

Chamber pots were used in ancient Greece at least since the 6th century BC and remained in common use in many parts of the world until the mid-20th century. In rural areas lacking indoor plumbing they are still in use today. They have also been modified to serve as bedpans for the ill and disabled.

The affectionate term 'potty' is often used with children especially during toilet training. The term potty is also used to describe the child-size chamber pot type toilets that are at the appropriate height with a child-size seat. When a child sits on an adult-size toilet seat there is a genuine fear of falling in, which can inhibit having a bowel movement.

Regular adult toilets, which have an opening that is normally too large and frightening for a child, may be used if a child seat adapter is provided. To remind you that their fear is not unjustified American adults suffer 40,000 toilet related injuries per year. Falling off a toilet directly contributed to the death of King George II of Great Britain. Because the height of the adult toilet does not allow the feet of children to touch the ground, a foot stool can be a great help. This gives their feet a place to rest and to assume the squatting posture. This eases the initiation of a bowel movement and can accelerate toilet training.

Chickenshit (see Manure)

Chicken shit, or more commonly chickenshit, is a slang term, usually regarded as a vulgar adjective. It has two meanings, the first signifying a lack of courage and cowardice. The second is to describe something as being petty or insignificant.

The term was first used as an insult for cowardice early in the twentieth century. The color yellow, typically associated with cowardice, is the color of young chicks before they mature into adulthood. Some sources suggest that chickenshit has military roots in its use as a derogatory for petty mindedness. Chickenshit is used instead of more substantial horse, bull, or elephant shit, as chickenshit is described as something small-minded that takes the trivial seriously.

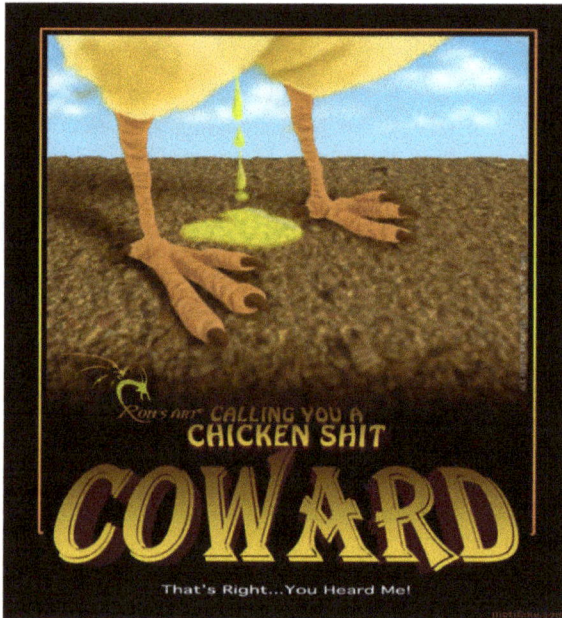
CALLING YOU A
CHICKEN SHIT
COWARD
That's Right...You Heard Me!

mofosquad.blogspot.com

Close Stool (see Groom of the Stool)

A close stool, also called a necessary or night stool, was in popular use for nearly five hundred years from the sixteenth century until the advent of indoor plumbing. It was an enclosed cabinet at chair height with an opening in the top often covered by a lid. It contained a pewter or earthenware chamber pot. In the nineteenth century it was referred to as a night commode, and in the twentieth century the commode euphemism was extended to the flush toilet.

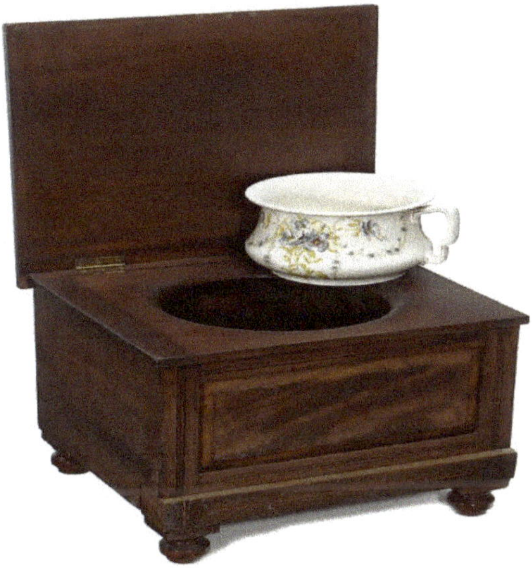

www.liveauctioneers.com

Clyster (see Enema)

Colon (see Digestion)

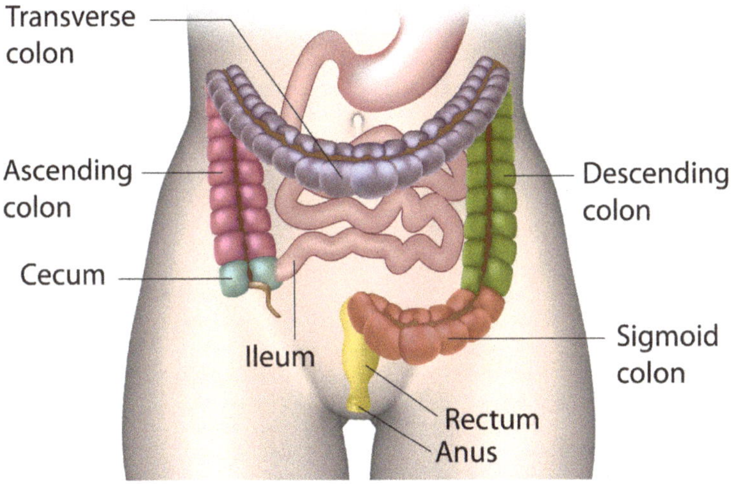
Transverse colon
Ascending colon
Cecum
Ileum
Descending colon
Sigmoid colon
Rectum
Anus

shutterstock/AlilaMedicalMedia

The colon is also known as the large intestine or large bowel. Unlike the small intestine, it is less involved in the digestion of foods and nutrients. It is primarily involved in the absorption of water and sodium as well as some fat-soluble vitamins such as vitamin K. The colon removes the excess moisture from the watery chyme, and the stool solidifies as it transits the gut. It is stored in the rectum and sigmoid colon awaiting the right opportunity to be eliminated through defecation. A process or illness that impairs the colon's absorption of water will lead to more fluid stool and diarrhea. If the elimination is delayed, moisture continues to be absorbed and the stools can become harder resulting in constipation.

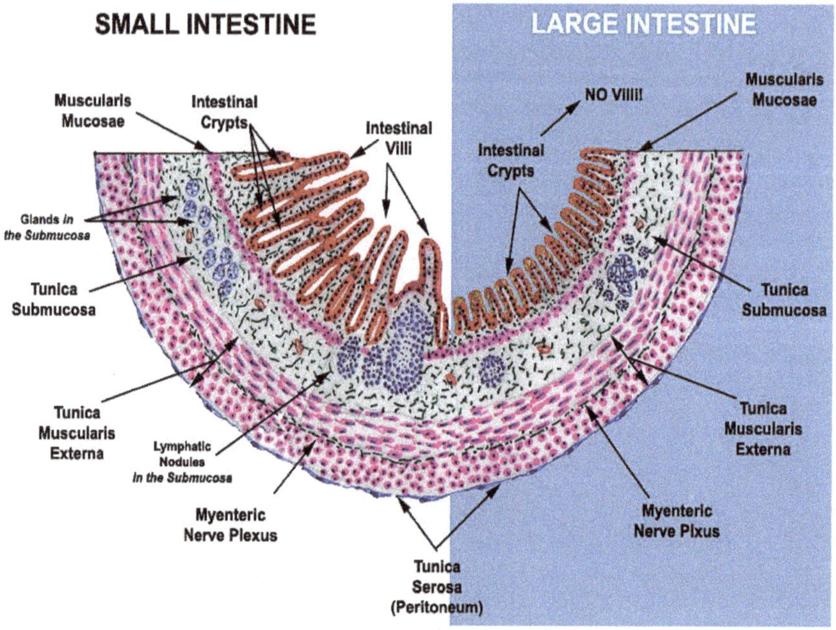
SMALL INTESTINE
LARGE INTESTINE
Muscularis Mucosae
Intestinal Crypts
Intestinal Villi
NO Villi!
Intestinal Crypts
Muscularis Mucosae
Glands in the Submucosa
Tunica Submucosa
Tunica Submucosa
Tunica Muscularis Externa
Lymphatic Nodules In the Submucosa
Myenteric Nerve Plexus
Tunica Serosa (Peritoneum)
Myenteric Nerve Pixus
Tunica Muscularis Externa

www.vetmed.vt.edu

Colon Hydrotherapy (see Enema)

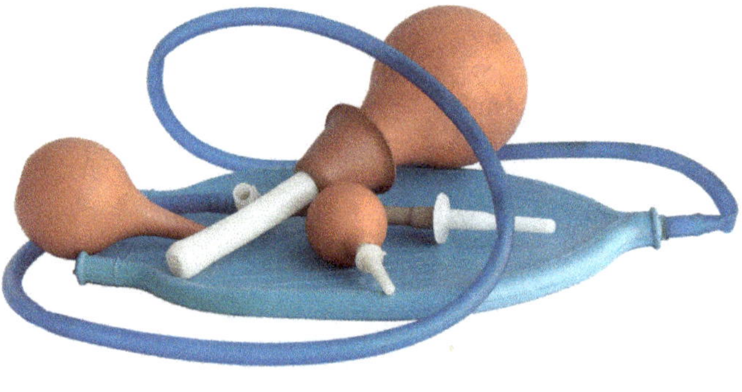

shutterstock/FradkinaVictoria

Colonic Hydrotherapy, Proctoclysis

Prior to the development of convenient access for intravenous administration, fluids and medication were commonly administered by proctoclysis or rectoclysis, also known as the Murphy drip after its developer, American surgeon John Murphy. The rationale for its use, particularly when oral intake could not be accomplished, remains valid although it is rarely used today. Although it may not be aesthetically pleasing, the bottom line is that the administration of fluids can be lifesaving in severe dehydration.

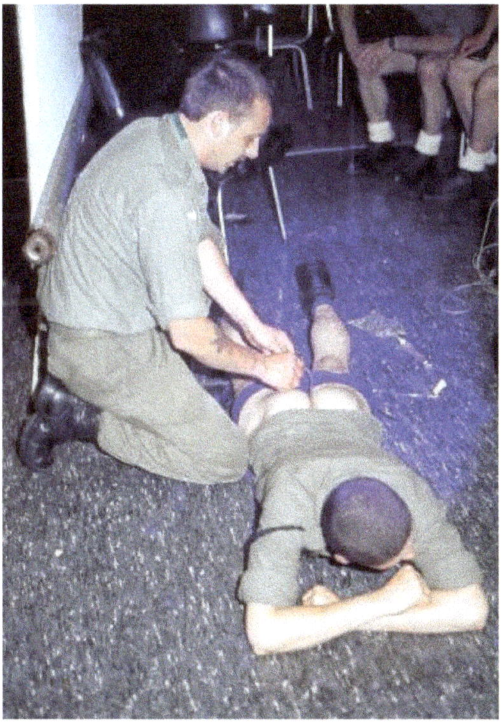

The colon is the primary organ for the absorption of fluids and electrolytes. It's rich blood supply and absorptive capacity makes it a suitable route for the administration of fluids and medicines. Proctoclysis is an easy, safe and effective way to provide fluid replacement. It does not require sterile fluids, specialized equipment, or advanced training, and it is very useful when alternative routes are not available such as remote locations away from access to medical care. Suppositories have the additional advantage of avoiding the portal circulation and bypassing metabolism in the liver. liver. Hypodermoclysis, the subcutaneous administration of fluids, was also used as an alternative and continues to be popular in veterinary medicine.

Colonography

Colonography is also known as virtual colonoscopy and uses the technology of computed axial tomography to generate images of the internal aspects of the colon. Computed axial tomography (Greek tomos (slice) graphein) (CAT scan) is an imaging procedure that uses computer-processed X-rays to produce images that appear as cross sectional slices of specific areas of the body.

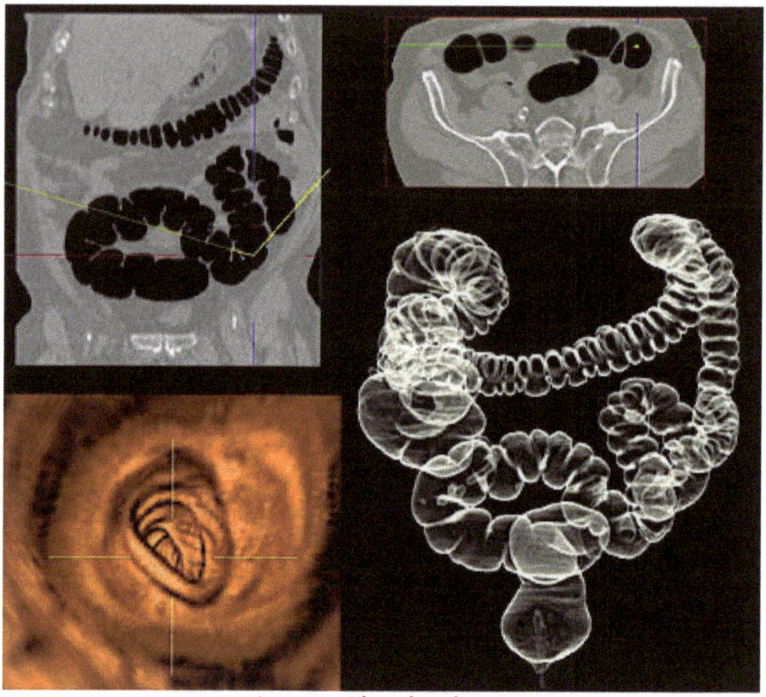

www.journey-with-crohns-disease.com

Colonography is regarded as a moderate to high radiation diagnostic technique. Further refinement has led to computed axial tomography angiography to view vascular anatomy. A computed axial tomography scan colonography, also known as virtual colonoscopy, was also developed and may be used as a screening method for detecting colon polyps and cancer.

The ionizing radiation in the form of x-rays used in computed axial tomography scans may damage cellular genetic material (DNA) if not corrected properly by cellular repair mechanisms. Such damage has the potential of leading to the development of cancer in the tissue. The most common cancers thought to be caused by radiation exposure are lung, breast, thyroid, stomach, and the blood cell lines of leukemia.

Virtual colonoscopy, also called Computed Axial Tomography (CAT) Colonography, is a medical imaging procedure that has great potential. It utilizes x-rays or magnetic imaging and computers to produce two- and three-dimensional images of the colon. The procedure may be used to diagnose colon and bowel disease, including polyps, diverticulosis and cancer. It holds great promise as a potential screening study for colon polyps and colon cancer. A virtual colonoscopy can provide three-dimensional reconstructed endoluminal views of the bowel. The patient may also be given a solution designed to coat any residual feces, which may not have been cleared by the laxative preparation used to empty the colon prior to the study. This is called 'fecal tagging' and avoids otherwise false positive results where remaining feces could falsely appear to be a polyp or cancer. The examination takes about ten minutes and does not require sedatives.

A thin tube is inserted into the rectum and air is pumped in to inflate the colon for better viewing. This can be uncomfortable but lasts for only a few minutes. The patient is asked to hold their breath occasionally during the scan to provide the clearest images. After the examination, the images produced by the scanner are processed by computer software into a three-dimensional image, which the radiologist evaluates to identify any abnormalities. The patient may resume normal activity after the procedure, but if abnormalities are found and the patient needs conventional colonoscopy, it may be performed the same day.

Virtual colonoscopy is more comfortable than conventional colonoscopy and does not require sedation. The patient can return to their usual activities after the procedure. The lack of sedation also lowers the risk of the procedure in avoiding side effects from the medication as well as a reduction in the risk of perforation. It is a faster procedure than visual colonoscopy and can see the entire colon which visual colonoscopy may not have accomplished in up to ten percent of patients. Virtual colonoscopy provides clearer more detailed images than the older conventional x-ray using a barium enema, also called a lower gastrointestinal (GI) series. Virtual colonoscopy provides a secondary benefit of revealing diseases or abnormalities outside the colon.

The main disadvantage to virtual colonoscopy is that a radiologist cannot take tissue samples (biopsy) or remove polyps during virtual colonoscopy, so a conventional colonoscopy must be performed if abnormalities are found. Virtual colonoscopy does not show as much detail as a conventional colonoscopy, so polyps smaller than between two and ten millimeters in diameter may not show up on the images. Furthermore virtual colonoscopy performed with computed axial tomography exposes the patient to ionizing radiation.

Optical colonoscopy and virtual colonoscopy are complementary studies in screening the colon for polyps and cancers. Other modalities may also be used such as stool test for blood, and DNA markers of polyps and cancers. Screening for colon cancer is suggested for men and women at age fifty, and younger if there is a family history of colon cancer, polyps, or personal history of inflammatory bowel disease or polyps.

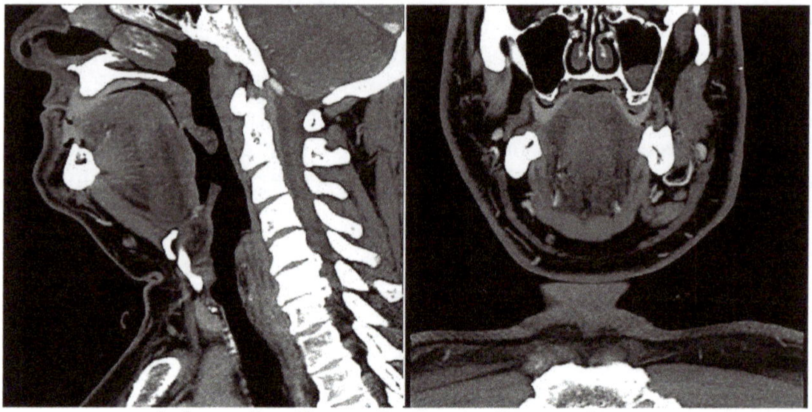

Author en:User:ChumousRex Creative Commons License

Colonoscopy

Colonoscopy is an endoscopic procedure that allows the visual inspection of the lower bowel, including the colon and the terminal ileum. Endoscopy is the procedure of using an instrument to allow the visual inspection of the internal organs, usually through a natural orifice.

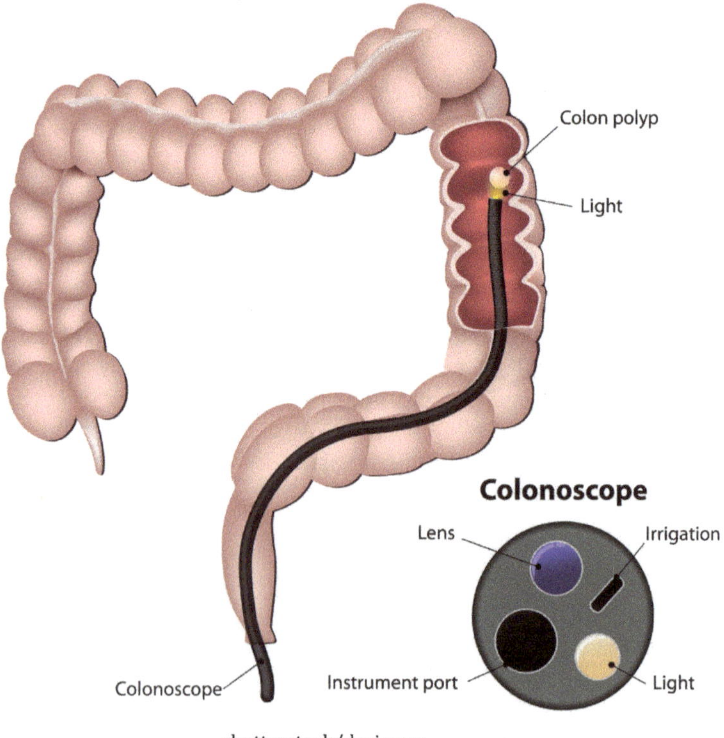
Colon polyp
Light
Colonoscope
Lens
Irrigation
Instrument port
Light
Colonoscope

shutterstock/designua

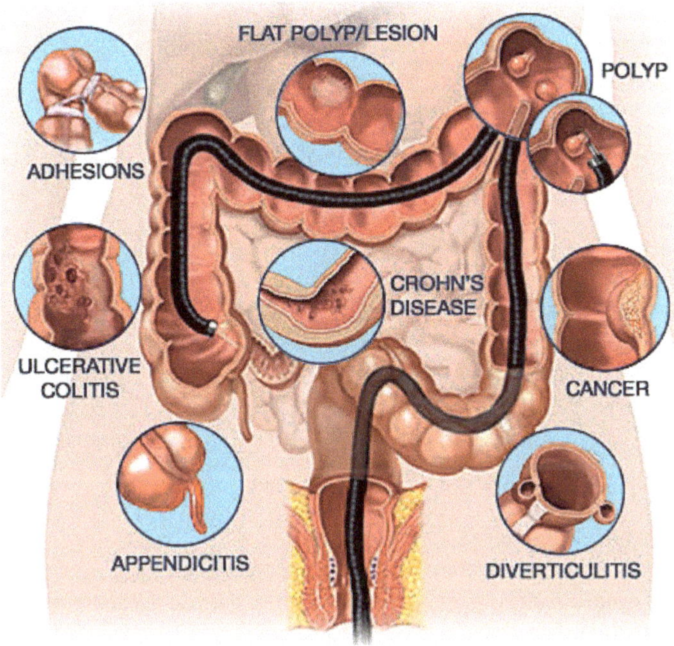
FLAT POLYP/LESION
POLYP
ADHESIONS
CROHN'S DISEASE
ULCERATIVE COLITIS
CANCER
APPENDICITIS
DIVERTICULITIS

hwww.tabletprep.com Creative Commons License

In the field of gastroenterology the major endoscopic examinations include esophagoscopy, gastroscopy, duodenoscopy, all often combined as esophagogastroduodenoscopy also abbreviated as EGD or simply referred to as endoscopy. Enteroscopy, the evaluation of the small intestine, requires a very long specialized instrument or the examination may be performed during abdominal surgery with the assistance of a surgeon manipulating the small intestine while the endoscope is inside the bowel.

The instruments have evolved from rigid instruments with limited visibility, to flexible instruments using fiber optics, to very slender instruments using charge coupled device (CCD) video chips, and the newest generation of higher resolution, spectroscopic, magnification, and capsule endoscopes. The addition of ultrasonography to endoscopy has added additional diagnostic capabilities as the ultrasound probe can now be brought to the closer proximity of the lesion. Further advancements in diagnostic and therapeutic technology are anticipated.

The technology and terminology is modified for use in several specialties including pulmonary (bronchoscopy), urology (cystoscopy), gynecology (colposcopy, hysteroscopy, falloposcopy), surgery (laparoscopy), otolaryngology (rhinoscopy and laryngoscopy), orthopedics (arthroscopy) etcetera. A similar approach is used in other fields such as the borescope evaluation of jet engines, complex machinery, pipelines, etcetera.

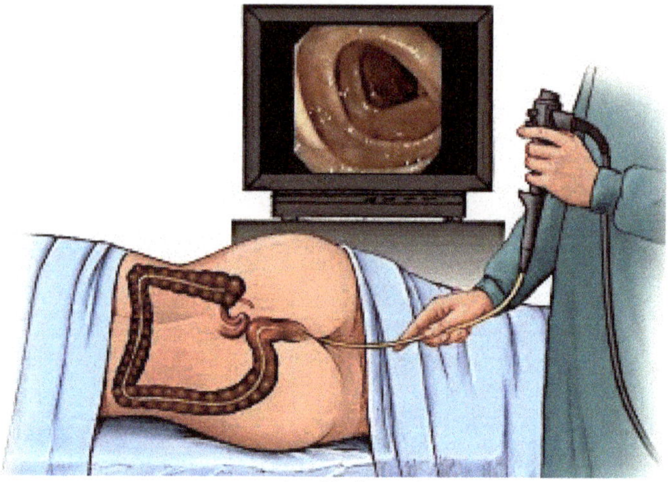

www.daviddarling.info

Capsule enteroscopy has become the diagnostic study of choice for evaluating most of the small intestine. Anoscopy (anus), proctoscopy (rectum), sigmoidoscopy (sigmoid colon and rectum), colonoscopy (colon and rectum, and often the distal ileum, and ileoscopy (ileum), are commonly performed as well to evaluate for colorectal or ileal disorders. Besides visual inspection, all of the endoscopic procedures offer the ability to obtain biopsy or cytology specimens, and aspirate fluids for examination or culture. Therapeutic options are also available to control bleeding, destroy lesions with electrocautery or lasers, to suture or to cut, to retrieve foreign bodies or gallstones, to inject medications or therapeutic agents, dilate areas of stenosis or stricture, etcetera

The risks of perforation of the organ being examined, bleeding, infection, and adverse reactions to sedative medication or therapeutic maneuvers are significant but fortunately very infrequent. The specific risks are dependent on the nature of the procedure and should be discussed with the health care provider. Having performed several thousand endoscopic procedures, and having been on the receiving end of a few of the procedures myself, they are rarely felt or remembered when sedative medication is administered. I wish I could say the same for the bowel cleansing preparation for colonoscopy. There is certainly room for improvement in this area and a number of specialists are beginning to recognize the ease and value of colon hydrotherapy as an alternative.

Colonoscopy is the endoscopic examination of the large bowel and the distal part of the small bowel with a CCD video or fiberoptic camera on a flexible tube passed through the anus. It can provide a visual diagnosis and provides the opportunity for biopsy or removal of colorectal lesions. The instrument is typically less than a half inch in diameter, much narrower than the normal caliber of stool. The discomfort with the procedure is the clearing preparation and the air insufflation and distention.

Most procedures can be completed in about thirty minutes with a ninety-five percent success rate of inspecting the full length of the colon. It takes about sixty to ninety minutes for the medication to wear off. Aspirin should be avoided for about a week before the procedure. If a polyp is found and removed the risk of bleeding is about one percent, and the risk of perforation is less than one in a thousand. In extremely rare occurrences in the past intra-colonic gasses, due to the bowel preparation administered, have ignited with the electric snare removal of polyps.

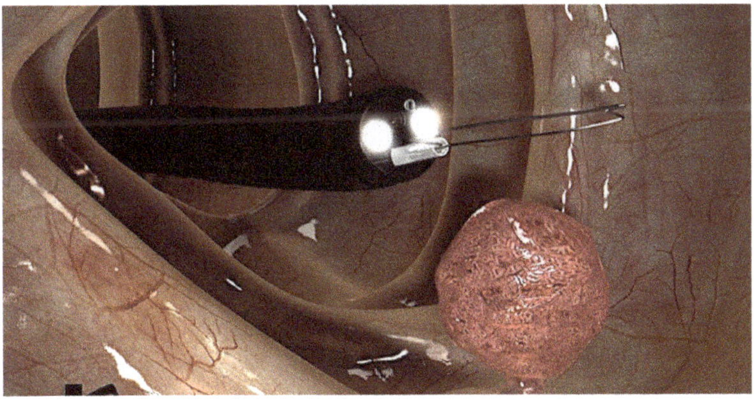

In the image above a colonoscope is approaching a colon polyp with a wire snare that will lasso the polyp, and cauterize the base with electric current. Following the polypectomy the polyp will be retrieved and examined under the microscope by a pathologist to determine if any cancer cells have developed within the polyp. The larger the polyp the greater the chance of colon cancer. Removing polyps before they develop into a cancer has proven to be effective in reducing the incidence of colon cancer.

During the procedure the patient is often given sedation intravenously with midazolam and an analgesic fentanyl. About sixty to ninety minutes time elapse for the medication to wear off sufficiently to be fully awake. Substituting propofol as the sedative agent gives the patient a very fast recovery and is gaining wider use, but requires closer monitoring of respiration. Air release after the procedure is expected and clears rapidly.

Computed axial tomography (Greek tomos (slice) graphein) (CAT scan) is an imaging procedure that uses computer-processed X-rays to produce images that appear as cross sectional slices of specific areas of the body. It is regarded as a moderate to high radiation diagnostic technique. Further refinement has led to computed axial tomography angiography to view vascular anatomy. A computed axial tomography scan colonography (virtual colonoscopy) was also developed and may be used as a screening method for detecting colon polyps and cancer.

The main disadvantage to virtual colonoscopy is that a radiologist cannot take tissue samples (biopsy) or remove polyps during virtual colonoscopy, so a conventional colonoscopy must be performed if abnormalities are found. Virtual colonoscopy does not show as much detail as a conventional colonoscopy, so polyps between two and ten millimeters in diameter may not show up on the images. Furthermore, virtual colonoscopy performed with computed axial tomography exposes the patient to ionizing radiation.

Optical colonoscopy and virtual colonoscopy are complementary studies in screening the colon for polyps and cancers. Other modalities may also be used such as stool test for blood, and DNA markers of polyps and cancers. Screening for colon cancer is suggested for men and women beginning at age fifty, and younger if there is a family history of colon cancer, polyps, or personal history of inflammatory bowel disease or polyps.

Composting Toilet

A composting toilet is a dry toilet that uses managed aerobic decomposition to treat human waste. They are an alternative to flush toilets where there is a limited water supply or no waste treatment facility is available. The human excrement is normally mixed with sawdust, coconut coir, or peat moss to encourage aerobic decomposition, absorb liquids, and to control odor. The decomposition process is typically faster than the anaerobic decomposition used in wet sewage systems such as septic tanks. Urine can contain ninety percent of the nitrogen, fifty percent of the phosphorus, and seventy percent of the potassium present in human excreta. In healthy individuals the urine is sterile and thus pathogen free. Undiluted urine may contain inorganic salts and organic compounds toxic to plants.

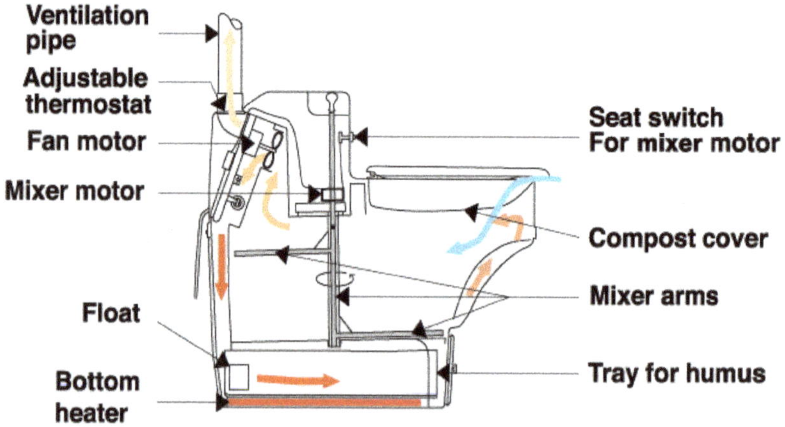
Ventilation pipe
Adjustable thermostat
Fan motor
Mixer motor
Float
Bottom heater
Seat switch For mixer motor
Compost cover
Mixer arms
Tray for humus

www.watersavingsystem.com/composting-toilet.php

The requirement critical for aerobic microbial action is sufficient oxygen. Some units require manual methods for periodic aeration of the solid mass. Significant reductions in the volume of waste occur through the process, with only ten percent of the inputs coming out as a humus-like material, which can be used as a soil amendment.

Constipation

Constipation may be defined as three or fewer bowel movements per week, staining with twenty-five percent or more of bowel movements, hard stools type 1 or 2 on the Bristol Scale, or incomplete bowel evacuation. It is estimated to affect twelve percent of the population worldwide, with some studies suggesting a figure as high as thirty percent. Severe constipation with the failure to pass gas as well as stool is called obstipation (Latin obstīpātiō, from ob- (intensive) + stīpāre to press together).

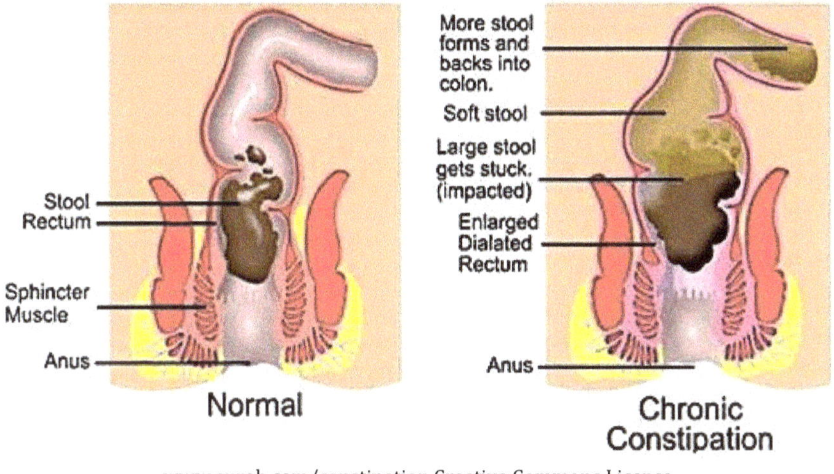
Stool
Rectum
Sphincter Muscle
Anus
Normal
More stool forms and backs into colon.
Soft stool
Large stool gets stuck. (impacted)
Enlarged Dialated Rectum
Anus
Chronic Constipation

www.auroh.com/constipation Creative Commons License

Constipation can also be defined by stool appearance as outlined in the Bristol stool scale or chart, developed by Dr. Ken Heaton at the University of Bristol. It classifies human feces into seven stool types based on appearance and consistency.

Constipation is a symptom with two main categories. The first includes mechanical obstruction such as colon cancer or fecal impaction. The second is colonic hypomotility with inadequate colon emptying such as hypothyroidism or medication side effects. Additional causes may include inadequate physical activity, inefficient fiber in the diet, inadequate fluid intake, neuromuscular disorders like Parkinson's Disease, multiple sclerosis, muscular dystrophy, cystic fibrosis, hypercalcemia, diabetes, etcetera. Hirschsprung disease is a consideration in infants with constipation. The presence of higher levels of methane in intestinal gas has been associated with decreased gastrointestinal motility and constipation. The colonic flora of the gut microbiome in conjunction with diet plays an important role.

While constipation and narrowing of stool caliber may be a later sign of cancer of the colon these findings are typically localized to the left side of the colon involving the descending colon, sigmoid colon, or rectum. Cancers of the transverse colon and right side of the colon are less likely to cause obstructive symptoms and signs because the stool is less well formed and can more easily pass the cancer. Many medications may be constipating include narcotic pain medications, psychoactive medications, calcium, iron, and a very wide therapeutic range of drugs. A review of the medications being taken, including over the counter preparations, nutritional supplements, vitamins, minerals, and anything else taken in by mouth should be considered possible sources of constipation.

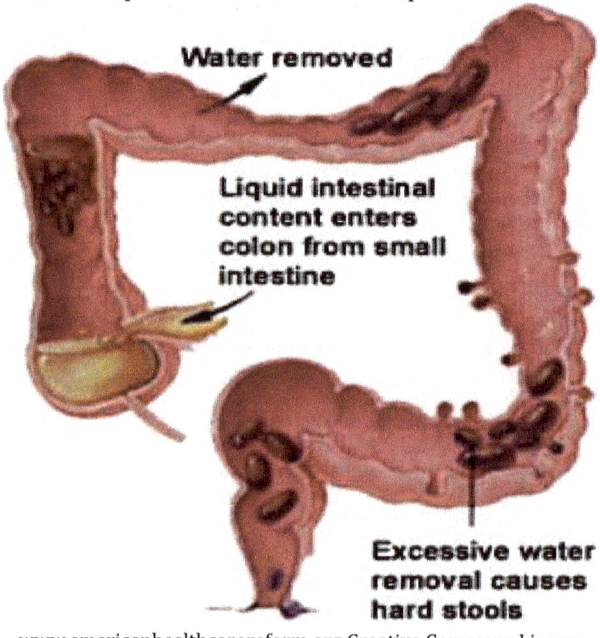
Water removed
Liquid intestinal content enters colon from small intestine
Excessive water removal causes hard stools

www.americanhealthcarereform.org Creative Commons License

Laxatives and purgatives are foods, compounds, chemicals, drugs, or plant based products taken to loosen the stool and increase the frequency of bowel movements. They may be taken in oral form or as a suppository and a number of products contain combinations of laxatives. Stimulant, lubricant and saline laxatives are often used to evacuate and cleanse the colon in preparation for diagnostic or therapeutic bowel procedures and examinations.

Treatments are directed to address the underlying cause and may include changes in diet, physical activity, supplements, laxatives, or enemas. The first choice in treatment is the increased intake of fiber and fluids. Enemas can be used to stimulate a bowel movement, and mild laxatives such as milk of magnesia may be helpful. Other products such as polyethylene glycol, lactulose, prucalopride, lubiprostone, and newer prokinetic agents may be necessary. In general stimulant laxatives are avoided to prevent dependency.

Naloxegol (Movantik) may help to restore bowel function in patients who have chronic illness and receive opioids or narcotics for pain relief. This prescription product recently approved by the Food & Drug Administration (FDA) is a mu-opioid receptor antagonist and decreases the constipating effect of the opioids or narcotics on the gut. Because naloxegol is a pegylated derivative of naloxone, it has limited ability to cross the blood-brain barrier so it does not interfere with the central analgesic effect desired. Another product available for managing chronic severe pain with an opioid or narcotic is marketed as Targin, Targinact, or Targiniq ER an extended release combination of oxycodone and naloxone. The naloxone is a narcotic antagonist and reduces the risk of dependence and constipation by its effect on the gut after absorption, but before its metabolism in the liver.

Humans can defecate in a number of defecation postures. The two most common are the squatting posture and the sitting posture. The squatting posture is used for squat toilets and is also commonly used for defecation in the absence of toilets or other devices. It is commonly used in non-Western cultures. The sitting defecation posture is used in Western toilets with either a leaning forward posture or a ninety-degree sitting upright posture. The posture chosen appears to be largely a cultural decision although there is evidence that the squatting posture is more efficacious and induces the least bodily strain

The Bristol Stool Scale illustrated below has become a standard to define the nature and consistency of the bowel movement.

Type 1: Separate hard lumps, like nuts (hard to pass)
Type 2: Sausage-shaped, but lumpy
Type 3: Like a sausage but with cracks on its surface
Type 4: Like a sausage or snake, smooth and soft
Type 5: Soft blobs with clear-cut edges (passed easily)
Type 6: Fluffy pieces with ragged edges, a mushy stool
Type 7: Watery, no solid pieces. Entirely liquid

The transition from constipation at Type 1 to diarrhea as Type 7 is indicative of stool moisture content and its effect on morphology.

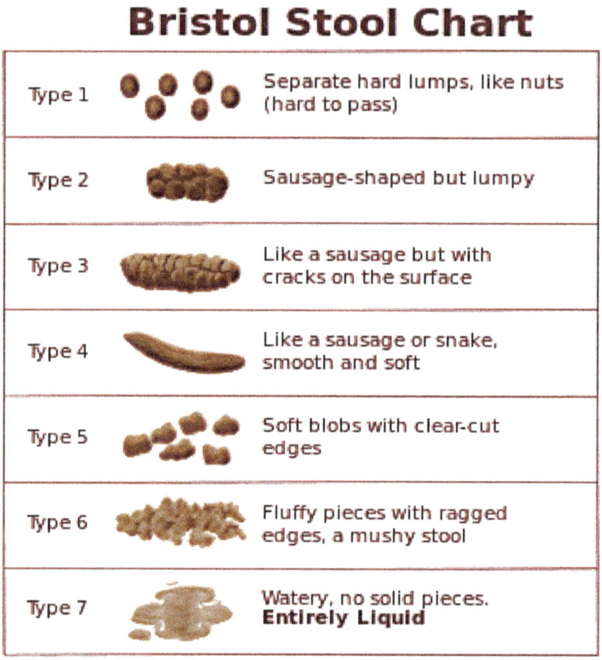
Bristol Stool Chart
Type 1
Separate hard lumps, like nuts (hard to pass)
Type 2
Sausage-shaped but lumpy
Type 3
Like a sausage but with cracks on the surface
Type 4
Like a sausage or snake, smooth and soft
Type 5
Soft blobs with clear-cut edges
Type 6
Fluffy pieces with ragged edges, a mushy stool
Type 7
Watery, no solid pieces.
Entirely Liquid

Bristol Stool Chart 2011 Author Kyle Thompson Creative Commons License

The sitting position can cause the defecating human being to repeat the Valsalva maneuver many times and with great force. This can lead to diverticulosis, hemorrhoids, hernias and cardiovascular stress and defecation syncope. For those with underlying cardiac disease the additional stress induced by defecating in the sitting position as opposed to the more natural squatting position may be surprisingly life threatening. The degree of straining during defecation is at least three times greater when sitting on a toilet than with the squatting posture.

Difficulty with the seated position is particularly true if the feet cannot reach the floor as is commonly seen when small children are placed on adult height toilets. The affectionate term 'potty' is often used with children especially during toilet (potty) training. The term potty is also used to describe child size chamber pot type toilets that are at the appropriate height and have a child size opening to sit on.

Regular adult toilets have an opening that is too large and frightening for a child who could accidentally fall in if not assisted. To remind you that their fear is not unjustified American adults suffer 40,000 toilet related injuries per year. Falling off a toilet directly contributed to the death of King George II of Great Britain. Child size seats are available that can be placed on an adult seat to accommodate a child.

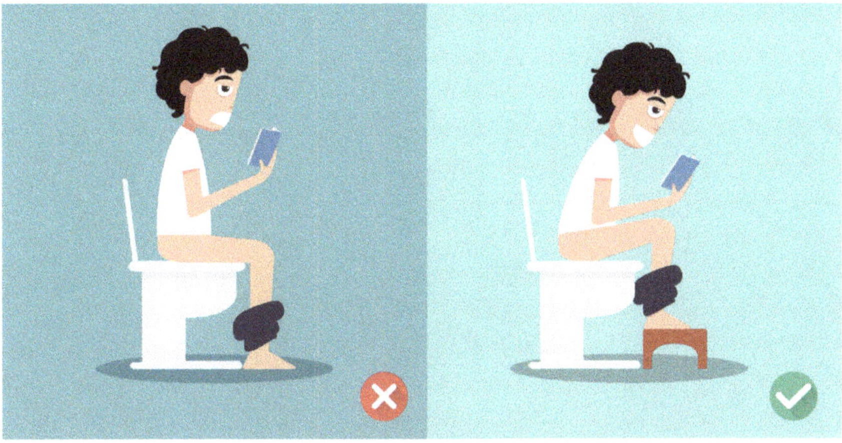

shutterstock/jehsomwang

The height of the adult toilet does not allow the feet of children to touch the ground to assist in the squatting maneuver that assists defecation. A footstool to give their feet a place on which to rest can assist squatting. This may ease the initiation of a bowel movement and can accelerate toilet training. An adult may become frustrated that it is taking the child so long to defecate, not realizing that not being able to brace their feet against a solid surface is a problem. They may need a stepstool to apply resistance so that they are able to generate the intra-abdominal pressure needed to promote defecation.

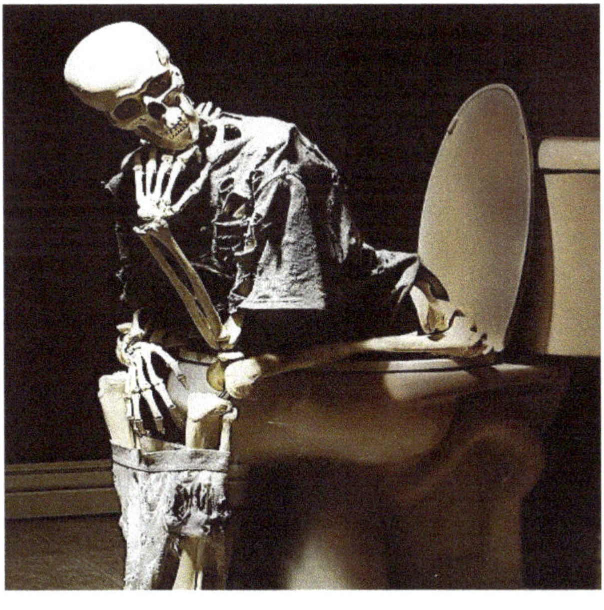

Constitutional

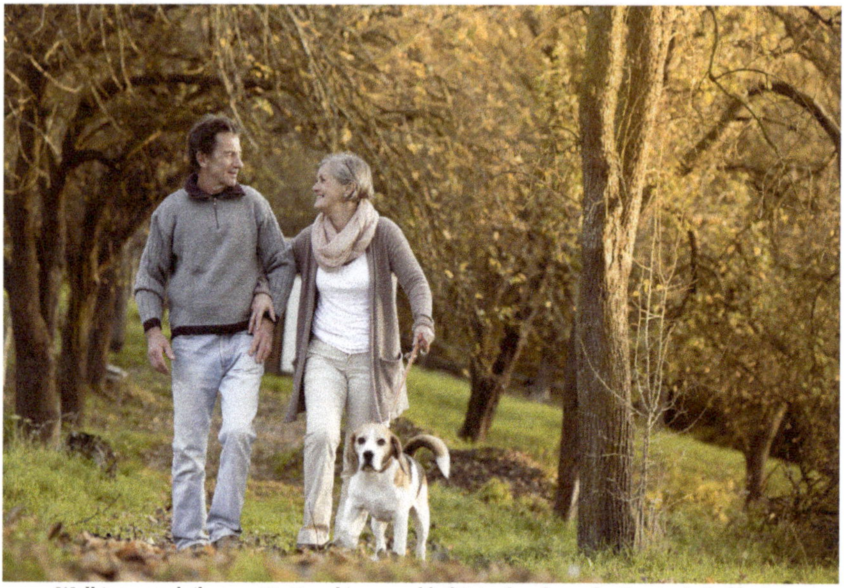

Walking as a daily constitutional is a good habit to develop. shutterstock/halfpoint

Constitutional is a term used for an activity that is conducive to general good health. It usually refers to exercise in some form such as walking. Physical activity has an association with stimulation of gastrointestinal motility, sometimes to the extreme such as is seen in the condition known as 'runner's trots'. The term morning constitutional and daily constitutional also became used as euphemism for having a bowel movement, often referring to the first bowel movement of the day.

Continence, Fecal

Fecal continence is the control over defecation leading to the voluntary evacuation of bowel contents. The most common causes of the loss of continence, referred to as fecal incontinence, are damage from childbirth, complications from prior anorectal surgery, and altered bowel habits. An estimated two-point-two percent of adults are affected.

The primary symptom is a lack of control over bowel contents, which may worsen without treatment. Secondary symptoms that are the result of leakage include the intense itching of pruritus ani, the irritation and inflammation of perianal dermatitis and urinary tract infections. There is often reduced self-esteem, depression, humiliation, and avoidance of enjoyable activities. Unfortunately it is a mistakenly stigmatized genuine medical condition. There are too many people who may be too embarrassed to seek medical help and deal with the frustrating symptoms in secrecy for prolonged time periods. It is generally very treatable with a variety of dietary, pharmacologic, or surgical options.

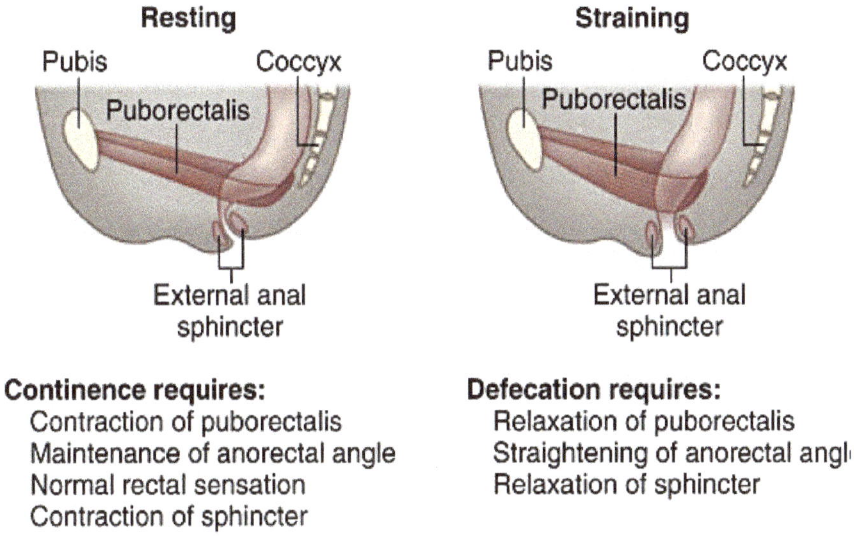
Resting
Pubis
Coccyx
Puborectalis
External anal sphincter
Straining
Pubis
Coccyx
Puborectalis
External anal sphincter
Continence requires:
Contraction of puborectalis
Maintenance of anorectal angle
Normal rectal sensation
Contraction of sphincter
Defecation requires:
Relaxation of puborectalis
Straightening of anorectal angl
Relaxation of sphincter
www.cixip.com/Public Creative Commons License

The evaluation of fecal incontinence is multifactorial. Some of the factors that are considered in evaluation and treatment include the nature and magnitude of the incontinence. It may be limited to or include the passage of flatus, mucus, liquid stool, or solid stool. The volume passed may be minor staining of underwear, increasing to soilage, seepage, or full bowel movements. There may a sensation of urgency and impending passage implying that the sensory pathway is intact and the message can be detected, or passive release without sensation. There may be a reduction in the ability of the rectum to distend normally to store and accommodate stool prior to evacuation. The internal anal sphincter, external anal sphincter, or both may be impaired.

The description of fecal incontinence may not be incontinence at all. It may be a rectal discharge of mucus and blood from various causes ranging from inflammatory bowel disease and local infections to radiation proctitis and rectal stercoral ulceration. There may be a perianal fistula such as frequently seen in the inflammatory bowel disease of Crohn Disease. A perianal abscess or rectal prolapse may cause drainage mistaken for incontinence. Anal fissures, hemorrhoids, anal warts, anal cancer, hemorrhoids, abscess, and fistula may also prevent complete and continent closure of the anus. There may be a condition causing diarrhea, which is harder to maintain continence of compared to solid stool. Constipation as well as fecal impaction can cause an overflow incontinence where liquid stool bypasses the obstructing constipated stool.

There are a number of interrelated mechanisms and factors that contribute to normal continence. In up to eighty percent of patients with continence issues there is more than one contributing factor. The puborectalis sling forming the anorectal angle is responsible for gross continence of solid stool. The internal anal sphincter is an involuntary muscle that contributes about fifty-five percent of the resting anal pressure. Together with the hemorrhoid vascular cushions the internal anal sphincter maintains continence of flatus and liquid during rest.

The external anal sphincter is a voluntary muscle, doubling the pressure in the anal canal during contraction. The rectoanal inhibitory reflex is an involuntary internal anal sphincter relaxation in response to rectal distention. This allows a sampling of some of the rectal contents to descend into the anal canal. Here it is brought into contact with specialized sensory mucosa to detect consistency. The rectoanal excitatory reflex is an initial semi-voluntary contraction of the external anal sphincter and puborectalis, which returns tone following the rectoanal inhibitory reflex.

Other factors include the specialized anti-peristaltic function of the last part of the sigmoid colon, the sensory ability of the lining of the rectum and the anal canal to detect the consistency and quantity when of stool present, and the normal rectoanal reflexes and defecation cycle that completes evacuation. Problems affecting any of these mechanisms and factors may be contributing to incontinence. Reduced rectal storage capacity with either a reduction in rectal volume or rectal compliance for distention may lead to urge incontinence. It may be caused by surgery such as a lower anterior resection, radiation therapy of the rectum, or inflammatory bowel disease all of which may cause scarring and reduced compliance of the rectum. Tumors and strictures may impair reservoir function. A rectocele may cause an incomplete evacuation of the rectum with post defecation leakage.

Caffeine can contribute by relaxing the anal sphincter tone. Pharmaceuticals that can reduce sphincter tone pressure and contribute to incontinence include nitrates, calcium channel antagonists, beta-adrenoceptor antagonists (beta-blockers), sildenafil, selective serotonin reuptake inhibitors like fluoxetine (Prozac), antibiotics, topical drugs applied to anus including glyceryl trinitrate ointment, diltiazem gel, bethanechol cream, botulinum toxin A injection, vitamin C, magnesium, phosphorus, calcium, and a large number of others.

Beyond a thorough history and physical examination including close examination of the anorectal area, additional studies may be undertaken. Anorectal physiology tests assess the functioning of the anorectal anatomy. Anorectal manometry records the strength and tone of the anal sphincters and puborectalis during rest and during contraction. Electromyography tests for anal nerve damage which is often associated with a difficult obstetric delivery. Pudendal nerve terminal motor latency tests for damage to the pudendal motor nerves. Dynamic pelvic MRI is replacing defecography as the most informative study of the anorectal anatomy and defecation function. Proctosigmoidoscopy of the anal canal, rectum and sigmoid colon inspects for inflammation, tumors, or scar tissue. Endoanal ultrasound evaluates the structure of the anal sphincters, and may detect occult sphincter tears.

Historically, bowel management has been a practical approach to manage fecal incontinence or constipation. The definition of fecal incontinence is the inability to voluntarily hold feces in the rectum. This can lead to significant disruption in social activities and reduction in the quality of life. Bowel management is the purposeful clearing of colonic contents on a schedule that prevents uncontrolled bowel movements. Daily enemas, laxatives, and a controlled diet may be components of a bowel management regimen. For those dependent on a daily enema as part of the regimen a creative approach has been the development of an operation to convert the appendix to an access port for the administration of fluid into the colon. Called a continent appendicostomy or Malone procedure, a catheter to administer the enema fluid is inserted into a small orifice usually located near the belly button. This allows full control of the enema process to the individual to maintain independence. Even more dramatic advances have taken place in both the surgical techniques and technology widening the therapeutic options.

There have been very significant advances in the diagnosis and management of fecal incontinence. A clear and accurate diagnosis of the underlying contributing factors leads to the treatment and management, which generally provides considerable improvement. Conservative measures are always the preferred approach but there have been great advances in the surgical management as well. Dietary modifications, avoidance of caffeine, checking for contributing medications are a basic first step. Drug treatment, anal and pelvic floor exercises, biofeedback, and perineal hygiene and pads or plugs may be used during the course of treatment.

Nerve stimulators may be helpful in increasing sphincter tone and are available in a variety of approaches ranging from intra-anal to sacral implants. The injection of material that closes the anal opening at rest has shown promising results and continues to be refined and improved. Newer pharmacologic agents to enhance sphincter tone are being investigated. If necessary, surgical procedures ranging from sphincter repair to replacement with a neosphincter or artificial anal sphincter have been successfully developed.

Perhaps the most remarkable advance is leaving the realm of science fiction and getting closer to reality, the use of stem cells to repair or create a new sphincter. Successful replacement of a number of human tissues has already been accomplished including the replacement of the trachea in several different medical centers. Additional organs successfully regenerated and transplanted into humans include tear ducts, vagina, and urinary bladder. Regenerated nose, ear, coronary artery, urethra, and bile duct are now ready. The work on anal sphincters has already taken place in animal models, and holds great promise.

Pseudo-incontinence or overflow incontinence is actually due to underlying constipation and fecal impaction with liquid stools bypassing the blockage. When the impaction and constipation are corrected continence can once again be achieved. The phrase is commonly heard, but can you really 'scare the shit' out of someone? This phrase actually has a physiological basis and can be taken literally as true. It is part of the survival response to stress called the fight-or-flight response. It occurs in response to a perceived threat to survival, and results in the generalized discharge of the autonomic and sympathetic nervous system and the hormonal releases of adrenaline (epinephrine), norepinephrine, and other catecholamines.

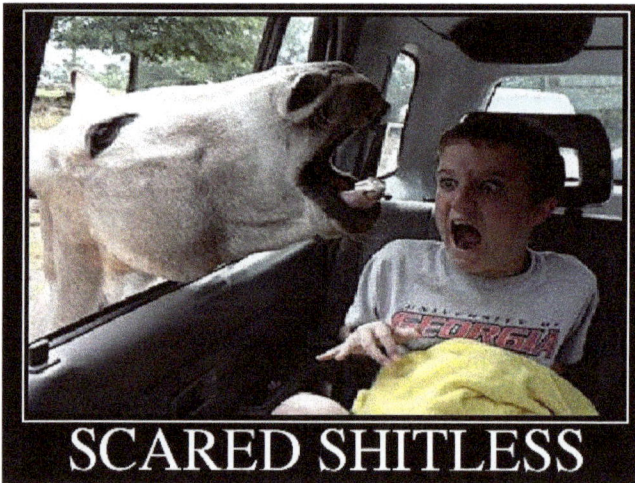
SCARED SHITLESS

The heart rate races, the pupils of the eye dilate, and the respiratory rate quickens. You become super alert with a discharge of cortisol and glucose into the bloodstream, increased blood flow to the muscles and away from digestion, and yes the anal sphincter and urinary sphincters can suddenly give way to a mass evacuation of feces and urine to lighten your load if you needed to sprint to safety. The generalized body shaking and knocking of knees is also reality, not fiction. The story of hanging victims losing bowel and bladder control could either be the fear factor if it occurs just prior to hanging, or the consequence of decerebrate posturing with the broken neck and quadriplegia that results from the hanging action. In states where capital punishment is carried out by hanging the victim is provided with rubber pants and diapers, not so much as not to embarrass themselves but to make the job easier for care of the body after the execution.

The Far Side cartoonist Gary Larson had one, of his early cartoons rejected from publication by his syndicate because they considered it in poor taste. A spider with a paper bag over its head approaches another spider in the web that has just released his entire internal supply of web silk into a large pile on the ground underneath the web. The caption reads: "Did I scare you, or what?

Coprolith

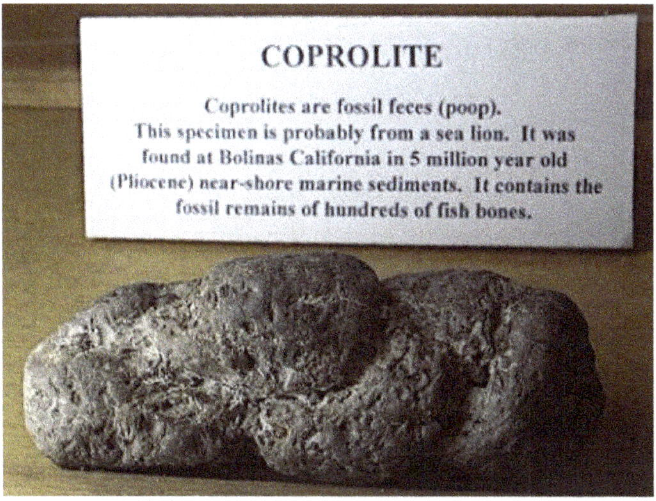
COPROLITE
Coprolites are fossil feces (poop).
This specimen is probably from a sea lion. It was found at Bolinas California in 5 million year old (Pliocene) near-shore marine sediments. It contains the fossil remains of hundreds of fish bones.

s4.hubimg.com/u/ Creative Commons License

A coprolith or coprolite (Greek κόπρος kopros - 'dung' and λίθος lithos - 'stone') is fossilized feces by which paleontologists can determine whether the diet of the animal was herbivorous or carnivorous. It is similar to a fecaloma or fecalith in concept, but with the advanced passage of time so that it is basically petrified or fossilized feces. Human coprolites can identify cannibalism, parasites, migratory patterns and domestication of animals. Coprolites have been recorded in deposits ranging back to the Cambrian period and are found worldwide in sizes up to two feet across (sixty centimeters).

Paleofeces are ancient human feces often identified at sites of previous habitation including caves and sites of archaeological exploration. When the feces are found in caves or in areas with an arid climate they provide information about the diet and health of the humans who produced it.

Analyses of seeds, bones, parasite eggs, DNA, and other markers have made ancient feces a treasured find for paleoarcheologist. When the ancient feces becomes fossilized it is described as a coprolite or coprolith. William Buckland first described coprolites in the early nineteenth century; prior to this they were known as "fossil fir cones" and "bezoar stones". Coprolites from dinosaurs have been identified, and can shed insight into their diet and behavior.

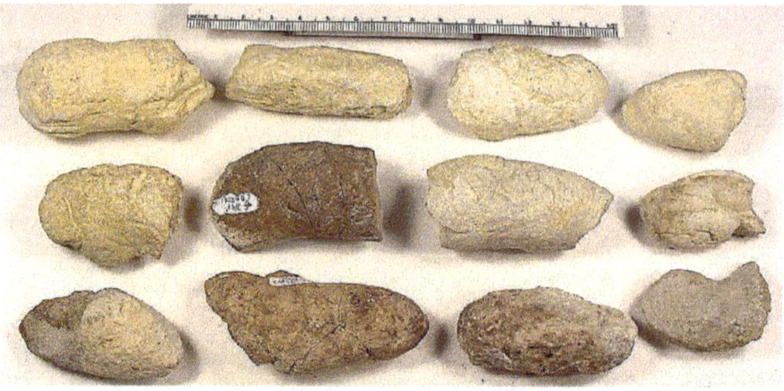

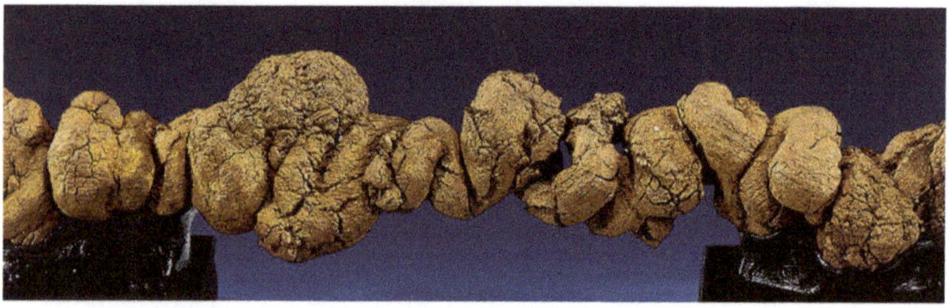

A forty inch coprolith described as being the longest ever discovered sold at auction in Beverly Hills, California in 2014 for over fourteen thousand dollars. Noted experts questioned its authenticity as a true coprolith but the collector was not dissuaded, as its age of twenty million years left no witnesses to challenge the theory that it was dropped by a dinosaur.

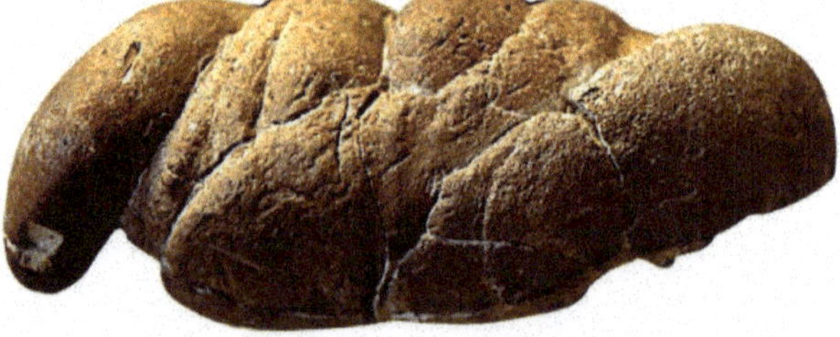

Fossilized dinosaur dung is a treasure house of information for the paleontologist. This specimen found in San Juan County, New Mexico is housed at the New Mexico Museum of Natural History and Science a Division of the New Mexico Department of Cultural Affairs. Image by David Baccadutre.Bryant, Vaughn M. and Glenna W. Dean Archaeological coprolite science: The legacy of Eric O. Callen (1912–1970). *Palaeogeography, Palaeoclimatology,*

Palaeoecology 237(1):51-66

Coprographia

Coprographia (Greek κόπρος feces γραφή (graphê) drawing or writing) is the creation of vulgar writings or drawings. Wolfgang Amadeus Mozart (1756 - 1791) was a musical child prodigy who maintained a juvenile sense of humor throughout his relatively short but incredibly prolific and talented life. Some of his musical notes suggest the playing of a human wind instrument. He was obsessed with jokes about farts, farting, feces, analingus, and coprophilia.

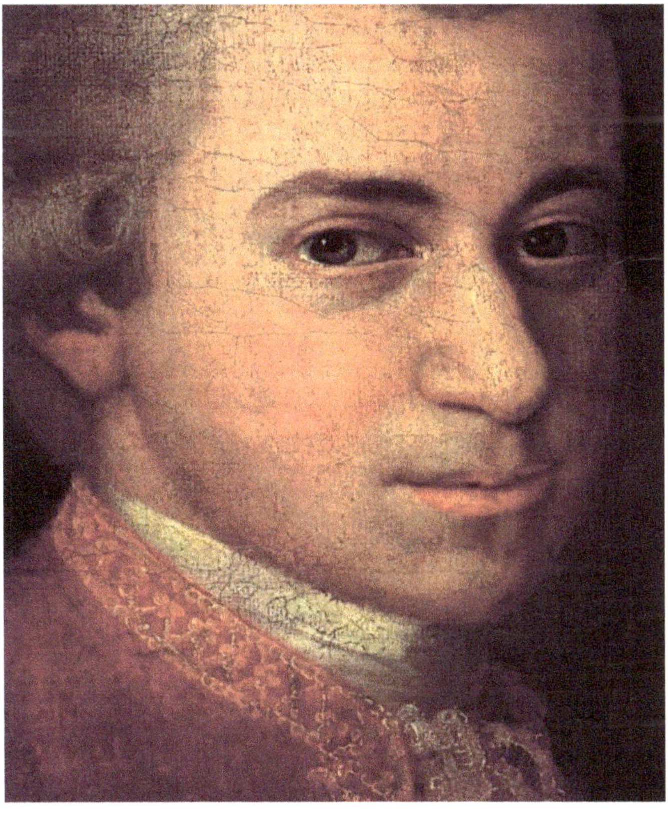

Detail of the face of Wolfgang Amadeus Mozart. Cropped version of the painting where Mozart is seen with Anna Maria (Mozart's sister) and father, Leopold, on the wall a portrait of his deceased mother, Anna Maria. Artist Johann Nepomuk della Croce (1736-1819) Mozart House Salzburg, Austria Public Domain

Mozart wrote the following poem for his dear mother in letter from 1778:
"Oh mother of mine:
Butter is fine.
Praise and thanks be to Him,

We're alive and full of vim.
Through the world we dash,
Though we're rather short of cash,
But we don't find this provoking
And none of us are choking.
Besides, to the people I'm tied
Who carry their muck inside
And let it out if they are able,
Both before and after the table.
At night of farts there is no lack,
Which let off, forsooth, with a powerful crack.
The king of farts came yesterday
Whose farts smelt sweeter than the may.
His voice, however, was no treat
And he himself was in a heat.
Well, now we've been over a week away
And we've been shitting everyday.
Wendling, no doubt, is in a rage
That I haven't composed a single page;
But when I cross the Rhine once more,
I'll surely dash home through the door
And, least he call me mean and petty,
I'll finish off his four quartetti.
The concerto for Paris I'll keep, tis' more fitting.
I'll scribble it there someday when I'm shitting.
Indeed I swear 'twould be far more fun
With the Webers around the world to run
Then go with those bores, you know whom I mean.
When I think of their faces, I get the spleen.
But I suppose it must be and off we shall toddle,
Though Weber's arse I prefer to Ramm's noodle.
A slice of Weber's arse is a thing
I'd rather have than Monsieur Wendling.
With our shitting God we cannot hurt,
And least of all if we bite the dirt.
We are honest birds, all of a feather,
We have summa summarum eight eyes together
Not counting those on which we sit.
But now I must rest a bit
From Rhyming. Yet this I must add,
That on Monday I'll have the honor, egad,
To embrace you and kiss your hands so fair.
But first in my pants I'll shit, I swear.
Your faithful child, With distemper wild.
Trazom."

Coprolalia

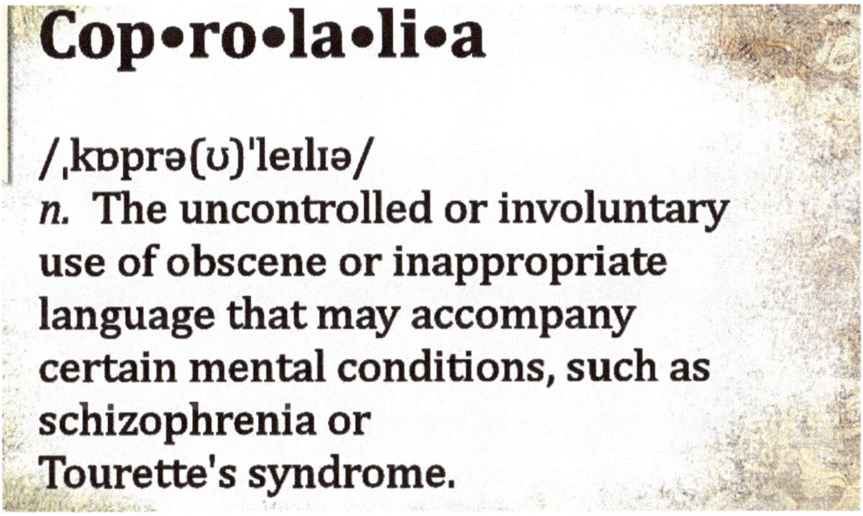
Cop•ro•la•li•a
/ˌkɒprə(ʊ)ˈleɪlɪə/
n. The uncontrolled or involuntary use of obscene or inappropriate language that may accompany certain mental conditions, such as schizophrenia or Tourette's syndrome.

Coprolalia (Greek κόπρος (kopros) feces and λαλιά (lalia) talk) is the involuntary utterances of obscene swear words or socially inappropriate and derogatory remarks. Often seen and heard in schizophrenia, coprolalia is one of the symptoms of Gilles de la Tourette syndrome, but is not a required feature of the condition and is seen in as few as ten percent of patients. Tourette Syndrome is not as rare as once thought and may exist in up to one percent of the population. The incidence of Tourette in those with autism may be as high as thirty percent. The offensive phrases uttered do not necessarily reflect the thoughts or opinions of the person. When a person with coprolalia uses offensive language in their mind, rather than saying it out loud, it is called sub vocalizations. Even though it is not uttered out loud they may find the occurrence very distressing.

Coprology

Scatology or coprology Greek σκώρ 'feces' is the study of feces that can be used to determine diet, parasites, and migratory patterns. In psychology the term is used to describe the study of obsessions with excretion or excrement. In literature, 'scatological' is a term to describe works that make particular reference to excretion or excrement, as well as to toilet humor. Feces are seventy-five percent water, while bacteria are the main component when measured by dry weight. The residue is indigestible, unfermented fiber and excreted compounds. The fecal output can vary markedly depending on the dietary intake, particularly of fiber. A range between 20 and 280 g over 24 hours would be considered normal.

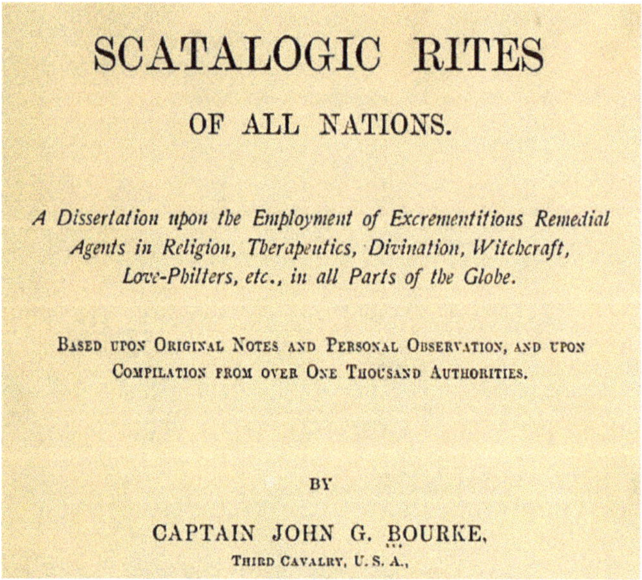

SCATALOGIC RITES

OF ALL NATIONS.

A Dissertation upon the Employment of Excrementitious Remedial Agents in Religion, Therapeutics, Divination, Witchcraft, Love-Philters, etc., in all Parts of the Globe.

Based upon Original Notes and Personal Observation, and upon Compilation from over One Thousand Authorities.

BY

CAPTAIN JOHN G. BOURKE,

Third Cavalry, U. S. A.,

Classic volume on scatology by Captain John G. Bourke, 1891. See Chapter 11 for more details.
Public Domain

Coprophagia

Coprophagia (Greek κόπρος copros, "feces" and φαγεῖν phagein, "to eat") is the ingestion of feces. Many animal species practice coprophagia, especially early in life, presumably to populate their digestive tract with a healthy gut flora. Coprophagous insects, such as the dung beetle and common fly, consume the feces of large animals that contain semi-digested food. Pigs will eat feces, including their own, if it contains semi-digested matter. Human consumption of feces would nowadays be considered a paraphilia or psychiatric disturbance. Surprisingly, the tasting of patients feces for diagnostic and therapeutic purposes was occasionally practiced by physicians' centuries ago.

Ttongsul, or feces wine, is a Korean traditional wine made from human feces, preferably from a young child. Ttongsul has an alcohol content of nine percent and is traditionally produced by submerging a bamboo stick in a chamber pot which contains feces and rice alcohol. It is fermented for several months and then extracted from the bamboo. Its reported benefits include treatment of epilepsy and broken bones. Medicinal compounds produced from feces have a long history in China, Korea, Japan, and the Middle East. In Tang Dynasty chicken manure was used, in Japan, horse manure was believed to have medicinal properties dating from the Sengoku period. In the Middle East camel dung was preferred. Feces of various animals including flying squirrels, bats, hare, sparrows, and silkworms have also been used in medicines.

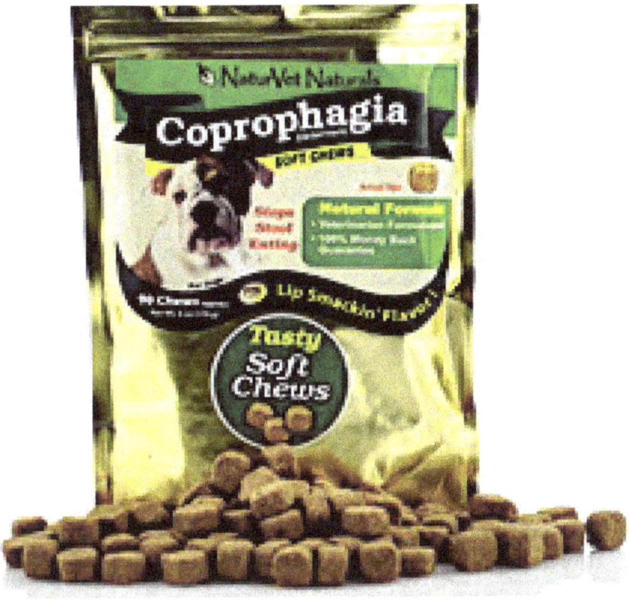
Coprophagia
Tasty
Soft
Chews

Coprophagia is very common in dogs and other animals. The product illustrated above is designed to discourage dogs from eating their own stool but the product certainly resembles what it is supposed to discourage. It doesn't say if the smell and taste have also been modeled on the stool original . www.bestbullysticks.com

Enemas of feces from healthy people were used as a treatment for food poisoning and diarrhea in China dating back to 300 AD. In recent times in North Africa Bedouins would consume fresh warm camel feces for the treatment of dysentery. German soldiers confirmed the efficacy of this remedy during WWII. In Ayurveda the ingestion of panchagavya, a product that includes cow feces, is sometimes advocated for medicinal purposes.

The first use of a fecal enema to treat pseudomembranous colitis was reported in the American medical literature in 1958. Further understanding of the importance of the gut flora, and the rest of the human microbiome, is changing the approach to a number of digestive conditions. Fecal transplants either by insertion of feces into the rectum or by ingesting capsules of fecal material with a healthier mix of microbes are under clinical investigation.

A number of organisms ingest fecal material on a regular basis. This may be in part to balance their gut flora and microbiome, but also because feces actually have residual nutritional value. Human ingestion of fecal contaminants and feces occurs with surprising regularity. Fecal-oral route (fecal-oral contamination) is the transmission of a disease pathogen via feces particles that are ingested by the now infected host. The process of transmission may be by gross contamination as described by the term coprophagia, but much more often the transmission is less visible or microscopic (although it technically remains coprophagia). Examples may include a scenario where a fly that had been feeding on feces lands and feeds on open food at a picnic, which it contaminates by the feces residue on its feet.

Swimming in a pool that had an undisclosed recent toddler 'accident' is another occurrence of hidden coprophagia. One more common example is poor hand washing after a bowel movement with less than perfect toilet paper wiping, then eating finger foods such as potato chips or popcorn from a common bowl.

The degree of fecal-oral contamination that takes place on a daily basis in even the most sophisticated and highest levels of socioeconomic achievement are sobering. An illness that is easily transmitted by purely fecal-oral contamination will infect nearly all members of any closely living household within a matter of days. The number of infectious particles we are exposed to each and every day is astronomical.

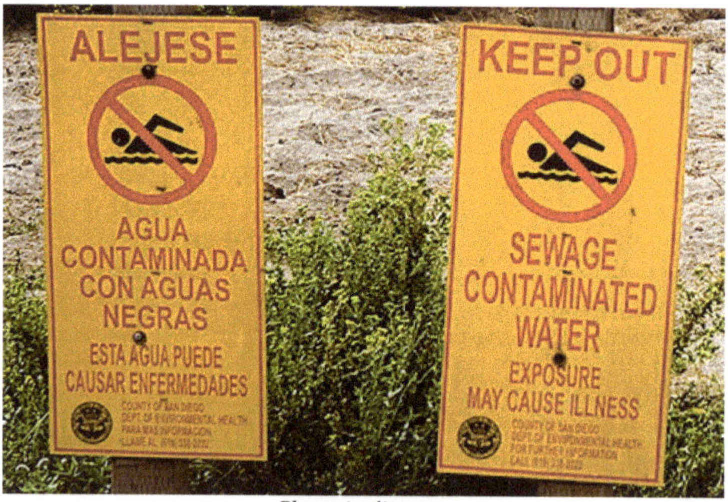
ALEJESE
AGUA CONTAMINADA CON AGUAS NEGRAS
ESTA AGUA PUEDE CAUSAR ENFERMEDADES
KEEP OUT
SEWAGE CONTAMINATED WATER
EXPOSURE MAY CAUSE ILLNESS

Blog.epicedits.com

Rotavirus is transmitted by the fecal-oral route and is the most common cause of severe diarrhea among infants and young children. Nearly every child in the world has been infected with rotavirus at least once by the age of five. It is estimated to cause about forty percent of all hospital admissions due to diarrhea among children less than five years of age worldwide. Rotavirus causes one hundred million episodes of acute diarrhea that result in 350,00 to 600,000 child deaths each year.

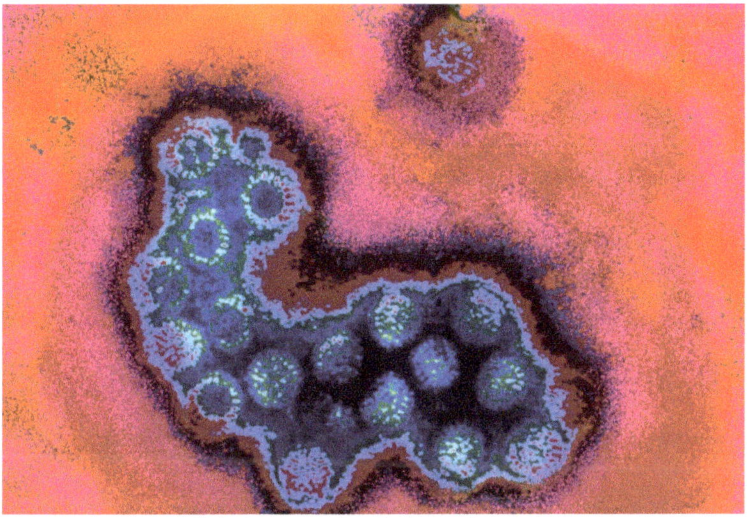
Rotavirus, scanning electron microscopy

The number of infectious viral particles in one gram (less than 1/30 of an ounce) of feces from a child with rotavirus is more than ten trillion (10,000,000,000,000). One child in a household has more than enough viral particles in a thimble of stool to infect every human on the planet Earth and another ten thousand planets with the same population. Most transmission of pathogens is via the fecal to oral route is usually accomplished by way of the hands. The average human stool contains three trillion microorganisms. Wiping with toilet paper nearly guarantees that the hands will come into contact with fecal microorganisms. After wiping it is not uncommon to find brown streaks on underwear because of inadequate anal hygiene

Some of the diseases that can be passed via the fecal-oral route include poliomyelitis, norovirus acute gastroenteritis, giardiasis, hepatitis A, hepatitis E, rotavirus, shigellosis (bacillary dysentery), typhoid fever, *Vibrio parahemolyticus* infections, enteroviruses, cholera, *Clostridium difficile*, cryptosporidiosis, ascariasis, and many others. The development of antibiotic associated colitis and diarrhea from the pathogenic bacteria *Clostridium difficile* has led to the development of therapeutic fecal transplants. The standard approach is to use an enema of feces with healthy gut flora to displace the pathogens.

A novel approach is to swallow capsules containing healthy feces and gut flora. The capsules are sealed and dissolve in the small intestine and colon where they release the healthy feces bacteria. Strange as it may be, coprophagia has become one of the latest advances in medical therapeutics. Perhaps even stranger yet are the references to coprophagia found in the writings of biblical era prophets. "And thou shalt eat it as barley cakes, and thou shalt bake it with dung that cometh out of man, in their sight." (Ezekiel

4:12-13) Hath he not sent me to the men which sit on the wall, that they may eat their own dung, and drink their own piss with you?" (II Kings 18:27) (See also Isaiah 36:12). " Behold, I will corrupt your seed, and spread dung upon your faces, even the dung of your solemn feasts; and one shall take you away with it." (Malachi 2:2-3)

Coprophagia - Housefly

After a mammal, such as a human, consumes their diet the digestive process removes only a portion of its nutrient value. Feces can and does serve as a nutritious food of choice for many organisms and microbes, including insects and animals. When they ingest the feces they extract additional nutrient value and also aid in its decomposition and recycling.

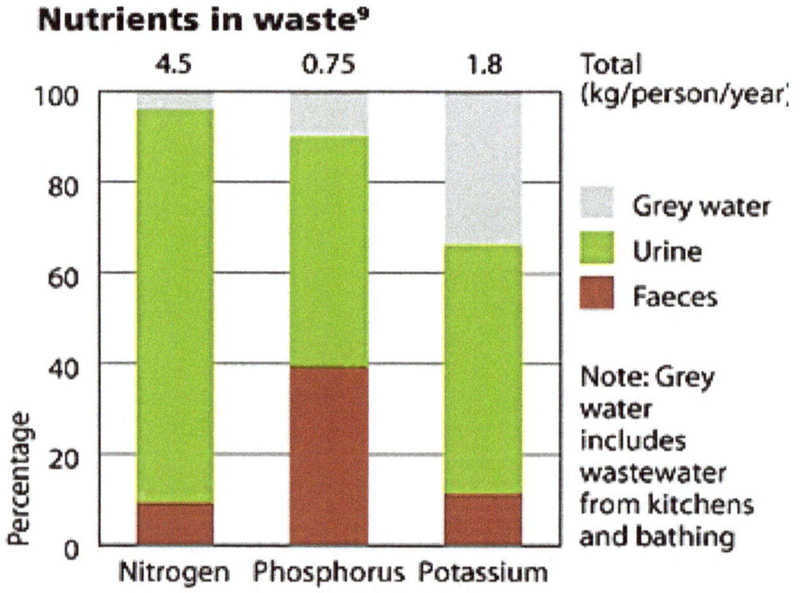
Nutrients in waste[9]
4.5
0.75
1.8
Total (kg/person/year)
100
80
60
40
20
0
Percentage
Grey water
Urine
Faeces
Note: Grey water includes wastewater from kitchens and bathing
Nitrogen
Phosphorus
Potassium

New Internationalist.

If you find coprophagia hard to stomach, you may have already been a participant. Although we are most familiar with the domestic housefly *Musca domestica*, there are some ninety thousand different species of flies in the world with different feeding strategies. Houseflies secrete saliva whenever they attempt to feed and they drool onto their food. They do not spread disease from their drool. The disease comes from their feet when they land on your food after having feasted on feces or rotting matter laden with microbes. Even if the flies on the outdoor buffet have been shooed away before the guests arrive, they probably left footprints of feces on the food, which you ingest and become an unwitting participant in the world of coprophagia.

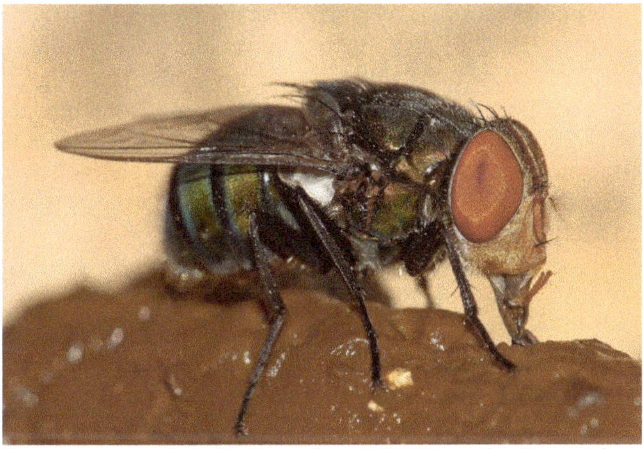

A female *Chrysomya megacephala* feeding on feces. 2009 Pictured in Dar es Salaam, Tanzania Muhammad Mahdi Karim (www.micro2macro.net) Creative Commons License

The degree to which fly populations are dependent on the supply of horse manure to feed on is surprising. In the late 1800's most forms of transportation were dependent on the horse. In New York City alone the horse population in 1880 was between 150,000 and 175,000 horses. The quantity of horse manure deposited on the city streets was estimated at between three million and four million pounds per day, along with forty thousand gallons of horse urine. In 1900 it was estimated that in the United States three billion flies were hatched in horse manure each day. Swarms of flies transmitted the organisms responsible for dozens of infectious diseases including typhoid and infant diarrheal diseases. Outbreaks of disease were closely linked to spikes in the fly population.

Coprophagia, Shrimp

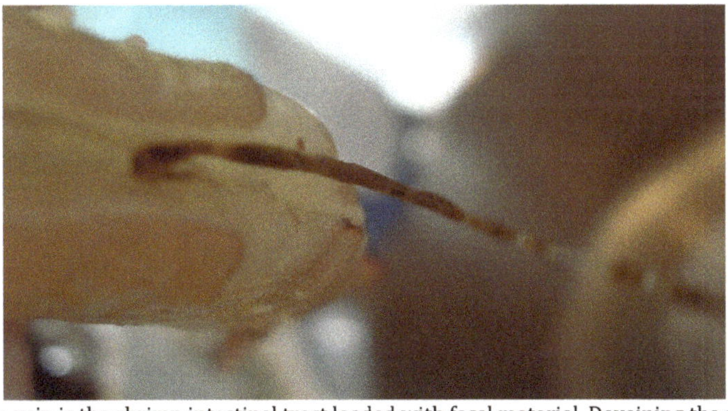

Shrimp vein is the shrimp intestinal tract loaded with fecal material. Deveining the shrimp reduces the degree of coprophagia to go along with the appealing 'appetizer'. www.blahblahblagher.com

It is called a vein for marketing purposes, yet many people know the truth and they eat it anyways. It is the shrimp intestinal tract, and although the shrimp dorsal vein does travel along the intestinal tract, the black line is shrimp feces that may add a gritty texture. The shrimp intestine is transparent and if you look closely you can see that the black line looks like a series of intermittent dots and dashes. These are the equivalent of shrimp turds traveling down its intestinal tract. Shrimp are scavengers so the shrimp turds actually started as decaying organic material and if that makes them sound less appealing to you, you can always increase the amount of cocktail sauce to mask the flavor.

Accidental involuntary coprophagia is nearly universal. When it comes to eating shrimp that have not been deveined, it brings the coprophagia to a new level of being a conscious purposeful decision. Surprisingly, it is very commonly accepted practice amongst shrimp consumers including those who are otherwise fastidious about hygiene.

<u>Coprophagia, Holy Feces</u>

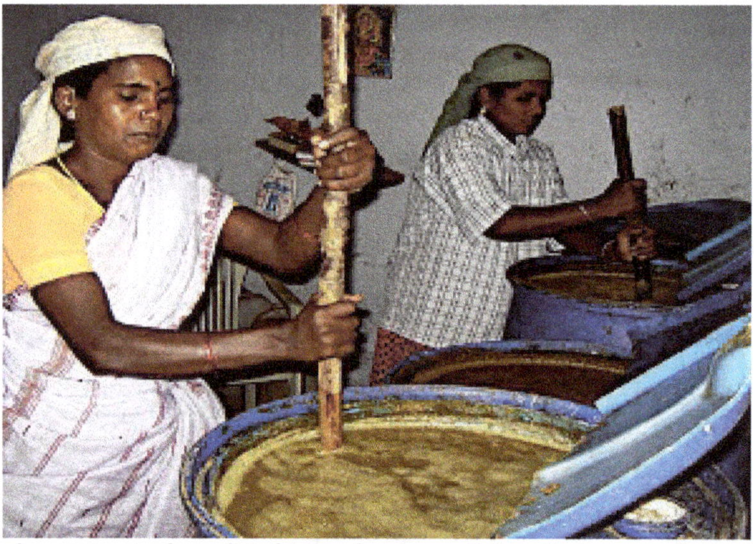

Panchagavya is eaten for medicinal Ayurveda purposes. Its ingredients are cow feces, urine, milk, curd, and ghee. www.newseq.blogspot.com

Panchagavya, also known as panchakavyam, is a concoction of five cow products. Its ingredients include cow feces, cow urine, milk , curd, and ghee. Although usually used as a growth stimulant for plants it has also been advocated for its medicinal benefits to both animals and humans. It is considered cowpathy and a medical treatment regimen according to Ayurveda, the system of medicine developed in ancient India.

In the tradition of Tibetan Buddhism some consider the feces of the Holy Lama holy itself. There have been historical reports that the dried and powdered feces, known as 'big fragrance of the lama are collected for distribution to the faithful who eat it and drink lama urine, known as 'little fragrance', for medicinal and religious purposes. There is another explanation for the ritual of the ingestion of what are commonly thought of as unclean substances. These include five kinds of meat (bull, dog, elephant, horse, and human) as well as five kinds of body tissues (feces, brain, sexual fluids, blood, and urine). The rationale is that the ingestion practice allows one to obtain practical knowledge that nothing in nature is clean or unclean, and that such concepts are based on false abstractions.

Coprophagia, Kopi Luwak

Kopi luwak, or civet coffee, is made from the beans of coffee berries that have been eaten by the Asian Palm Civet (*Paradoxurus hermaphroditus*). After passing through a civet's digestive tract the beans are searched for and collected from the animal's feces. In the 18th century the Dutch established coffee plantations of Arabica coffee from Yemen in their colony on the Indonesian islands of Java and Sumatra. The native plantation workers were prohibited from picking coffee beans for their own use. The wild Asian Palm Civet ate the ripe coffee berries and the coffee beans were collected from their droppings, cleaned, roasted and ground them to make their own coffee beverage.

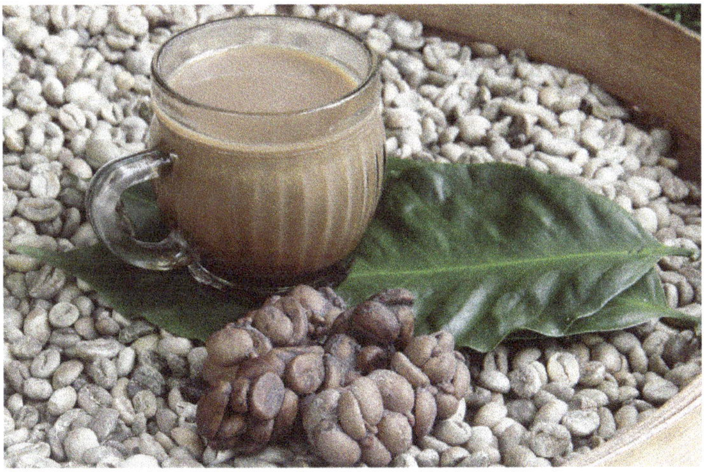

Kopi Luwak shutterstock/LucyLiu

The civet's digestive proteolytic enzymes seep into the beans generating shorter peptides and amino acids. The reputation of the unique flavor and aroma of civet coffee spread from the natives to the Dutch plantation owners. Because of its rarity and unusual processing it was the most expensive coffee, even in colonial times. The collecting and processing of feces from wild civets have been supplemented by caged farming methods where civets are force fed coffee beans. The natural selection of especially ripe coffee berries by the civet is not a part of the commercial farming method and for aficionados the special flavor is lost. Most experts in the coffee industry consider farmed kopi luwak abusive to the animals and a gimmick or novelty item. Tim Carman, the food critic for the *Washington Post* described a taste test of civet coffee as "Petrified dinosaur droppings steeped in bathtub water. I couldn't finish it".

Kopi luwak made by collecting coffee beans eaten by wild civets remains the most expensive coffee in the world, with prices over $1,300 a pound reported ($3,000 kg). In 1995 a Kopi luwak processor was awarded an Ig Nobel Prize, a parody of the Nobel Prize granted for useless scientific 'advances'. The inability to guarantee the authenticity of wild civet feces coffee versus caged civet feces coffee has led to a great deal of deceptions and fraud. Kopi luwak was also given notoriety in the movie *The Bucket List* (2008) as the character played by Morgan Freeman reveals to the one played by Jack Nicholson that the coffee they had just tasted came from the feces of a jungle cat. Nicholson exclaims "You're shitting me!" and Freeman replies "No, the cats beat me to it!"

Copraphagia - Black Ivory Coffee

Black Ivory Coffee is a brand of coffee produced in northern Thailand from Arabica coffee beans consumed by elephants and collected from their feces. The taste of Black Ivory coffee reportedly has less bitterness because of the activity of elephants' digestive enzymes on the coffee bean reducing their protein content. The coffee beans are digested within 15 to 70 hours, and are digested in the presence of other plants since the elephant is an herbivore. Civets who the animal used to digest coffee beans in making Kopi Luwak are omnivores, which may give the coffee a different characteristic.

Black Ivory coffee has been described is among the world's most expensive coffees, at US $1,100 per kilogram. In spite of its reputation as being very smooth and without bitterness, the market and supply of Black Ivory coffee is very limited. Found at a few luxury hotels in Thailand, the Maldives, and Abu Dhabi it is available at the price of US $50 a cup. Availability is dependent on the appetite of the elephants, and the ability of the mahouts and their wives to recover intact beans. 33 kilograms (72 pounds) of raw coffee cherries results in 1 kilogram (2 pounds) of the finished product since most of the beans are crushed by the elephants chewing and cannot be recovered from its feces.

The coffee is produced by Black Ivory Coffee Co. Ltd. at the Golden Triangle Asian Elephant Foundation in Chiang Saen, Thailand. Approximately 20 elephants at the foundation rescued elephant refuge produce the coffee. It costs approximately $1000 per month to care for an elephant so a percentage of Black Ivory Coffee Company sales are donated back to the Golden Triangle Asian Elephant Foundation to support the elephant refuge. Veterinary tests concluded that caffeine is not absorbed from the coffee cherries they consume, and there is no harm to the elephants.

The creative force behind Black Ivory Coffee is Blake Dinkin, a Canadian previously involved in the production of Kopi Luwak from civet cats. He describes the elephant diet as an herbivore and slow digestion as being an advantage over the omnivorous civet cat. The elephant may eat bananas, sugar cane and other plants that impart a unique earthy and fruitful flavor to the coffee. Black Ivory Coffee states they use pure Arabica beans hand-picked by hill-tribe women from a small mountain estate. The wives of elephant mahouts collect the dung, pick out the coffee beans, which are thoroughly washed and then brought to a gourmet roaster in Bangkok. Much like civet coffee, which has its aficionados, the elephant coffee has also become the butt of jokes. Dinkin's favorites include Crap-accino, Good to the last dropping, and Elephant poop coffee. Black Ivory's initial production of 70 kilograms (150 pounds) has sold out. Dinkin sees a market targeted to the relatively affluent, open-minded, adventurous, with a desire to tell a good story. For the tea drinkers feeling smug about keeping their distance from feces, the world's most expensive green tea is fertilized with the droppings of panda bears.

Coprophagia - Kudu Dung Spitting

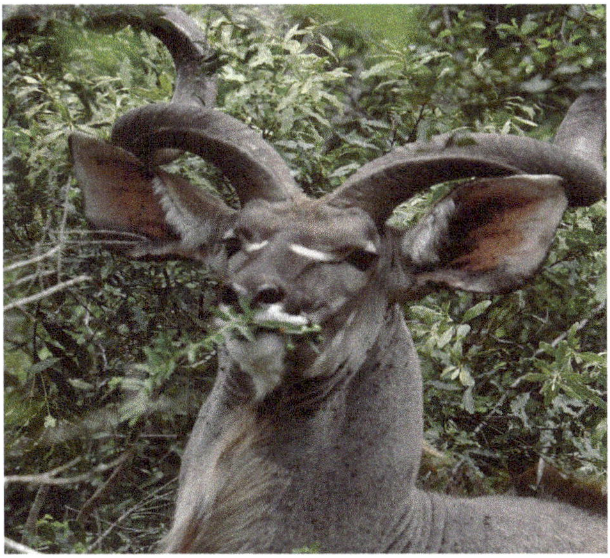

A large male Kudu eating in preparation for producing dung to be used in a championship kudu dung spitting competition. Author Ozten Austin King Creative Commons License

Kudu dung spitting is a formal sport practiced by the Afrikaner community in South Africa. The competition involves placing a small, hard pellet of kudu (an antelope native to Africa) dung in the mouth and spitting it out to the greatest distance. The distance is measured from the starting point to the place the dung pellet comes to rest, not where it initially hit the ground. The knowledge that they have dung in their mouth might be useful in encouraging the greatest effort at expectoration.

Coprophilia

Coprophilia (from Greek κόπρος, kópros—excrement and φιλία, filía—liking, fondness), also called scatophilia (Greek: σκατά, skatá-shit) is the condition of deriving pleasure (often of a sexual nature) from feces.

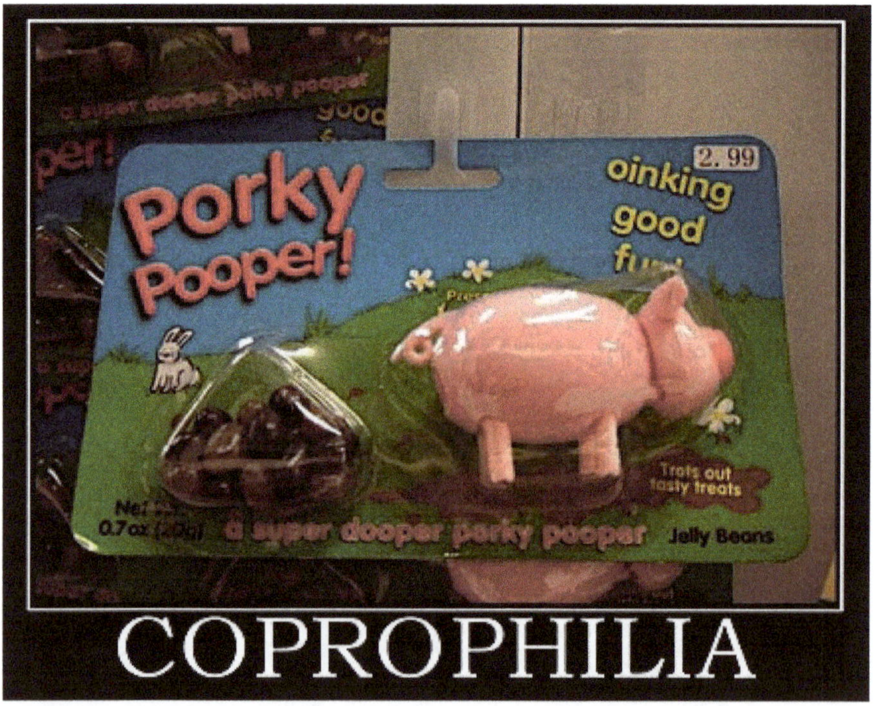
Porky Pooper!
2.99
oinking
good
Trots out tasty treats
a super dooper porky pooper
Jelly Beans
COPROPHILIA

Copropraxia

Copropraxia (Greek κόπρος feces and πράξις action) is the involuntary performance of obscene gestures, such as the familiar upright middle finger seen in Western societies. Occasionally, especially with international travel, an inadvertent hand gesture imitates what the locals consider an obscene gesture. This can be problematic when the viewer is not aware that the gesture was simply accidental, and not

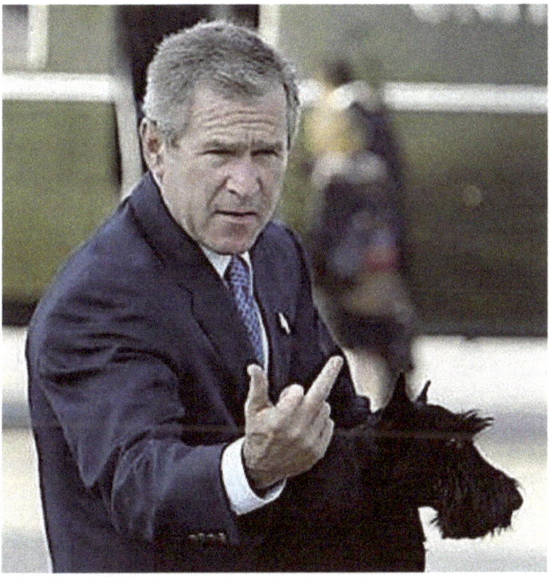

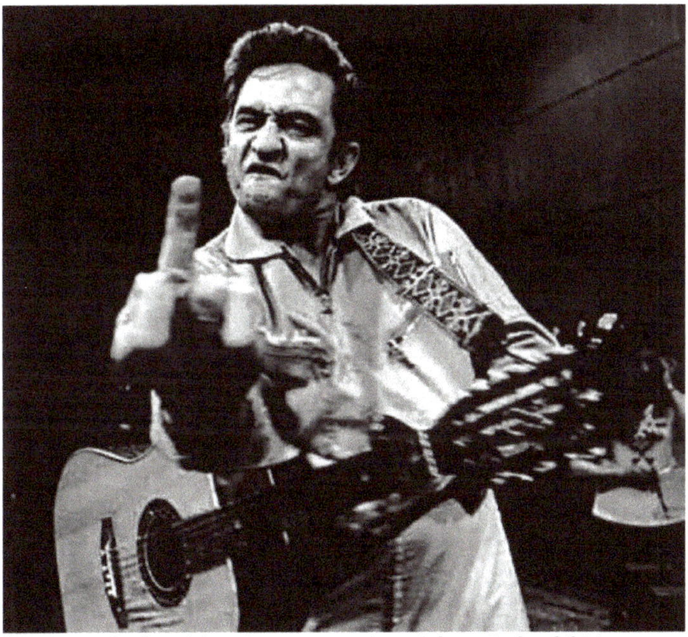

President George Bush and American country singer Johnny Cash exhibiting copropraxia behavior of 'giving the finger'. Public Domain

Defecation

Defecation, a bowel movement often referred to simply by its abbreviated initials BM, is the elimination of fecal waste material from the digestive tract via the anus. The stimulus to defecate is the distention of the rectum or sigmoid colon with feces. This reflex can be triggered by manual digital stimulation of the rectal wall stretch receptors. Voluntary control of defecation is part of the toilet training process and is typically mastered during childhood. The voluntary control can be lost again with neurological, psychological or senescent changes. The involuntary release of fecal material is fecal incontinence, often called encopresis in children.

Defecation is a complex reflex coordination of neuromuscular activity that relaxes the puborectalis muscle straightening the anorectal angle, which is normally at ninety-degree angle. This initiates the relaxation of the internal anal sphincters. There is a strong urge to defecate but the external anal sphincter contracts to prevent defecation until voluntarily released to initiate the process. Colonic contractions, along with increased intra-abdominal pressure by performance of the Valsalva maneuver (attempting to exhale against a closed epiglottis) allows the individual to propel the fecal material out of the rectum via the anus.

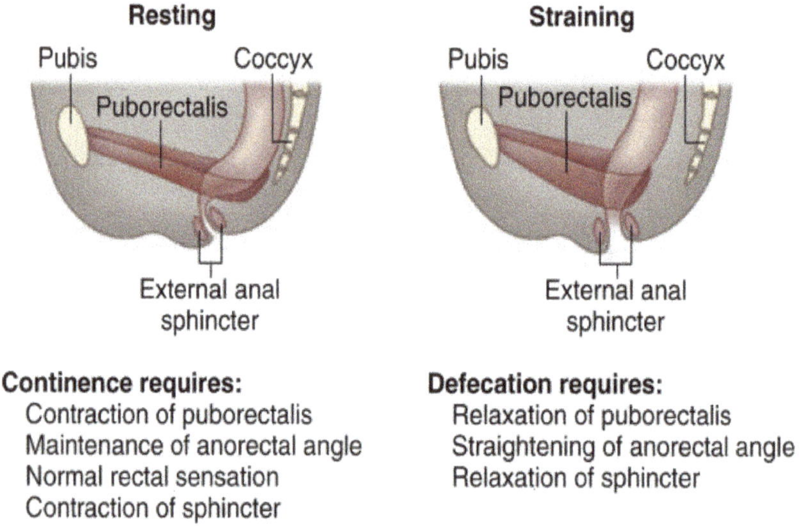
Resting
Pubis
Coccyx
Puborectalis
External anal sphincter
Straining
Pubis
Coccyx
Puborectalis
External anal sphincter
Continence requires:
Contraction of puborectalis
Maintenance of anorectal angle
Normal rectal sensation
Contraction of sphincter
Defecation requires:
Relaxation of puborectalis
Straightening of anorectal angle
Relaxation of sphincter

www.cixip.com/Public Creative Commons License

The frequency range of normal bowel movements is quite variable, and can range from two bowel movements per day to once per week, often dependent on diet. The squatting position is most conducive to defecation. Using Western style sitting toilets, as opposed to squat toilets found in non-Western locales, can be problematic especially if the feet cannot reach the ground as in young children. An elevated footrest to allow the thighs and legs to be flexed can greatly assist in the ease of elimination for both children and adults.

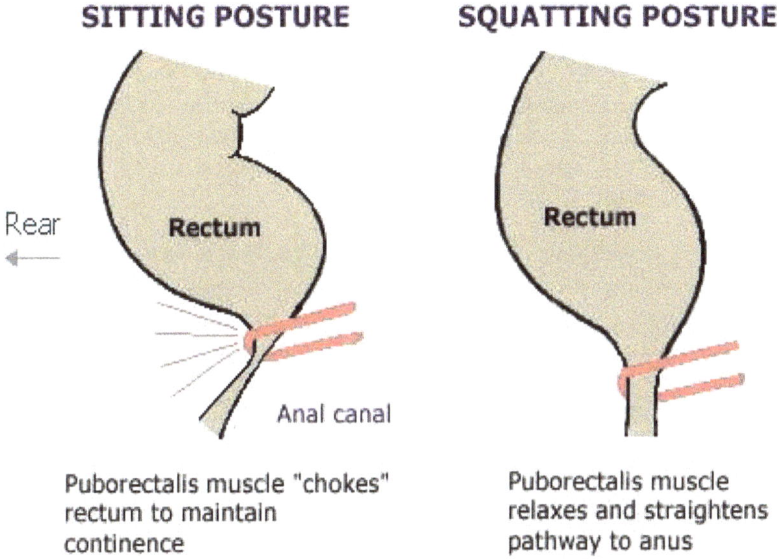
SITTING POSTURE
SQUATTING POSTURE
Rear
Rectum
Rectum
Anal canal
Puborectalis muscle "chokes" rectum to maintain continence
Puborectalis muscle relaxes and straightens pathway to anus

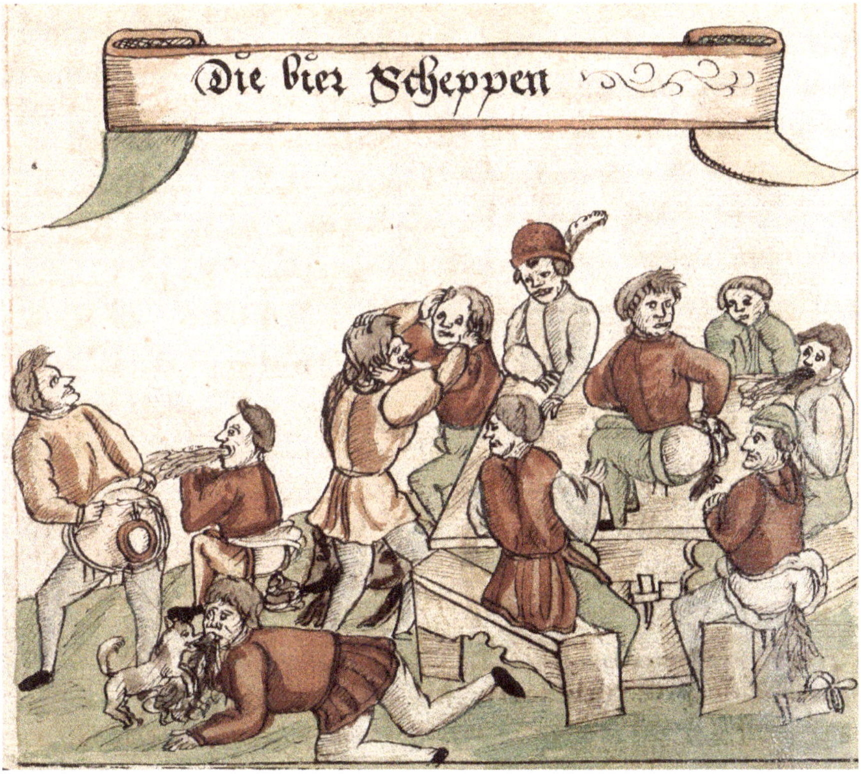
Die bier Scheppen

The puborectalis sling forming the anorectal angle is responsible for gross continence of solid stool. The internal anal sphincter is an involuntary muscle that contributes about fifty-five percent of the resting anal pressure. Together with the hemorrhoid vascular cushions, the internal anal sphincter maintains continence of flatus and liquid during rest. Parasympathetic stimulation causes the sphincter to relax allowing the passage of material.

The internal anal sphincter is a muscular ring that surrounds about 2.5-4.0 cm of the anal canal just proximal to the external anal sphincter. Its action is entirely involuntary and it is in a state of continuous contraction to prevent the passage of feces and intestinal gas. The internal anal sphincter is an involuntary sphincter surrounding the superior two-thirds of the anal canal. It is a thickening of the circular muscle layer. Its contraction (tonus) is stimulated and maintained by sympathetic fibers from the superior rectal (periarterial) and hypogastric plexuses; its contraction is inhibited by parasympathetic fiber stimulation, both intrinsically in relation to peristalsis and extrinsically by fibers passing through the pelvic splanchnic nerves.

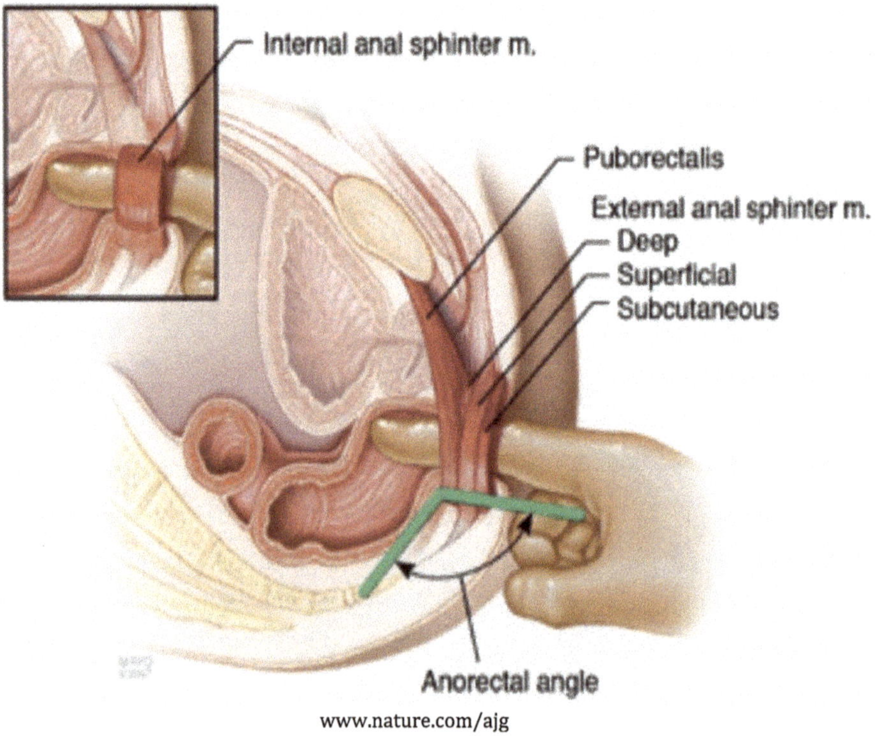
Internal anal sphinter m.
Puborectalis
External anal sphinter m.
Deep
Superficial
Subcutaneous
Anorectal angle

www.nature.com/ajg

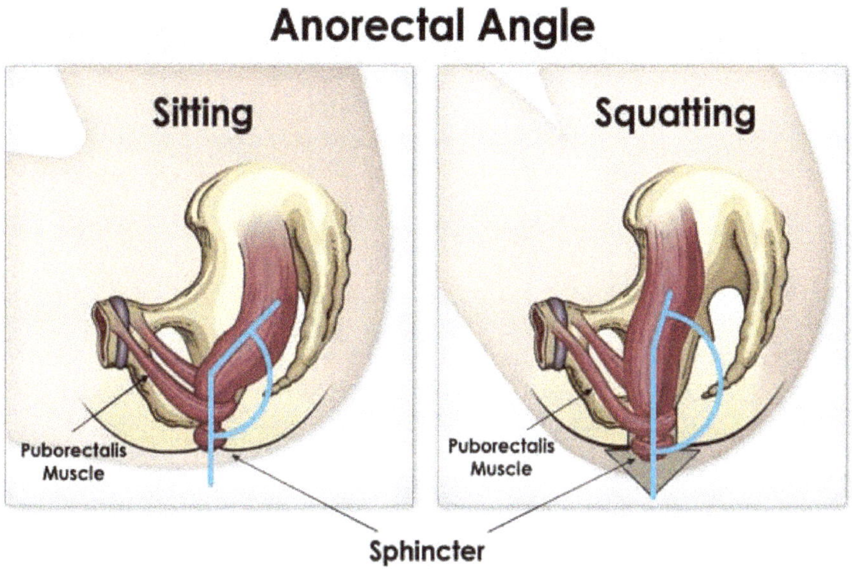
Anorectal Angle
Sitting
Squatting
Puborectalis Muscle
Puborectalis Muscle
Sphincter

Squatting is the most natural defecation posture. Creative Commons License

This sphincter is tonically contracted most of the time to prevent leakage of fluid or flatus; however, it is inhibited and relaxes temporarily in response to distension of the rectal ampulla by feces or gas. When the internal anal sphincter is relaxed voluntary contraction of the puborectalis and external anal sphincter is required if defecation or flatulence is not to occur. The ampulla relaxes after initial distension when peristalsis subsides. The tone returns until the next peristalsis or until a threshold level of distension occurs, at which point inhibition of the sphincter is continuous until distension is relieved.

The external anal sphincter is a voluntary muscle, doubling the pressure in the anal canal during contraction. The rectoanal inhibitory reflex is an involuntary internal anal sphincter relaxation in response to rectal distention. This allows a sampling of some of the rectal contents to descend into the anal canal. Here it is brought into contact with specialized sensory mucosa to detect consistency.

The rectoanal excitatory reflex is an initial semi-voluntary contraction of the external anal sphincter and puborectalis, which returns tone following the rectoanal inhibitory reflex. Other factors include the specialized anti-peristaltic function of the last part of the sigmoid colon, the sensory ability of the lining of the rectum and the anal canal to detect the consistency and quantity when of stool present, and the normal rectoanal reflexes and defecation cycle that completes evacuation.

Humans can defecate in a number of defecation postures. The two most common are the squatting posture and the sitting posture. The squatting posture is used for squat toilets and is also commonly used for defecation in the absence of toilets or other devices. It is commonly used in non-Western cultures. The sitting defecation posture is used in Western toilets with either a leaning forward posture or a 90-degree sitting upright posture. The posture chosen appears to be largely a cultural decision, although there is evidence that the squatting posture is more efficacious and induces the least bodily strain.

The sitting position can cause the defecating human being to repeat the Valsalva maneuver many times and with great force. This can lead to diverticulosis, hemorrhoids, hernias and cardiovascular stress and defecation syncope. With underlying cardiac disease the additional stress induced by defecating in the sitting position as opposed to the more natural squatting position may potentially be life-threatening. The magnitude of straining during defecation is at least three times greater in the sitting posture than with the squatting posture.

Difficulty with the seated position is particularly true if the feet cannot reach the floor as is commonly seen when small children are placed on adult height toilets. The adults may become frustrated that it is taking the child so long to defecate not realizing that without being able to brace their feet and apply resistance that are unable to generate the intra-abdominal pressure needed to promote defecation.

The affectionate term 'potty' is often used with small children especially during toilet (potty) training. The term 'potty' is also used to describe child size chamber pot type toilets that are at the appropriate height and have a child size opening to sit on. Regular adult toilets have an opening that is too large and frightening for a child who could accidentally fall in if not assisted.

To remind you that their fear is not unjustified American adults suffer 40,000 toilet related injuries per year. Falling off a toilet directly contributed to the death of King George II of Great Britain. The height of the adult toilet does not allow their feet to touch the ground to assist in the squatting maneuver that assists defecation. A footstool to give their feet a place on which to rest can assist squatting, which eases the initiation of a bowel movement and can accelerate toilet training.

Defecography

Defecography, also known as defecation proctography, is a radiology study of the anorectum and pelvic floor to evaluate defecation disorders. It usually utilizes fluoroscopy or videography of the defecation of barium contrast material that has been introduced to distend the rectum.

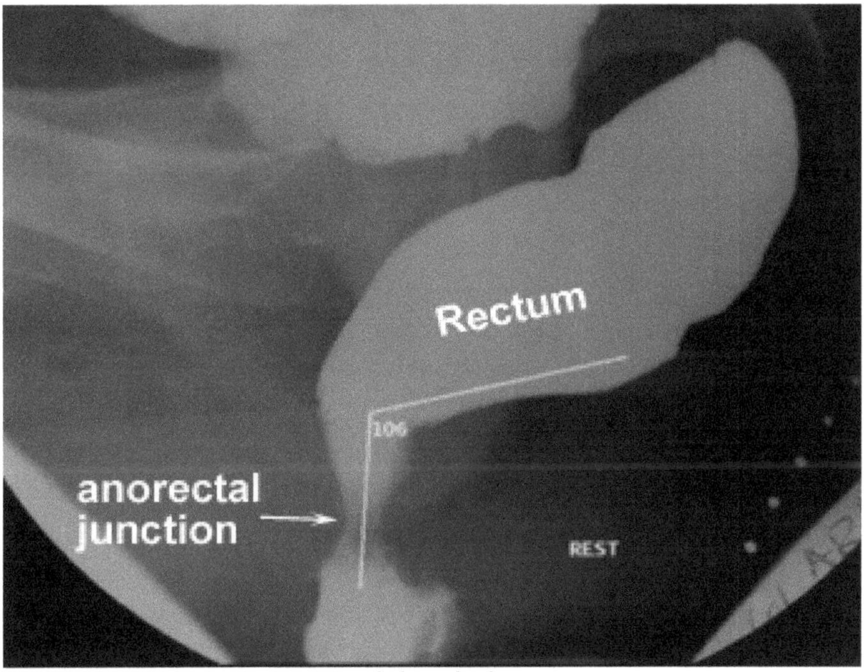
Rectum
106
anorectal
junction
REST

www.radiologyschools.com

Dentate Line

The dentate (pectinate) line is an embryological demarcation line that divides the upper two-thirds of the anal canal derived from the hindgut, from the lower one-third of the anal canal derived from the proctodeum. It is an important anatomical landmark and has several distinctions, which have clinical relevance. They have different lymphatic drainage, arterial blood supplies, and venous drainage.

The upper two-thirds has columnar intestinal type epithelium and the lower one-third has stratified squamous epithelium. The squamous epithelium is non-keratinized until Hilton's white line, where the anal verge becomes continuous with the perianal skin containing keratinized epithelium.

The inferior comb-shaped limit of the anal valves forms an irregular line called the pectinate line or dentate line. It demarcates the junction of the superior and inferior parts of the anal canal. The superior portion is visceral and derives derived from the embryonic hindgut. This portion has afferent nerve fibers that can sense distention and spasm but not the sensation of pain.

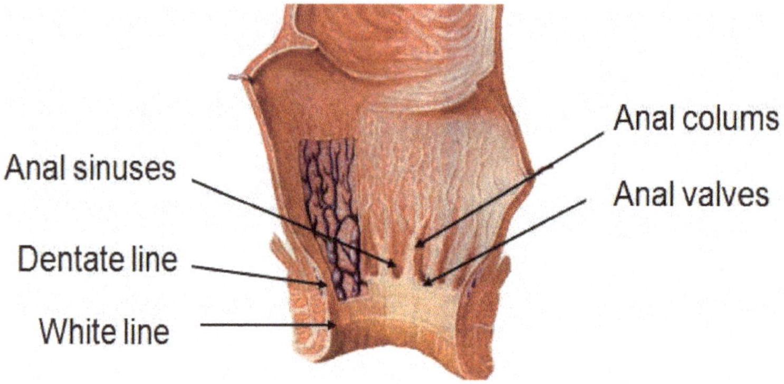
Anal colums
Anal sinuses
Anal valves
Dentate line
White line

3.bp.blogspot.com Creative Commons License

Internally, the dentate line demarcates the transition from visceral to somatic neurovascular supply and drainage. The canal is surrounded by superficial and deep venous plexuses, the veins of which normally have a varicose appearance. The treatment of internal hemorrhoids above the dentate line is painless because of the lack of somatic innervation. The inferior part is somatic and is derived from the embryonic proctodeum. Because the somatic portion is very sensitive to pain, thrombosed external hemorrhoids and its treatment as well as anal fissure, fistulas, perianal, and perirectal abscesses can be exquisitely painful.

The internal anal sphincter is above the pectinate line, while he external anal sphincter is below. Perhaps the most important distinction is the innervation as the upper two-thirds can only sense distention and spasm, while the lower one -third is richly enervated and can receive a wide variety of painful or pleasurable stimuli. This is why internal hemorrhoids above the dentate line are painless, and external hemorrhoids below the dentate line can be exquisitely painful.

Deoxyribonucleic Acid (DNA)

Deoxyribonucleic acid, most commonly known by its initials DNA, is a molecule, which serves as the primary means of transmitting genetic information. Most DNA molecules are in the form of complementary strands that form a spiral structure known as a double helix. Each nitrogen containing nucleotide base is attached to helix backbone of a monosaccharide sugar called deoxyribose alternating with a phosphate group. The bases of adenine with thymine, and guanine with cytosine, are bonded as pairs with hydrogen bonds. The matching pairs allows any single strand of DNA to duplicate its matching strand, which is the process by which DNA is transmitted to the next generation with cell division. The double helix structure of DNA was identified by Nobel Laureates James Watson & Francis Crick, who relied on the experimental work and data collected by Rosalind Franklin and Maurice Wilkins.

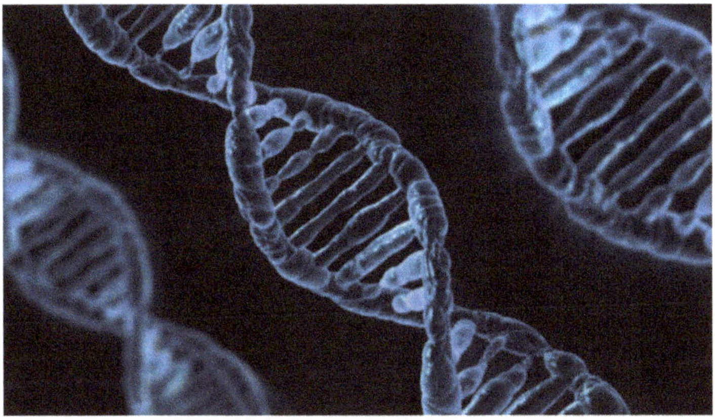

DNA double helix. Creative Commons License

The DNA on chromosomes of cells is often billions of base pairs long, and each three-letter sequence of base pairs may code for a specific amino acid that must be assembled in the proper sequence to manufacture a protein with a specific function. A mutation of a single letter in the sequence of base pairs may result in a defective or inactive protein that may have major consequences for the health or survival of the cell. There are a variety of mechanisms for self-repair of DNA, and with the astronomical number of cell divisions and duplications of DNA the efficiency and accuracy of the system is remarkable.

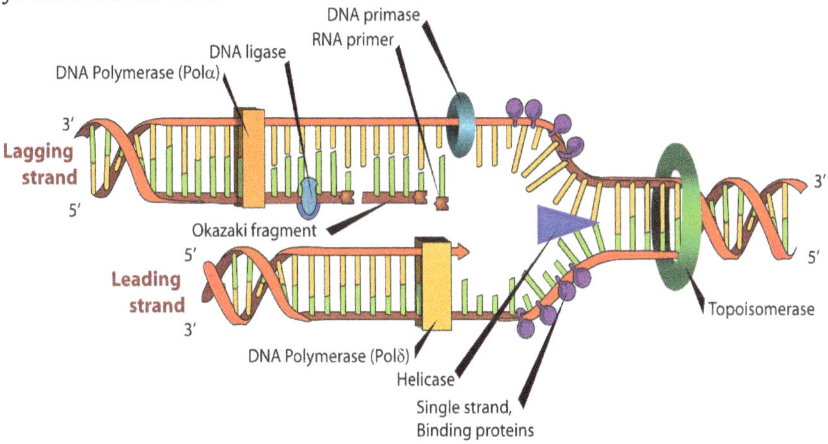
DNA primase
RNA primer
DNA ligase
DNA Polymerase (Polα)
3'
Lagging strand
5'
Okazaki fragment
5'
Leading strand
3'
3'
5'
Topoisomerase
DNA Polymerase (Polδ)
Helicase
Single strand, Binding proteins

DNA replication. Creative Commons License

Diarrhea

Diarrhea (Greek διάρροια "flowing through") is defined as having three or more loose or liquid bowel movements per day. The most common cause is gastroenteritis from a virus or bacteria, and it can result in life threatening dehydration and electrolyte disturbances. Diarrhea causes over 2.5 million deaths per year and is the second most common cause of infant deaths worldwide.

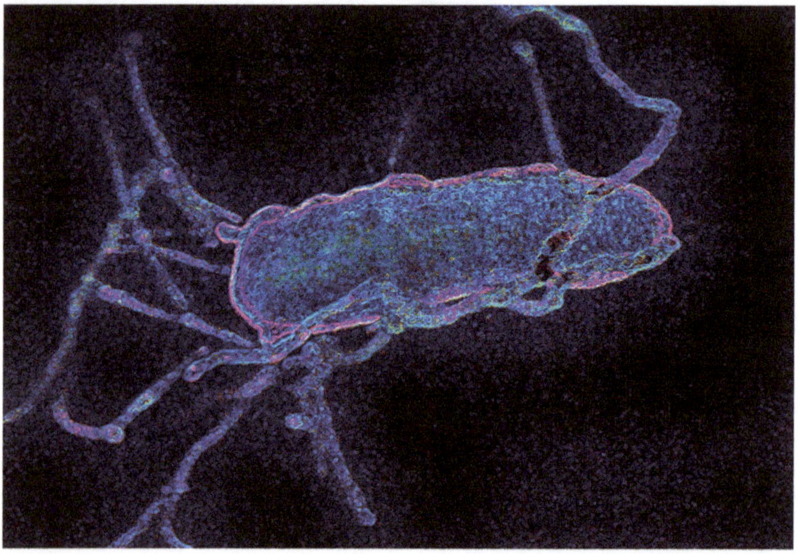

There are many different causes of diarrhea ranging from infections, inflammatory bowel disease, enzyme deficiencies, and ischemic bowel to gluten sensitivity, hormonal imbalance, irritable bowel, bile acid malabsorption, laxative abuse, carcinoid syndrome, and a wide variety of other causes. Defining the type of diarrhea often helps to narrow the differential diagnosis of possibilities.

Secretory diarrhea is an increase in the active secretion of ions such as chloride and sodium without structural damage to the bowel. The most common cause of this type of diarrhea is a bacterial product such as the cholera toxin. Osmotic diarrhea occurs when too much water is drawn into the bowels by the presence of excess sugars or nutrients. This is often seen in malabsorption from enzyme deficiencies, gluten sensitivity, or usage of osmotic laxatives.

Besides the number of pharmaceutical products that can cause adverse reactions and diarrhea, you need to keep an eye out for the unlabeled fillers often added to products for packaging or as volume filler in capsules. Mannitol and lactose are commonly used and can contribute to diarrhea, especially if the individual is lactose intolerant.

Inflammatory or exudative diarrhea occurs with inflammation with the presence of blood and pus in the stool. This occurs with inflammatory bowel diseases, and several intestinal infections. Motility-related diarrhea is caused by the rapid movement (hypermotility) of food and water through the intestines without enough time for absorption. This can be due to a vagotomy, diabetic neuropathy, hyperthyroidism, or prokinetic drugs. Short bowel and intestinal bypass syndromes can produce similar diarrhea. This type of diarrhea can be best treated with antimotility agents such as loperamide.

Laxative dependence abuse can lead to serious and potentially fatal fluid and electrolyte imbalances, including dehydration, hypokalemia, and metabolic alkalosis. Individuals with eating disorders such as anorexia nervosa and bulimia nervosa frequently abuse laxatives in an attempt to lose weight. The effects on body weight however are temporary losses of body water, rather than the desired prevention of calorie absorption. Chronic use of laxatives can lead to the bowels becoming dependent on their use, a condition known as a laxative gut.

Vaccines, probiotics, hand washing, sanitary sewage systems, and avoiding unwashed fruits and vegetables leads to a significant reduction of diarrhea. Oral rehydration solution may be used to prevent dehydration, which is a major cause of morbidity and mortality. Gastroenteritis (Latin gastro stomach, entero small intestine, itis inflammation) is an infectious diarrhea with inflammation of the gastrointestinal tract. It is commonly referred to as a stomach bug, virus, or flu. Gastroenteritis primarily affects children in the developing world, where hygiene is substandard and a clean and safe water supply is lacking.

Most transmission of pathogens is via the fecal to oral route is usually accomplished by way of the hands. The average human stool contains three trillion microorganisms. Wiping with toilet paper nearly guarantees that the hands will come into contact with fecal microorganisms. After wiping it is not uncommon to find brown streaks on underwear because of inadequate anal hygiene.

Gastroenteritis is an enormous public health issue that in this modern day and age causes disease and death in numbers hard to imagine. It is estimated that up to five billion cases of gastroenteritis each year result in nearly one and a half million deaths, primarily children and those in the developing world. In those less than five years of age there were about 1.7 billion cases resulting in 700,000 deaths, with over half the fatalities from rotavirus.

Cholera causes up to five million cases and kills approximately 100,000 people yearly. In the United States gastroenteritis is the most common infection after the common cold and results in up to 375 million cases of acute diarrhea and approximately ten thousand deaths annually. In the United States gastroenteritis as a whole is believed to result in costs of 23 billion US dollars per year, with that due to rotavirus alone resulting in estimated costs of 1 billion US dollars a year.

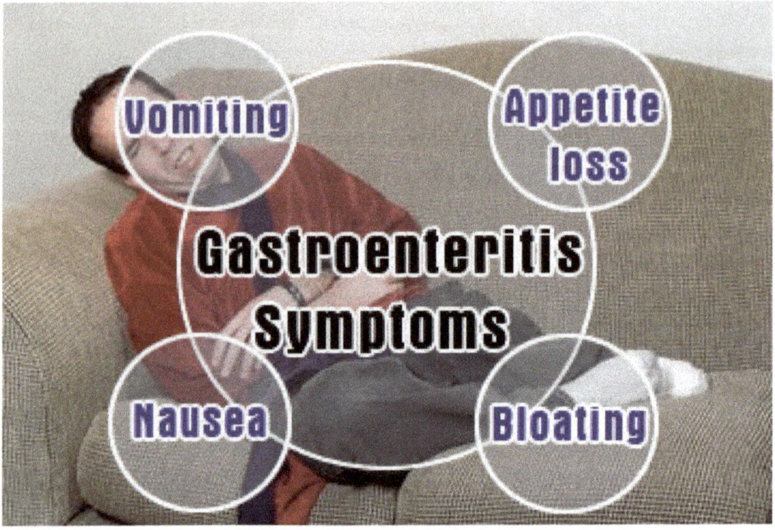
Vomiting
Appetite loss
Gastroenteritis Symptoms
Nausea
Bloating

healthprobs.com/wp

Viral gastroenteritis usually resolves within one week. In more severe cases intravenous fluids may be needed. Without adequate rehydration, gastroenteritis can lead to severe dehydration and death. A safe and effective vaccine has been available for years and the World Health Organization has embarked on campaigns to have children around the world immunized. In children the most common cause is a rotavirus, a self-limited infection that lasts from three to eight days. Signs and symptoms usually begin within 72 hours of ingestion of the infectious agent. For mild to moderate cases, oral rehydration solution prevents dehydration while the illness runs its course.

In adults the Norovirus is the causative agent in approximately ninety percent of cases. Norovirus is a genus of genetically diverse single-stranded RNA, non-enveloped viruses in the Caliciviridae family. The known viruses in the genus are all considered to be the strains of a single species called Norwalk virus. The viruses are transmitted by fecally contaminated food or water, by person-to-person contact, and via aerosolization of the virus and subsequent contamination of surfaces. Noroviruses are the most common cause of viral gastroenteritis in humans, and affect people of all ages. It often presents as a localized epidemic when groups of people are in close physical proximity to each other, such as on cruise ships, in hospitals, or in restaurants. People may remain infectious to others even after their diarrhea has ended. If blood is noted in the diarrhea a bacterial infection is the most likely cause.

Outbreaks of norovirus infection often make the news because they occur in closed or semiclosed communities, such as long-term care facilities, overnight camps, hospitals, prisons, dormitories, schools and cruise ships. The infection spreads very rapidly either by person-to-person transmission or through contaminated food. Many norovirus outbreaks have been traced to food that was handled by one infected person.

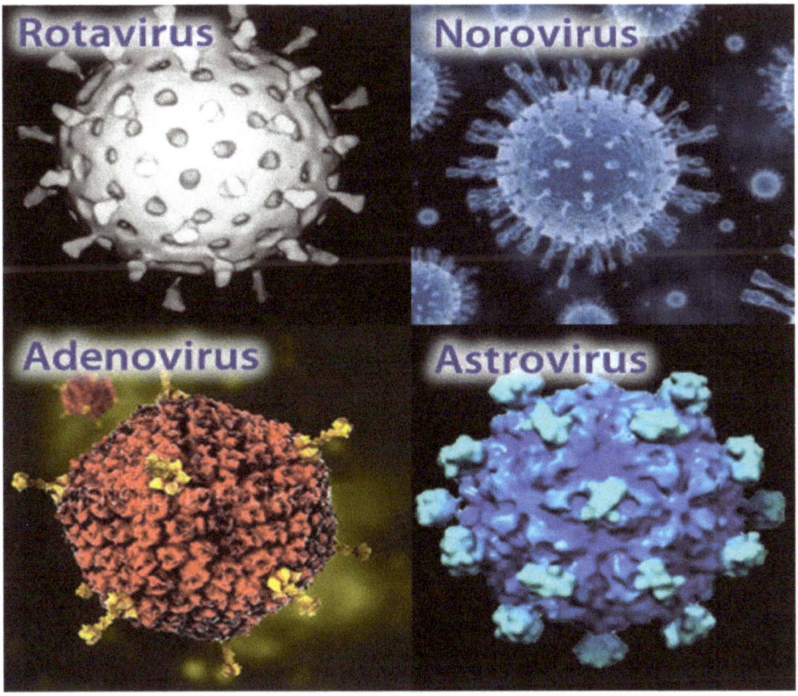
Rotavirus
Norovirus
Adenovirus
Astrovirus
www.tabletsmanual.com/img/wiki Creative Commons License

The genus name Norovirus is derived from Norwalk virus, the only species of the genus. The species causes approximately ninety percent of epidemic nonbacterial outbreaks of gastroenteritis around the world, and may be responsible for fifty percent of all foodborne outbreaks of gastroenteritis in the United States. The virus affects around 267 million people and causes over 200,000 deaths each year. These deaths are usually in less developed countries and in the very young, elderly and immuno-suppressed.

When a person becomes infected with norovirus, the virus begins to replicate within the small intestine. Symptoms may appear approximately one to two days later. The principal symptom is acute gastroenteritis that develops between twenty-four to forty-eight hours after exposure and lasts for twenty-four to sixty hours.

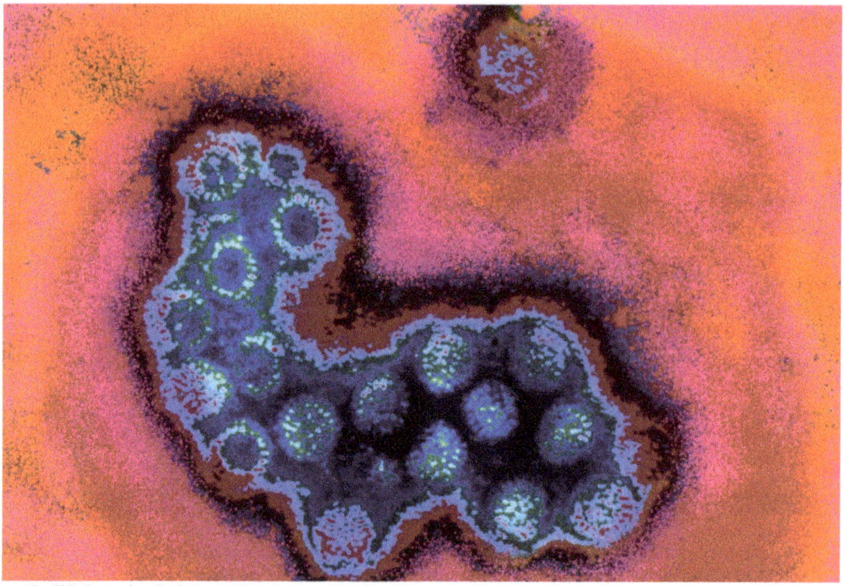

Shellfish and salad ingredients are the foods most often implicated in norovirus outbreaks. Ingestion of shellfish that have not been sufficiently cooked poses a high risk for norovirus infection.

The disease is usually self-limited and characterized by nausea, forceful vomiting, watery diarrhea, abdominal pain, and in some cases the loss of taste. General lethargy, weakness, muscle aches, headache, coughs, and low-grade fever may also occur. The number of deaths from norovirus in the United States is estimated to be around three hundred each year, with most of these occurring in the very young, the elderly, and persons with weakened immune systems.

Hand washing with soap and water is an effective method for reducing the transmission of norovirus. Alcohol rubs with over a sixty percent ethanol content are less effective than hand washing as the norovirus lacks a lipid viral envelope. The norovirus can survive for long periods outside a human host. It can survive for months and maybe even years in contaminated still water. The virus remained virulent on surfaces used for food preparation for over seven days after contamination. The common causes of a non-viral gastroenteritis include bacteria such as *Escherichia coli* and *Campylobacter jejuni*, bacterial toxins, and parasites. Transmission is usually via the fecal-oral route from contaminated food or water. A number of protozoans can cause gastroenteritis, most commonly *Giardia lamblia*, but *Entamoeba histolytica* and Cryptosporidium can also cause infection. A protozoan is responsible for about ten percent of gastroenteritis cases in children.

In the developed world *Campylobacter jejuni* is the primary cause of bacterial gastroenteritis, with half of these cases occurring from contaminated poultry. In children, bacteria are the cause in about fifteen percent of cases, with the most common types being *Escherichia coli*, Salmonella, Shigella, and Campylobacter species. If food becomes contaminated with bacteria and remains at room temperature the bacteria multiply rapidly and increase the risk of infection. Some foods commonly associated with illness include raw or undercooked meat, poultry, seafood, and eggs, raw sprouts, unpasteurized milk, soft cheeses, fruit, and vegetables. In the developing world, especially sub-Saharan Africa and Asia, cholera is a common cause of gastroenteritis and is usually transmitted through contaminated water.

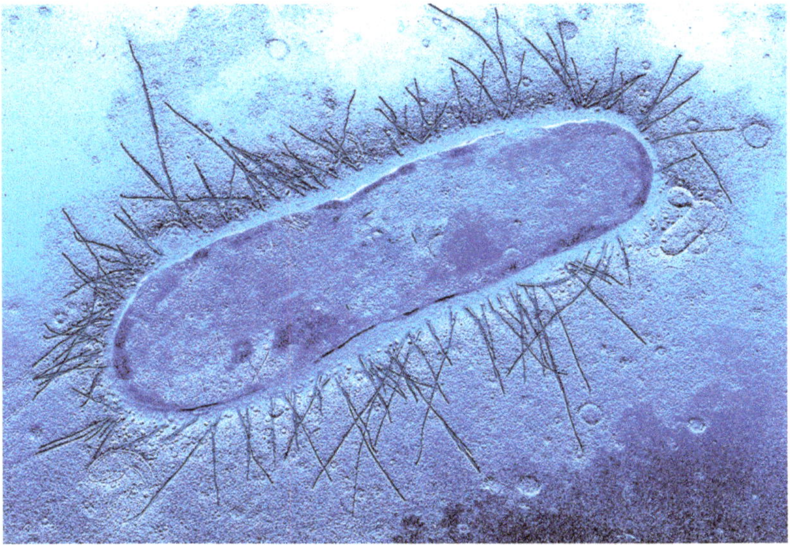

A large portion of the world population does not have access to a clean safe potable water supply, nor does it have adequate sanitation for the safe disposal of potentially infective human waste. Ironically in the U.S. clean drinking water is used for flushing toilets. Over one-quarter of the drinkable household water usage goes down the toilet bowl to be mixed in with sewage. The irony is similar to the problem of hunger and malnutrition in the underdeveloped world, and obesity and metabolic disorders in the best described as overdeveloped world. A number of nonprofit and charitable organizations are trying to address these issues.

Probiotics may be beneficial in reducing the duration and severity of illness. They may also be useful in preventing and treating antibiotic associated diarrhea. Supplementation with the micronutrient zinc appears to be effective in both treating and preventing diarrhea among children in the developing world. Acid-suppressing medication appears to increase the risk of infection by eliminating the natural defense of gastric acid destroying most bacteria. The risk is greater in those taking proton pump inhibitors than with H2 antagonists, as the degree and length of time of effective acid suppression is increased.

Diphenoxylate is an opioid agonist that works by decreasing the speed and amplitude of peristalsis, increasing the gut transit time. This allows more time for water and electrolytes to be absorbed by the colon solidifying the stool. It crosses the blood–brain barrier and tolerance and dependence can develop with chronic or excessive use. Diphenoxylate is produced in combination with atropine (Lomotil, Pfizer) to deter abuse.

Loperamide is an opioid agonist that acts on the μ-opioid receptors in the myenteric plexus of the large intestine. It decreases the peristaltic activity of the smooth muscles of the intestinal wall. This increases the gut transit time and allows the colon more time to absorb water and electrolytes making the stool less liquid. It also decreases colonic mass movements and suppresses the gastro-colic reflex.

Kaopectate is literally no longer the product it used to be, and it is a very different product in the United States than it is in Canada. The active ingredient in Kaopectate has changed since its original creation. Kaolinite clay as an absorbent in combination with pectin as an emollient had been a very popular remedy for diarrhea. Attapulgite (a type of absorbent clay) replaced the kaolinite in the 1980's, but was found to be unproven as to effectiveness by the FDA. As a consequence bismuth subsalicylate has been used as the active ingredient in U.S. marketed products. In the U.S. Kaopectate is now the equivalent of Pepto Bismol.

Children should not take medication with bismuth subsalicylate while recovering from influenza or chicken pox. The use of salicylate containing medications during certain viral infections may be associated with the onset of Reye's syndrome, a serious liver condition. For the same reason, it is typically recommended that nursing mothers not use medication containing bismuth subsalicylate because small amounts of the medication are excreted in breast milk and pose a theoretical risk of Reye's syndrome to nursing children. Bismuth will also turn the stools a black color that can be misinterpreted as melena, a sign of internal bleeding. In Canada, McNeil Consumer Healthcare continues to market Kaopectate using attapulgite as the active ingredient.

Dietary Fiber

Dietary fiber, also referred to as roughage is the indigestible component of plants consumed as food. Fiber is advocated to enhance bowel regularity, and to avoid constipation. It can also be helpful in irritable bowel syndrome where the additional bulk reduces the pressure on the intestinal wall. This sounds counterintuitive, but the distention of the bowel reduces the pressure on the colonic wall in accordance with the laws of physics.

Laplace's Law states that the pressure on the wall of a cylinder is inversely proportional to the diameter of the cylinder. There are two main types, differentiated by their solubility in water. Soluble fiber, which dissolves in water, is readily fermented in the intestinal tract producing gases and byproducts. It is further divided into viscous fiber and prebiotic fiber. It is commonly found in oat bran, beans, peas, and most fruits.

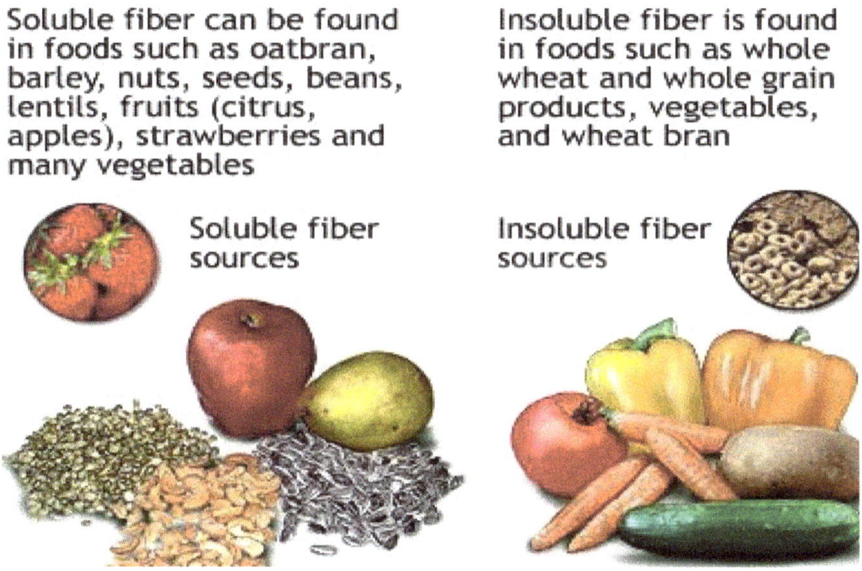
Soluble fiber can be found in foods such as oatbran, barley, nuts, seeds, beans, lentils, fruits (citrus, apples), strawberries and many vegetables
Insoluble fiber is found in foods such as whole wheat and whole grain products, vegetables, and wheat bran
Soluble fiber sources
Insoluble fiber sources

Insoluble fiber does not dissolve in water. It is further divided into fiber that is metabolically inert and simply provides added bulk and fluid retention, or prebiotic which is metabolically fermented by the gut flora. The bulk enhancing fibers ease defecation both by adding moisture to the stool as well as stimulating gut peristalsis and colonic mass movements. The added bulk also reduces the incidence of spasmodic contractions of the bowel. These spasms may contribute to the pain and discomfort of irritable bowel syndrome, previously known as a spastic colon or spastic colitis. Insoluble fiber is the type of fiber found in wheat bran and some vegetables.

Dietary fiber is comprised of non-starch polysaccharides such as arabinoxylans, cellulose, resistant starch, resistant dextrins, inulin, lignin, waxes, chitins, pectins, beta-glucans, and oligosaccharides.
Lignin, a major dietary insoluble fiber source, may alter the rate and metabolism of soluble fibers. Lignin is found in high concentrations in tree bark and its difficulty in being digested and decomposed played a major role in the Carboniferous era when tree bark was a multiple of the thickness it is today. On the other hand, insoluble fibers like the resistant starches are fully fermented.

Fiber Content Of Popular Foods

Food Source	Soluble Fiber (g)	Insoluble Fiber (g)	Total Fiber (g)
Apple (1 med)	0.9g	2.0g	2.9g
Banana (1 med)	0.6g	1.4g	2.0g
Orange (1 med)	1.3g	0.7g	2.0g
Broccoli (1 stalk)	1.3g	1.4g	2.7g
Carrots (1 large)	1.3g	1.6g	2.9g
Tomato (1 small)	0.1g	0.7g	0.8g
Potato (1 medium)	1.0g	0.8g	1.8g
All Bran (1/2 cup)	1.4g	7.6g	9.0g
Oat Bran (1/2 cup)	2.2g	2.2g	4.4g
Corn Flakes (1 cup)	0g	0.5g	0.5g
Rolled Oats (3/4 cup)	1.3g	1.7g	3.0g
Wheat Bread (1 slice)	0.3g	1.1g	1.4g
White Bread (1 slice)	0.3g	0.1g	0.4g
Green Peas (2/3 cup)	0.6g	3.3g	3.9g
Kidney Beans (1/2 cup)	1.6g	4.9g	6.5g
Lentils (2/3 cup)	0.6g	3.9g	4.5g

source: USDA/ARS Nutrient Data Laboratory

Public Domain

The main disadvantage of a diet high in fiber is the increased intestinal gas production with bloating and being a social outcast a possible consequence. The original definition of fiber was the components of plants that were not affected by digestive enzymes, a definition that includes lignin and polysaccharides. The definition was later expanded to include resistant starches, polysaccharides, lignin, and inulin with other oligosaccharides.

While dietary fiber is present in nearly all fruits and vegetables, the type and quantity of fiber varies widely. Persimmons have safety issues and if eaten unripe the soluble tannin shiboul can lead to gastric phytobezoars. In this condition a hardened wood like mass of fiber remains within the stomach for years or a lifetime.

Soluble fiber is present, in variable quantities, in plant food including legumes (peas, soybeans, lupins, beans), oats, rye, chia, and barley It is also found in some fruits and fruit juices (including prune juice, plums, berries, ripe bananas, apples, and pears), and certain vegetables such as broccoli, carrots, Jerusalem artichokes, root tubers and root vegetables such as sweet potatoes and onions (skins of these are sources of insoluble fiber also). Additional sources include psyllium seed husk (a mucilage soluble fiber), flax seeds, and nuts, with almonds being the highest in dietary fiber

Sources of insoluble fiber include, whole grain foods, wheat and corn bran, legumes such as beans and peas, nuts and seeds, potato skins, lignins, vegetables such as green beans, cauliflower, zucchini (courgette), celery, nopal, some fruits including avocado, and unripe bananas, the skins of some fruits, including kiwifruit, grapes and tomatoes. Vegetable gum fiber, such as guar gum and acacia Senegal gum, dissolve easily and have no aftertaste making them a popular fiber supplement additive.

Dietary fibers have three primary mechanisms: bulking, viscosity, and fermentation. As they can change the nature and transit of the intestinal contents they may impact how other nutrients and materials are absorbed. Some soluble fibers bind to bile acids preventing their normal reabsorption in the small intestine. This results in the interruption of the normal enterohepatic circulation of the bile from the small intestine to the liver, and results in the loss of cholesterol in the form of bile acids via the stool.

The cholesterol levels in the blood are subsequently lowered since the liver removes cholesterol from the circulation to synthesize replacement bile salts. Viscous soluble fibers may also inhibit the absorption of sugar, thus reducing the sugar insulin response after meals. Fatty foods and hypertonic solutions delay gastric emptying and gut transit time. The intestinal contents are called chyme once they leave the stomach. Chyme consists of food compounds, digestive enzymes, stomach acid and pancreatic and duodenal bicarbonate, bile acids, complex lipids in changing micellar, aqueous, hydrocolloid, hydrophobic, and hydrophilic phases all in a mixture of solid, liquid, colloidal and gas bubble phases. In other words, it is one chaotic churning, digesting, fermenting mass from which the gut may selectively absorb nutrients, ions and other products throughout the digestive process.

Non-absorbed carbohydrates such as pectin, gum Arabic, oligosaccharides and resistant starch, are fermented by the gut flora to short-chain fatty acids (mainly acetic, propionic and n-butyric), carbon dioxide, hydrogen and methane. The colon will absorb nearly all of the short-chain fatty acids with the butyric acid being utilized as the main source of energy for colonic cells.

Soluble and insoluble fiber both increases food volume without additional caloric content. The increased volume can provide greater satiety, which may lead to decreased food intake and weight loss. Intestinal fermentation can increase the production of beneficial short chain fatty acids. Soluble fiber absorbs water and forms a viscous gel, known as a hydrophilic mucilloid that slows gastric emptying and intestinal transit. The increased bulk may shield carbohydrates from enzymes, delay the absorption of glucose, and reduce the fluctuations of blood sugar levels that result. On the other hand the delayed transit allows more time for enzymatic activity as well as fermentation by the gut flora.

Insoluble fiber enhances gut motility and speeds transit time, as well as adding bulk and moisture to the stool promoting defecation and preventing constipation. Current recommendations for daily dietary fiber intake are thirty grams for the average adults. The average American consumes about half of that amount. Sugars and starches provide four calories per gram as the digestive system has enzymes to break them down into the simple absorbable sugars of glucose, fructose, and galactose. Insoluble fiber cannot be digested so no calories are absorbed. Soluble fiber is partially fermented, and the caloric intake is determined by the degree that it is broken down into absorbable nutrients.

As a result of the variability in calories generated there is controversy on their calorie count. Two calories per gram of soluble fiber is a reasonable compromise. Fibers with partial or low fermentability include cellulose, hemicellulose, lignans, plant waxes, and resistant starches. Fibers with high fermentability include beta-glucans, pectins, natural gums, inulins, oligosaccharides, and resistant dextrins.

Digestion

The gastrointestinal tract is also known as the alimentary tract or canal, digestive tract, intestinal tract, and gut. To understand the process of digestion it helps to understand how the digestive tract is organized. There are many organs and names, mentioned as a guide, and not to be memorized. It is normally considered to consist of the hollow tubular organs including the esophagus (also known as the gullet or food pipe), stomach, small intestine (also known as small bowel), large intestine (also known as large bowel or colon), and rectum.

The gastrointestinal system (also digestive system and alimentary system) include the accessory glands and organs that participate in the digestive process. This includes the mouth, teeth, salivary glands, tongue, pharynx, liver, gallbladder, bile ducts, and pancreas. The individual organs have names for specific sections that may be familiar, e.g. the appendix is part of the colon. The stomach has the antrum, body, pyloris, and fundus. The small intestine has three sections with different functions, the duodenum, jejunum, and ileum. The colon consists of the appendix, cecum, ascending colon, transverse colon, descending colon, sigmoid colon, and rectum. The anus, also known as the anal canal is functionally a part of the colon.

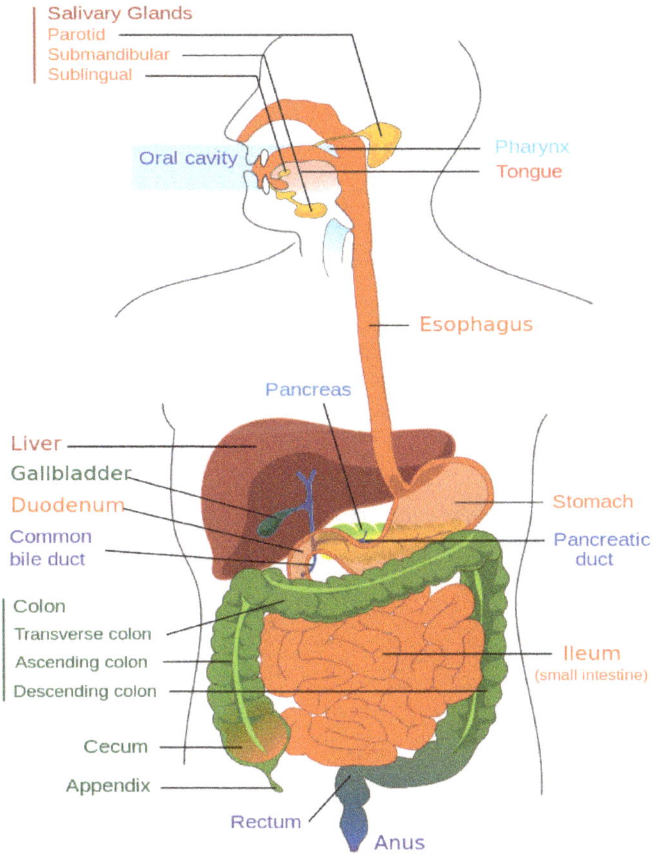
Salivary Glands
Parotid
Submandibular
Sublingual
Oral cavity
Pharynx
Tongue
Esophagus
Pancreas
Liver
Gallbladder
Duodenum
Common bile duct
Stomach
Pancreatic duct
Colon
Transverse colon
Ascending colon
Descending colon
Ileum
(small intestine)
Cecum
Appendix
Rectum
Anus

Mariana Ruiz LadyofHats, edited by Joaquim Alves Gaspar Creative Commons License

The teeth, jaws, and tongue work together in a remarkable and powerful dance with very few missteps of the equivalent of stepping on toes, the biting of the tongue. The incisors cut the food as you bite into an apple, the canines tear the food apart as you dig into your pastrami sandwich, and your molars crush and grind the salad and crunchy vegetables you have as a side dish. The grinding and crushing breaks the plant cell walls that would otherwise protect its internal nutritious content. The chewing process assures that the saliva and its active enzymes are well mixed with the food and can begin the process of breaking the carbohydrates and lipids into their basic components to ready them for further digestion and absorption.

The saliva also moistens the food and lubricates it for the coordinated motion of the tongue, teeth, palate and pharynx to roll it into an easy to swallow food bolus. The muscles of the swallowing process include those that protect the larynx and airway by having the epiglottis close off the passageway to the trachea, bronchi, and lungs to prevent aspiration. The coordinated activity is developed with age, which is why small children should avoid foods, such as nuts, grapes, and larger oval or rounded candies that if inappropriately swallowed into the airway can lead to fatal choking episodes. Tragically a number of children die because the oval or rounded shape can completely block the airway, as opposed to an irregularly shaped object, which can be life threatening but will allow some air to pass.

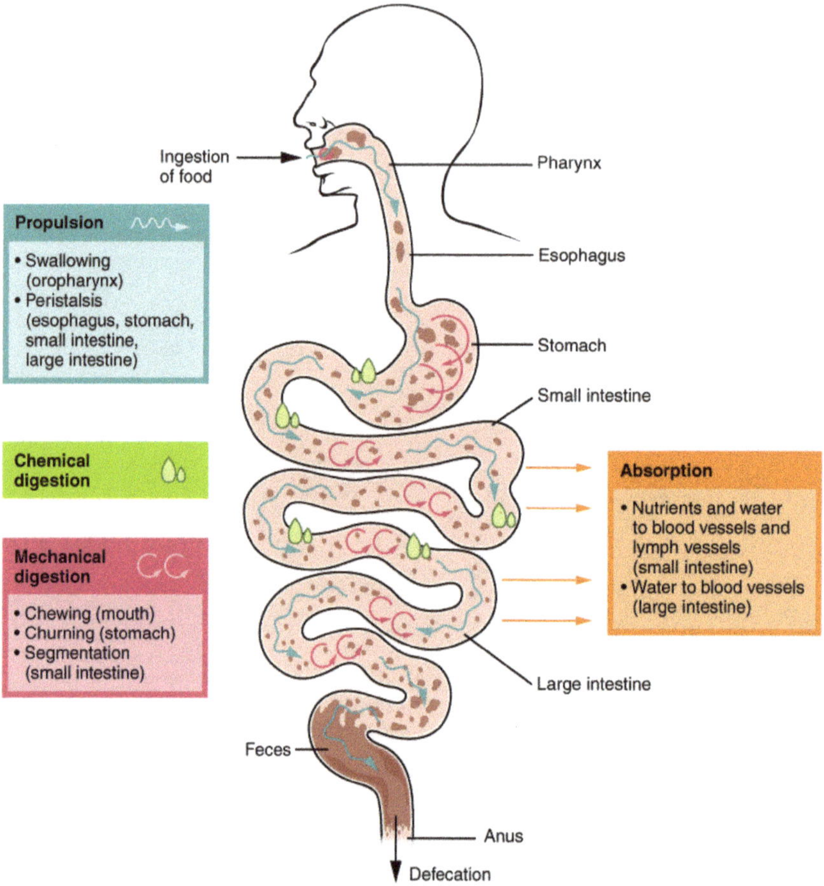
Ingestion of food
Pharynx
Esophagus
Stomach
Small intestine
Large intestine
Feces
Anus
Defecation
Propulsion
• Swallowing (oropharynx)
• Peristalsis (esophagus, stomach, small intestine, large intestine)
Chemical digestion
Mechanical digestion
• Chewing (mouth)
• Churning (stomach)
• Segmentation (small intestine)
Absorption
• Nutrients and water to blood vessels and lymph vessels (small intestine)
• Water to blood vessels (large intestine)
Openstax College philschatz.com Creative Commons License

The complicated swallowing neuromuscular coordination can also be affected by neurological disorders, stroke, surgery or other conditions, which may lead to the risk of aspiration. Once swallowed, the food bolus is propelled down the esophagus by coordinated snakelike muscular activity known as peristalsis. It is not recommended, but you can swallow against gravity while standing on your head. The muscular valve at the junction of the esophagus and stomach is called the lower esophageal sphincter (LES).

The LES is designed to allow food and fluid to enter the stomach with the door closed behind them once they leave the esophagus. If the valve opens at the wrong time gastric acid, digestive enzymes and food can flow back into the esophagus. This can lead to symptoms of heartburn or mucosal damage. If it occurs frequently gastroesophageal reflux disease (GERD) can predispose to a change in the tissue lining the esophagus. The development of intestinal type tissue is called a Barrett esophagus and has a higher incidence of cancer development.

The stomach is a churning cauldron of muscular mixing contractions, intense acid secretion, and more potent digestive enzymes. The vagus nerve and gut hormones play a role in the intricate balance of enzymes, acid, nutrients, and motility. When the conditions are right the pyloric channel out of the stomach opens to allow the acid, enzyme, and food mixture now called chyme to enter the first part of the small intestine called the duodenum.

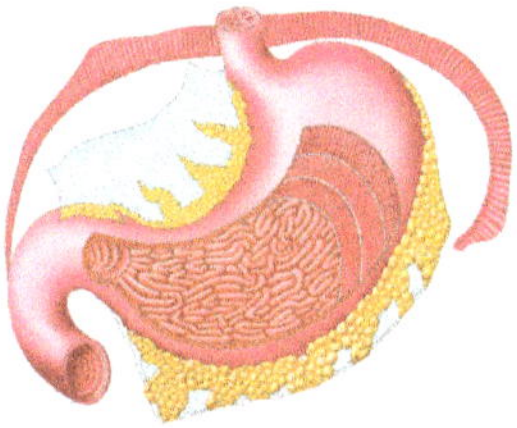

The structure of the wall of the stomach

Layers of the Stomach Wall

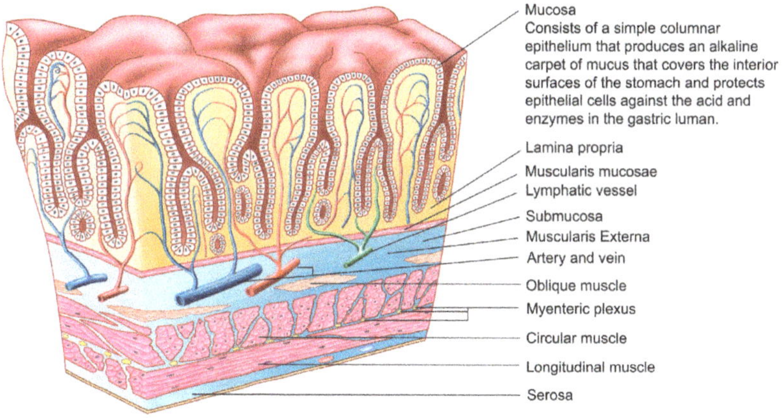
Mucosa
Consists of a simple columnar epithelium that produces an alkaline carpet of mucus that covers the interior surfaces of the stomach and protects epithelial cells against the acid and enzymes in the gastric luman.
Lamina propria
Muscularis mucosae
Lymphatic vessel
Submucosa
Muscularis Externa
Artery and vein
Oblique muscle
Myenteric plexus
Circular muscle
Longitudinal muscle
Serosa

In Greek duodenum means the width equivalent to twelve fingers, which is what its small size would measure using your digits. For a small area, it plays an amazing and complex role. The highly acid chyme would quickly damage the duodenum if it did not respond quickly with the pouring on, much like a fire extinguisher, of sodium bicarbonate. The sodium bicarbonate is produced in the duodenum itself as well as the pancreas, which releases it through the pancreatic duct, which empties into the duodenum.

The fire extinguisher analogy has a double story. Perhaps you actually made a fire extinguisher in a science class or home experiment by adding sodium bicarbonate and hydrochloric acid. This is the exact same reaction that takes place in the duodenum when the hydrochloric acid of the stomach meets the sodium bicarbonate released to neutralize it. When the two react water, sodium chloride (salt), and large quantities of carbon dioxide are released. The carbon dioxide is used as a fire extinguisher in the science experiment, but in the human duodenum it simply serves to bloat and distend the gut with gas. The body is pretty remarkable in getting rid of the bloat fairly quickly, in that it absorbs the carbon dioxide into the bloodstream where it travels to the lungs to be exhaled.

The bile ducts from the liver join the duct from the pancreas bringing digestive enzymes and bicarbonate and enter the duodenum through the sphincter of Oddi. If that sounds like a name from the *Wizard of Oz* that would be an appropriate analogy. The coordinated release of hormones, enzymes, motility, and vagal input is nothing short of wizardly. Subconsciously your body can sense exactly what type of nutrients you have ingested to release the right recipe of enzymes, acid in the stomach, bicarbonate in the duodenum, adjust the pH as necessary, add the right amount of bile to the mix, control the timing and volume of stomach emptying, and control the speed of transit and intensity of mixing contractions through the length of the intestinal tract. The majority of the sensing and control feedback takes place in the duodenum within the space the width of twelve fingers.

The breakdown products of the digestive process are absorbed through a the villi., They are the long finger like projections of the gut mucosal lining which dramatically increases the surface area for digestion and absorption. The villi are in continuous motion and are a major contributor to intestinal stirring and mixing. In spite of the relatively long length of the small intestine, its absorptive capacity would not be sufficient to maintain nutrition for an organism the size of a human without modifications to increase its surface area.

It looks like a field of waving wheat stalks, each upstanding villus ready to use its enzymes and absorptive capacity to absorb nutrients. If you looked under the microscope you would find that each villus has thousands of even smaller villi on its surface, of course given the appropriate name of microvilli. All of these folds of absorptive tissue, if flattened out, would be the equivalent absorptive capacity of a championship tennis court. This long tunnel of eagerly awaiting absorptive villi is about twenty feet long, and it does an amazing job of digestion and absorption.

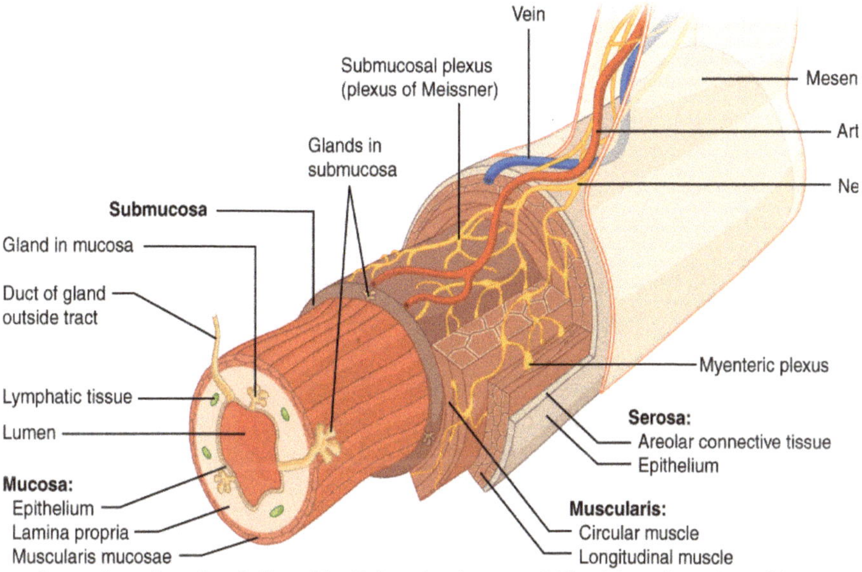
Vein
Submucosal plexus
(plexus of Meissner)
Mesen
Art
Ne
Glands in
submucosa
Submucosa
Gland in mucosa
Duct of gland
outside tract
Myenteric plexus
Lymphatic tissue
Lumen
Serosa:
Areolar connective tissue
Epithelium
Mucosa:
Epithelium
Lamina propria
Muscularis mucosae
Muscularis:
Circular muscle
Longitudinal muscle

Connexions, OpenStax College, Rice University, Anatomy & Physiology, Overview of the Digestive System Creative Commons License

If injured the ability of the small bowel is compromised. A condition that temporarily damages the small intestine, like diarrhea from a viral or bacterial gastroenteritis, often called a stomach flu, can cause a blunting or shortening of the villi. This will also lead to the loss of digestive enzymes that reside on the villi. This is one of the reasons people are often advised to avoid dairy products for a week or so after stomach flu to allow the villi and enzymes to recover. If you eat or drink lactose without waiting until the recovery is complete you may end up with symptoms of lactose intolerance such as gas and diarrhea.

When the liquid chyme leaves the jejunum and ileum of the small intestine for the colon it goes through the ileocecal valve. In the cecum of the colon lies the infamous appendix, which for thousands of years no one could figure out its purpose. It looks like its function has finally, and only very recently, been identified. It stores a reservoir of intestinal bacteria, representing the healthy gut microbiome, from which the gut flora can be replenished after a bout of intestinal dysentery. The gut microbiome is much more important than most people give it credit for. The microbes of the body far outnumber the number of human cells. The vast majorities are commensals, which means that they are engaged with us in a symbiotic relationship from which we both benefit.

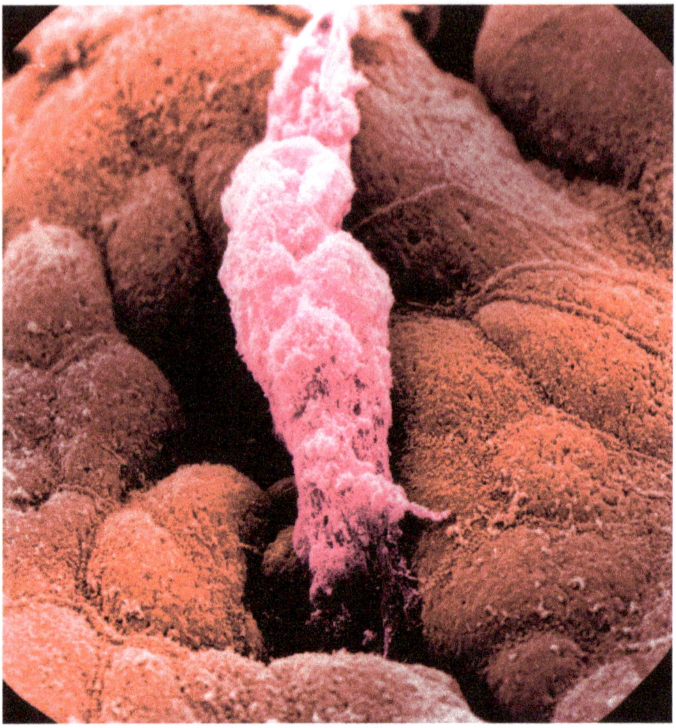

Mucus cell

The colon, unlike the small intestine, is less involved in the digestion of foods and nutrients. It is primarily involved in the absorption of water and sodium as well as some fat-soluble vitamins such as vitamin K. The colon removes the excess moisture from the watery chyme, and the stool solidifies as it transits the gut. It is stored in the rectum and sigmoid colon awaiting the right opportunity to be eliminated through defecation.

A process or illness that impairs the colonic absorption of water will lead to a more fluid stool and diarrhea. If the elimination is delayed, moisture continues to be absorbed and the stools can become harder resulting in constipation. The feces excreted can provide information about bowel health, but for most people going about their daily activities, the passage itself is the end of the story of digestion.

The three major classes of nutrients that undergo digestion are proteins, lipids (fats) and carbohydrates. Enzymes including pepsin, trypsin, chymotrypsin, carboxypeptidase, amino peptidase and dipeptidase digest proteins. The amino acid products are then absorbed by the small intestine. Lipids are digested by the enzyme lipase and bile acids into fatty acids, monoglycerides and glycerol, which are absorbed in the small intestine.

Dung (see Manure)

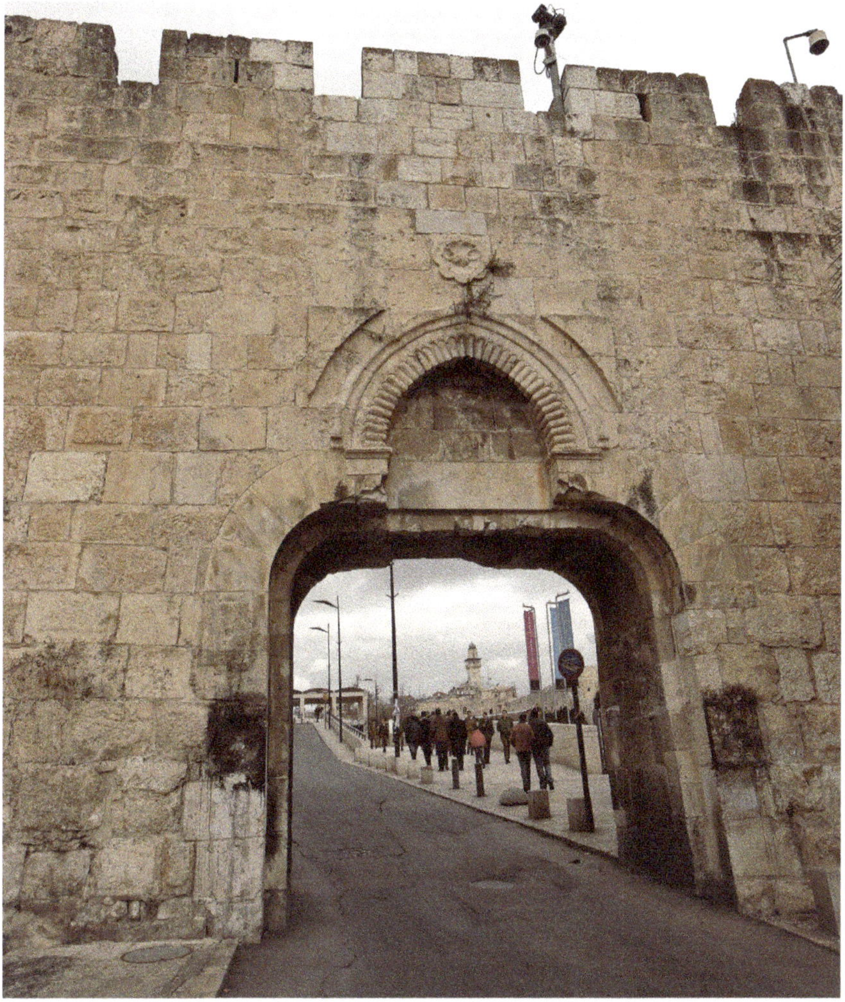

The Dung Gate entry into the walled city of Jerusalem

Dung Beetle

Dung beetles are beetles that feed partly or exclusively on feces. All the species belong to the superfamily Scarabaeoidea, which alone comprises more than five-thousand species. Many dung beetles, known as *rollers*, roll dung into round balls, which are used as a food source or brooding chambers. They can roll up to ten times their weight and some species can pull up to one-thousand times their weight.

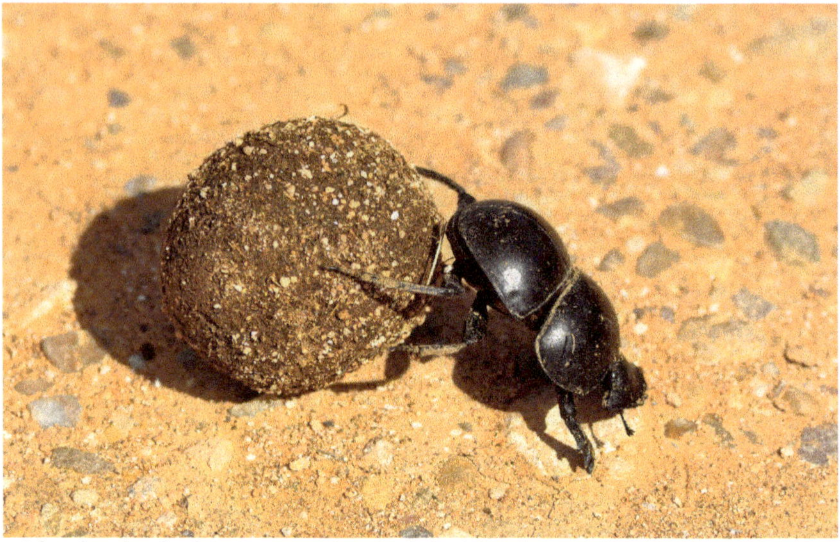

Other dung beetles, known as tunnelers, bury the dung wherever they find it. A third group, the dwellers, neither roll nor burrow: they simply live in manure. Dung beetles are currently the only animals, other than humans, known to navigate and orient themselves using the Milky Way. Shutterstock/JohnMichaelEvanPotter

Dung beetles play an important role in agriculture. By burying and consuming dung they improve nutrient recycling and soil structure. They also protect livestock, such as cattle, by removing the dung, which if left in the open could provide habitat for pests. Many countries have introduced the creatures for the benefit of animal husbandry and as an adjunct for improving standards of hygiene. Several species of the dung beetle, most notably the species *Scarabaeus sacer* often referred to as the sacred scarab, enjoyed a sacred status among the ancient Egyptians. The scarab was linked to Khepri ("he who has come into being") the god of the rising sun. The image of the scarab symbolizing transformation, renewal, and resurrection, is ubiquitous in ancient Egyptian religious and funerary art.

"Never did adventurers hurrying from the four corners of the earth display such eagerness," the French entomologist Jean-Henri Fabre once wrote. "They are there in the hundreds, large and small, of every sort, shape and size, hastening to carve themselves a slice of the common cake." Some grab what dung they can and cram it underground on the spot. Dung beetles have been known to steal treasured dung balls from each other. Others, the ball-rollers, embark on a journey that requires the heavens to navigate.

The ancients believed that the dung beetle was unique in that only the male gender existed, and that it reproduced by depositing semen into a dung ball. The supposed self-creation of the beetle resembles that of Khepri, who creates himself out of nothing. The dung ball rolled by a dung beetle resembles the sun. In ancient Greece Plutarch wrote "The race of beetles has no female, but all the males eject their sperm into a round pellet of material which they roll up by pushing it from the opposite side, just as the sun seems to turn the heavens in the direction opposite to its own course, which is from west to east".

The dung beetle has several appearances in the classical literature. In Aesop's fable *The Dung Beetle and the Eagle* the eagle kills a hare despite the beetle's appeals. The beetle takes revenge by twice destroying the eagle's eggs. The eagle, in despair, flies up to Olympus and places her latest eggs in Zeus's lap, beseeching the god to protect them. When the beetle finds out what the eagle has done, it stuffs itself with dung, goes straight up to Zeus and flies right into his face.

Zeus is startled at the sight of the unpleasant creature and jumps to his feet. The eggs are broken. Zeus then learns of the beetle's plea, which the eagle had ignored. He scolds the eagle and urges the beetle to stay away from the bird. But his efforts to persuade the beetle fail; so he changes the breeding season of the eagles to take place at a time when the beetles are not above ground. The ancient Greek playwright Aristophanes alluded to Aesop's fable several times in his plays. In *Peace*, the hero rides up to Olympus to free the goddess Peace from her prison. His steed is an enormous dung beetle, which has been fed so much dung that it has grown to monstrous size.

Dung Fuel

Dry animal dung is used as a fuel in many countries around the world. It is a source of Green fuel used by more than two-billion people, even though it does contribute modestly to air pollution. As a cheap, efficient, sustainable, and renewable bioenergy source it has gained growing interest. Its other advantages are that it allows the safe disposal of animal waste, and reduces the pressure of finding alternative wood resources.

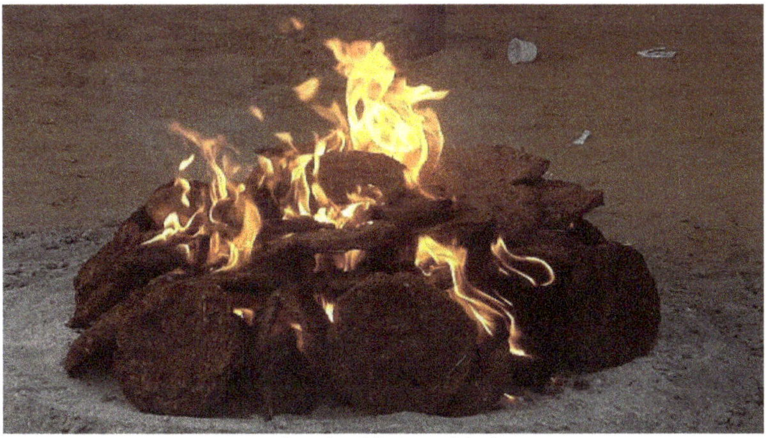

www.banglacricket.com/alochona

Dry dung (moisture content of less than thirty percent) is more popular, but moist dung may be also be used as a fuel. Animal dung commonly utilized includes cow, water buffalo, elephant, sheep, yak, camel, and others that may be readily available. Human waste is also utilized for the same purpose in many locations.

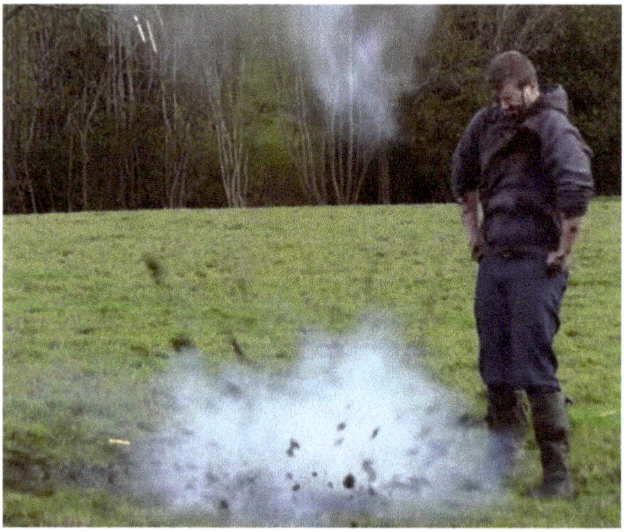

Lighting a match to a pile of cow dung is not a sign of higher intelligence. The methane and hydrogen generated by the microbes active in the dung pile may accumulate to explosive levels. youtu.be/bZI1eeV88lQ

On occasion dung and excrement can be more than just flammable, it can be explosive. The microorganism that produces hydrogen and methane that lead to ignitable farts continue their activity while sitting in a pile. For those foolish enough to light a match in a pile of cow dung to see what happens up close and personal the link to the video above should be convincing.

Methane and biofuels derived from feces propel public busses in several cities. The NASA space program uses various rocket fuels including hydrazine as a propellant. Even NASA can go green and rocket fuel from feces is technically a possibility. The bacteria *Candidatus brocadia anammoxidans* is the only organism capable of the anaerobic oxidation of ammonium and can create hydrazine from feces.

Methane is produced in the human intestinal tract by microbial organisms. Methanogens are microorganisms of the Kingdom Archaea, not bacteria as previously thought. They produce methane as a metabolic byproduct in anaerobic conditions when oxygen is not present. Methanogens have been found in a variety of extreme environments and can thrive and reproduce in boiling water as well as in ice cores taken miles down in arctic glaciers. They are common in wetlands, where they produce marsh gas, and in the digestive tracts of animals and humans where they generate the methane content of flatulence as well as the ruminant belch.

Hydrogen and Methane are combustible gasses. In the presence of oxygen and an ignition source you have a potent flammable commodity. When methane burns it has a characteristic blue flame that you may see in a pilot light if you have a gas stove or furnace. Adolescent males and those who remain as adolescents intellectually have a fondness for demonstrating their dragon like ability to be human flamethrowers by igniting their farts. This is not a recommended activity and severe injury has resulted from successful attempts to ignite farts.

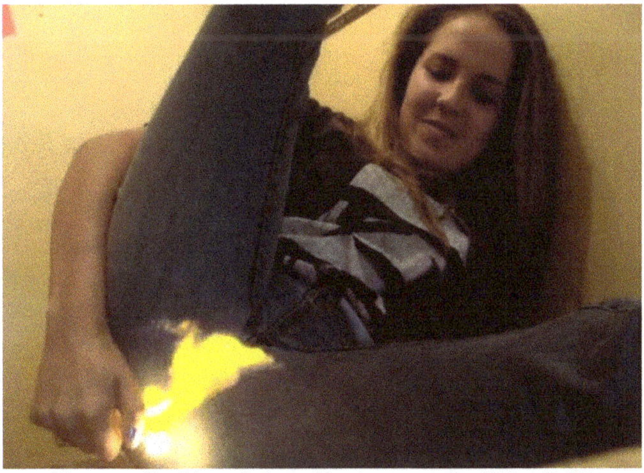

Moment of ignition of a fart, video is at youtu.be/Zt9rvaijpPY

Hydrogen and methane are the two flammable gasses that may be found in a fart making them flammable. Lighting a fart to see if one produces these gasses is actually a dangerous activity. Significant burns to the anogenital area have occurred as a result, especially when ignited without a clothing barrier. The popular television show *Mythbusters* filmed an episode confirming that many farts are indeed flammable. It appears that the network found the episode too provocative, and perhaps for liability concerns that children watching might attempt their own demonstrations decided to not 'air' the episode.

One of the more unusual injuries from a lit fart was second and third degree burns on the buttocks and a broken arm. The heavy gentlemen was sitting on the toilet defecating and farting extensively for a period of time. Being overweight his buttocks formed a firm seal around the toilet seat retaining all of the gasses in the enclosed space of the toilet bowl. He was smoking at the time and made a little space under his cheeks to innocently toss the lit cigarette into the toilet bowl. It promptly ignited blowing him off the seat, shattering the toilet bowl and causing extensive burn injuries to his buttocks. His wife called the paramedics and as he was being carried down the stairwell to the waiting ambulance he told them what caused the explosion. They laughed so hard they dropped the gurney thus breaking his arm.

Dysbiosis (see Gut Flora, Microbiome)

Encopresis

Encopresis is voluntary or involuntary fecal soiling in children who have usually been toilet trained. Up to three percent of four-year-olds have this disorder, which can be a source of discomfort, embarrassment, and stress. The disorder is six times more common in males than females.

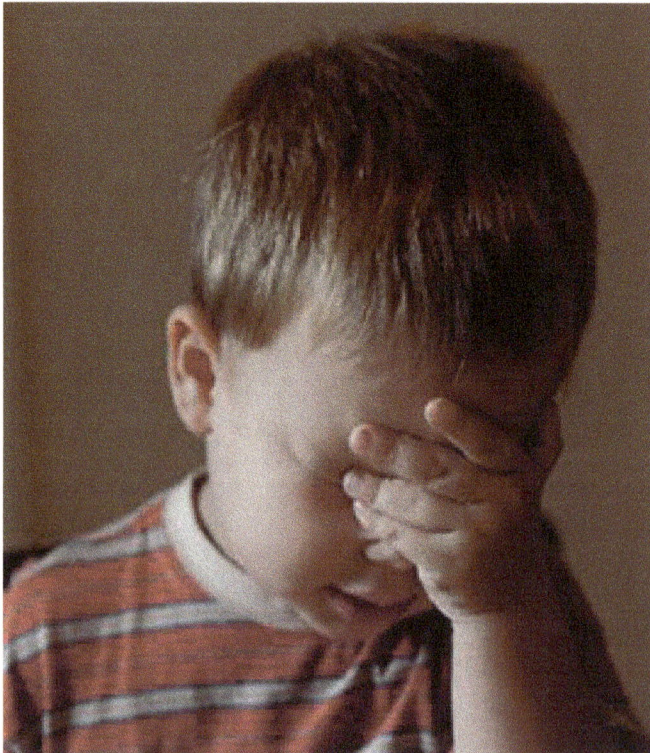

Encopresis, fecal soiling, can be a source of embarrassment and stress for both child and patents. www.buzzle.com

Encopresis may be caused by constipation, by reflexive withholding of stool after experiencing a painful bowel movement, or by various physiological, psychological, or neurological disorders. The colon removes excess water from feces. When the stool remains in the colon too long the stool becomes hard and painful to expel.

A vicious cycle may develop with the child avoiding a bowel movement in order to delay a painful toilet episode. Stool buildup stretches the colon and rectum to where the normal sensations associated with impending bowel movements are lost. Eventually softer stool leaks around the blockage resulting in an involuntary overflow incontinence. Treatment of encopresis associated with constipation usually involves behavioral therapy, stool softening agents, and scheduled toilet sitting times to establish a regular bowel pattern. The toilet time typically takes place after meals to take advantage of the gastrocolic reflex.

Enema (Clyster)

Enema (Greek ἐνίημι eníēmi "inject"), Clyster (Greek κλυστήρ klystḗr" wash"), and the colonic are all forms of irrigation of the large intestine for hygiene, evacuation of contents, comfort, or medicinal purposes. Historically medicine and physicians were closely associated with the administration of enemas, described as clysters in the past. The colonic enema has a long history in medical practice going back to the ancient Egyptians. The Ebers papyrus describes colonic irrigation prior to 1500 BCE.

The pharaoh's physician was called the guardian of the royal rectum, and enemas were the treatment of choice. Legend has it that the colonic was first initiated in Egypt because a native bird that has religious significance, the Ibis, would use its long narrow beak to insert the cleansing waters of the Nile River into its cloaca and rectum. Whether for hygiene or pleasure the Egyptians adopted the practice using hollow reeds from the Nile River banks.

In 600 BCE Babylonian and Assyrian cuneiform tablets include inscriptions on the use of enemas. In 400 BCE Hippocrates described using enemas in the treatment of fevers. In 124 BCE in Ancient Greece Asclepiades used the enema for intestinal worms as well for fevers as described by Hippocrates. In 30 AD Celsus, who was also the author of one of the first medical books *de Medicina* writes about the use of the enema. In 100 AD the prominent Greek physician Galen advocated the use of enemas. In 200 AD the Essene *Gospels of Peace* writes that Jesus was an advocate for colonics. In 500 AD the Greek physician Aetius recommended that pure water be used for enemas.

In 500 AD in Africa in Ivory Coast the natives administered enemas via a calabash filled with water while in other areas of the continent certain African tribes used a hollowed out cow horn. There is controversy over who deserves credit for the first specifically designed colonic administration instrument. The first enema syringe should either be credited to Avicenna

(980-1036 A.D.) or to Albucasis of Cordova (1013-1106). A preference would be to give the credit to Avicenna, as Cordova already has the distinction inventing the ear irrigation syringe. Further refinements developed an apparatus with a tube made of bone, reed or metal connected to a sleeve or animal bladder called the 'clyster purse'. Squeezing it between the two hands, often described as playing the bagpipes, emptied the bag.

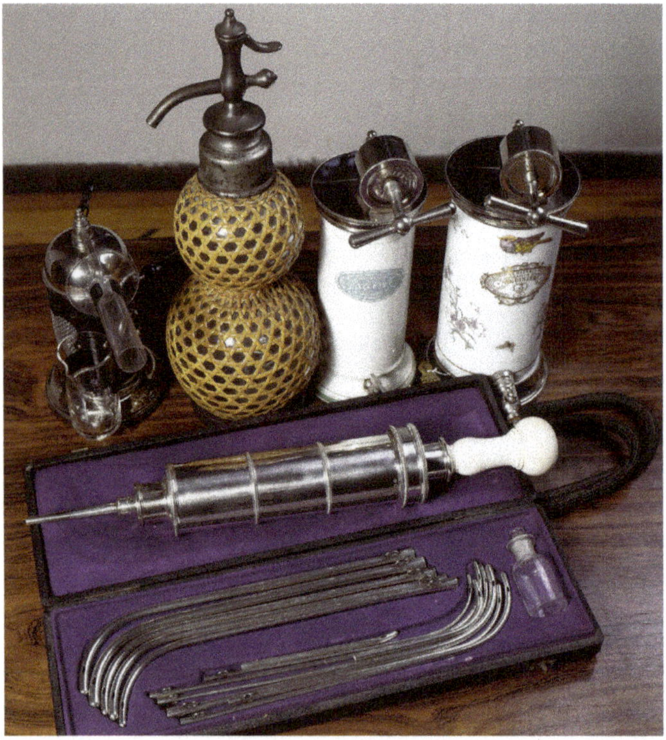

In the 1300's clysters and enemas were advocated and administered by the physicians to royalty and the aristocracy. In 1480, King Louis XI of France suffered an attack of apoplexy, which was treated by enemas prescribed by his physician, Angelo Catho. "The king became such an ardent advocate of clysters, that he even had his pet dogs clysterized when he thought they required it." In the 17th Century it was an acceptable practice in Parisian society to have as many as three or four enemas a day. The physicians of the day believed being that an internal washing or 'lavement' was conducive to good health. King Louis XIII had colonics performed at his royal court and had more than two-hundred enemas in one year.

With further refinements clyster syringes came in several styles. The clyster syringes were made of copper or porcelain, and the wealthy had fashionable syringes made of mother of pearl and silver. It was a status symbol to own several syringes and some aristocrats owned large collections of such instruments.

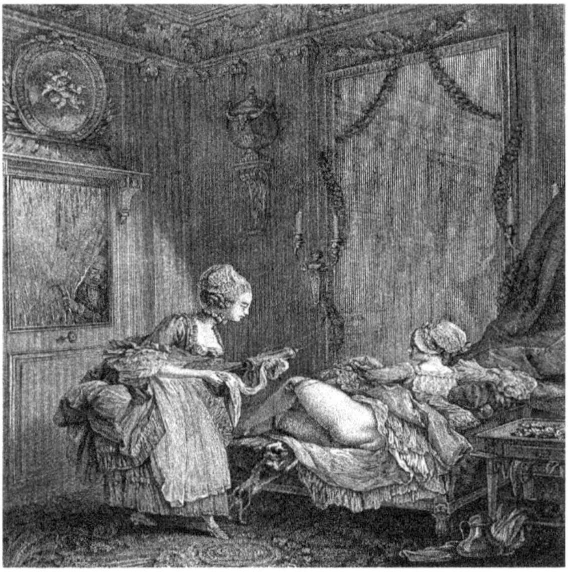

European culture embraced the clyster for medicinal and hygienic purposes. Molière has physicians and apothecaries recommending and prescribing clysters in several of his plays. The clyster reached the ultimate height of popularity in the early years of the reign of Louis XIV (1638-1715) who, it is reported, had over 2,000 enemas during his stay on the throne. He outdid his predecessor King Louis XIII by not only having colonics performed at royal court functions but by also receiving visitors during the procedure. I am curious if this is where the poker card game phrase 'Royal Flush' comes from.

In the 1700's Edward Jukes develops mechanical controls and instruments that are the precursors for colon hydrotherapy equipment today. Further developments in vulcanized rubber allowed more advanced technology making full colonic irrigation the preferred approach rather than limited enemas. Dr. John Harvey Kellogg medical director of the Seventh Day Adventist owned Battle Creek Sanitarium was a strong proponent of colonic irrigation. He was also a pioneer in probiotics therapy with irrigation of the colon with live yogurt culture.

Autointoxication was a popular theory at that time, but is now is outdated and disproved. It theorized that any fecal residue in the colon could lead to toxic consequences from their absorption. In the early twentieth century adherents underwent regular colon irrigations and high enemas. Other approaches were to increase the amount of fiber and roughage in the diet to speed the passage of fecal material through the bowel in the shortest amount of time.

The Plombieres by De Langenhagen apparatus allowed the colonic procedure to be performed in a more comfortable reclined position. In 1900 Vincent Priessnitz developed a systematic form of colonic therapy. In 1932, W. Kerr Russell, M.D., B.S., wrote a book entitled *Colonic Irrigation.* He popularized the term colonic irrigation, which was used interchangeably with colonic lavage. More books followed including *Chronic Intestinal Toxemia and its Treatment* by Dr. James W. Wiltsie in 1938 and *Scientific Intestinal Irrigation and Adjuvant Therapy* by Dr. E.G. Waddington in 1940.

The medical community and the American Medical Association embraced the use of prescription products and laxatives instead of colonics, which had become embraced by the advocates of alternative approaches. The AMA Department of Propaganda (they wisely later changed its name) led to a campaign equating colonics with hucksterism and quackery. In the book *Inner Hygiene* Whorton (2000) provides a detailed history of the story behind colonic irrigation.

Today manufacturers of eight different types of colon hydrotherapy devices are registered with the FDA. The vast majority of colon hygienists and therapists are well-trained and enthusiastic advocates of the procedure and its benefits. A few medical doctors are revisiting the blanket condemnation of the procedure that took place in the early twentieth century after thousands of years of its acceptance. With the lifesaving value of screening for cancer of the colon, and the requirement of a clean bowel for the most accurate examination, it is surprising that colonic irrigation as part of the preparation for colonoscopy has not been thoroughly assessed and considered. After drinking and experiencing the standard purgative solutions, colonic irrigation sounds like a relatively attractive alternative.

In other parts of the world the enema would independently be discovered and put into routine practice for hygienic, therapeutic, religious, or social purpose. In the Americas native people would deliver the smoke of hallucinogenic plants into the rectum to induce trances associated with their spiritual beliefs. Interestingly the application of smoke to the rectum was a standard medical practice in cases of drowning or near drowning. A bellow similar to that used to stoke a fire in a fireplace was used to draw up tobacco smoke and inserted into the rectum for the administration of the smoke. Apparently some near drowning victims regained consciousness, probably because someone shoved a bellow nozzle up their rectum and unrelated to the smoke installation. When it finally was recognized as a useless and bizarre therapy it gave rise to the phrase of 'blowing smoke up the ass' for a totally wasteful activity.

Although still used for some therapeutics, particularly for the administration of therapeutics for inflammatory bowel disease such as ulcerative colitis, it appears to have fallen out of favor with the medical profession. In the first half of the twentieth-century physicians commonly recommended enemas for therapeutic purposes of constipation and bowel health in general. Dr. John Harvey Kellogg became one of the leading advocates of a regimen of bowel health with several colonic enemas each day. He established the Battle Creek Sanatorium, which attracted celebrities and powerful politicians and industrialist from around the world who embraced his regimen and advocacy of colon health.

Although not offered in standard allopathic medicine, the rich history of therapeutic and health promoting colon hygiene remains available. Colon hydrotherapy is recognized, licensed, and professionally available from independent practitioners, as well as frequently at chiropractic or alternative health care providers. The technology has also evolved with mechanical devices with various safety features and disposable equipment to avoid the risk of infection or perforation. Fluid and electrolyte imbalance may occur if overused, but professionals are careful to avoid complications whenever possible.

Home use of colonics has always been an option, and as medicine sometimes goes through cycles, colonics may be making a bit of a comeback in allopathic circles. With the advent of colonoscopy and its utility in screening for colon cancer, colon cleansing is an important part of the procedures efficacy. The oral purgatives are a challenge to tolerate and the results are inadequate too often. The use of colonics to cleanse and prepare the bowel for colonoscopy is gaining some advocates as a gentler and more efficacious approach.

Enemas and colonics, while overall having an excellent safety record, have had adverse events reported. Ozone dissolved in the water used for colonics and enemas can cause mucosal damage and a microscopic colitis. Phosphate based enemas can cause electrolyte imbalance and phosphate toxicity with several fatalities have been reported. Intestinal infections from colonics have been reported prior to the institution of safety measures.

Cayenne pepper in enema fluid has been used as an alternate treatment for irritable bowel syndrome. I suspect if this approach were tested in a scientific approach that cayenne pepper placed up one's colon would be more irritating than calming. Besides, if pepper can trigger a violent sneeze in the nose, an equivalent sneeze from a rectum full of enema fluid is something I would rather keep my distance from.

The Battle Creek Sanitarium in Battle Creek, Michigan, United States, was a health resort based on the health principles advocated by the Seventh Day Adventist Church, and its prominent medical director John Harvey Kellogg.

The complex was purchased by the U.S. Army during World War II and converted into the Percy Jones Army Hospital. The facility later became the Hart-Dole-Inouye Federal Center.

It first opened in 1866 as the Western Health Reform Institute. In 1876, John Harvey Kellogg became the superintendent, and his brother, W. K. Kellogg the bookkeeper. After a fire in 1902 it was rebuilt, enlarged and renamed The Battle Creek Sanitarium. Kellogg modified the word sanatorium, which was then defined as a health resort for invalid soldiers. He was quoted as saying "A change of two letters transformed 'sanatorium' to 'sanitarium', and a new word was added to the English language".

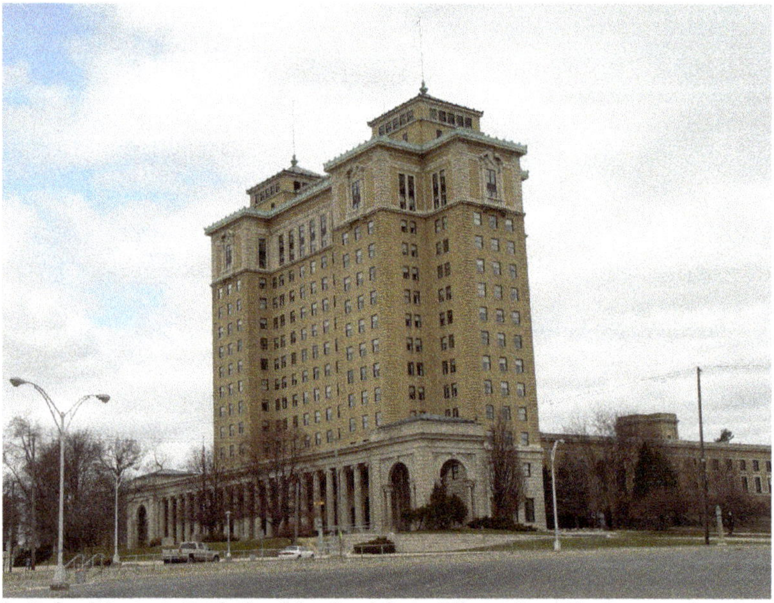

The Federal Center in Battle Creek has lived three different lives. The first was the original Sanitarium (World Health Reform Institute)where Dr. Kellogg invented cereal, then the Percy Jones Army Hospital, and now the Hart-Dole-Inouye Federal Center Uploaded by pixeltoo Author Battle Creek CVB Creative Commons License.

A healthy vegetarian diet, exercise, and vigorous colon irrigation were advocated at the sanitarium and it became a preeminent health spa destination for the rich and famous from around the world. The sanitarium and Kellogg were satirized in T. Coraghessan Boyle's 1993 novel *The Road to Wellville*, and the 1994 film adaptation. Kellogg believed that the health colon would empty itself between three to four times a day on average. He extrapolated the number of bowel movements that should occur each day based on observations of wild apes, infants, and institutionalized individuals with severe mental disorders. This calculation was the basis of the three to four times a day colonic cleansings each patron of the sanitarium was subjected to.

The story of the dry cereal enterprises with the famous names of Kellogg's and Post is intimately intertwined with their origins in Battle Creek, Michigan. The Battle Creek Sanatorium was an enormously famous and influential facility owned by the Seventh Day Adventist Church. Known for their health conscious regimen and vegetarian diet the sanitarium was frequented by presidents, celebrities, and the wealthy. Hundreds of thousands of others of more modest means made the pilgrimage to Battle Creek by the trainload. The medical director of the sanatorium was a graduate of the prestigious New York University (Bellevue) School of Medicine, John C. Kellogg.

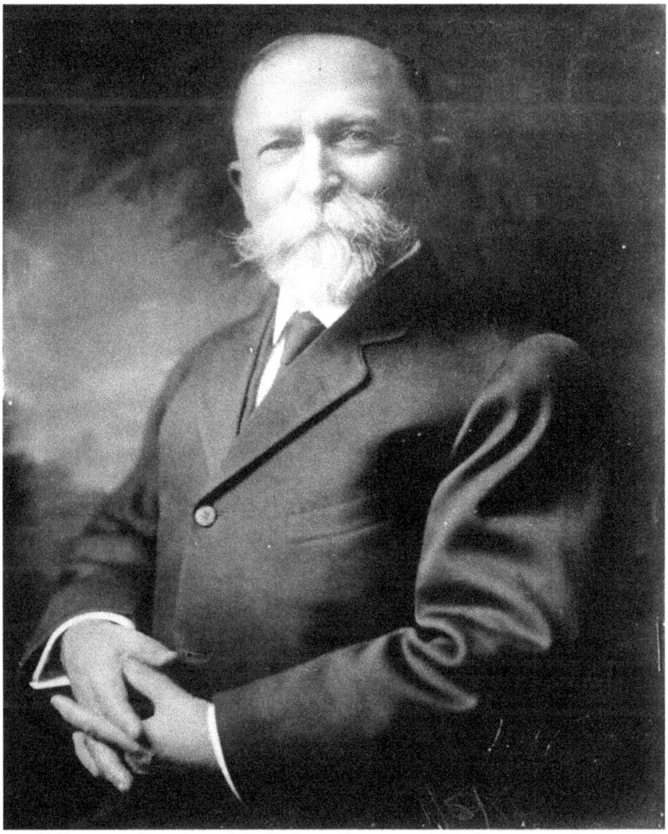

John Harvey Kellogg, co-founder of the Kellogg Company. This is a press photograph from the George Grantham Bain collection, which was purchased by the Library of Congress in 1948.

Dr. Kellogg was a firm believer in bowel cleanliness and health. Guests of the sanatorium were subjected to regular colonics, often times several times a day. He also advocated the use of probiotics well before it became fashionable to do so. Nobel Prize winning scientist Élie Metchnikoff had also advocated adding probiotic yogurt to the diet later, but Dr. Kellogg had a more direct way of changing the colonic flora. He instituted yogurt enemas to place the beneficial probiotics where they would do the most good.

Dr. Metchnikoff received the Nobel Prize in Medicine for his work on immunity, and identified the *Lactobacillus delbrueckii subspecies bulgaricus* organism in yogurt that is considered an ideal probiotic. His theory of aging being due to toxic bacteria, and that lactic acid producing organisms could prolong life, were very influential. His advocacy of probiotics was embraced by the Japanese scientist Minoru Shirota, who developed a stronger strain of the probiotic organism *Lactobacillus casei* found in Yakult and kefir.

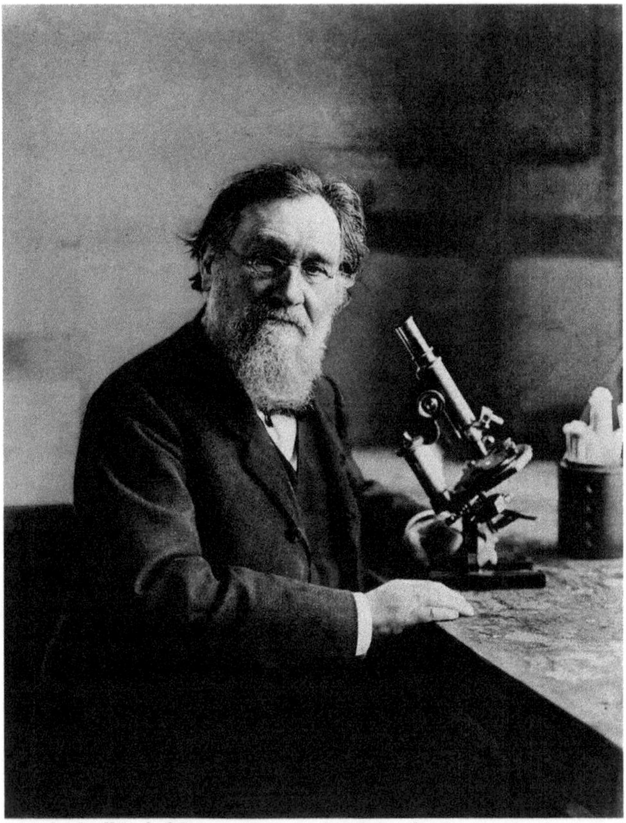

Élie Metchnikoff, Nobel Prize winning scientist at the Pasteur Institute in Paris

Kellogg made sure that the bowel of each and every patient was plied with water, from above and below. His favorite device was an enema machine that could rapidly instill several gallons of water in a series of enemas. Every water enema was followed by a pint of yogurt. Half was eaten, and the other half was administered by enema, "thus planting the protective germs where they are most needed and may render most effective service." The yogurt served to replace the intestinal flora of the bowel, creating what

Kellogg claimed was a squeaky-clean intestine. Kellogg believed that most disease is alleviated by a change in intestinal flora and that bacteria in the intestines can either help or hinder the body. He proposed that pathogenic bacteria produce toxins during the digestion of protein that poison the blood and that a poor diet favors harmful bacteria that could then infect other tissues in the body.

Following the concepts of Metchnikoff he advocated that the intestinal flora is changed by diet, and is generally changed for the better by a well-balanced vegetarian diet favoring low-protein, laxative, and high-fiber foods. Kellogg believed that this natural change in flora could be sped by enemas seeded with favorable bacteria, or by various regimens of specific foods designed to heal specific ailments.

He was also a highly skilled surgeon who often performed colectomies to remove the organ that can harbor pathogens. He was known as a very caring and generous man who often performed surgeries without charge to those who could not afford his fees and supported over forty foster children although he and his wife never had any biological children. His campaign for sexual abstinence applied to his honeymoon as well where he wrote his major work on the evils of masturbation. His fierce advocacy of sexual abstinence led to his development of several extreme surgical procedures to remove sexual desire by removing the source of sexual pleasure. He influenced Sylvester Graham to create the Graham Cracker.

The fiber added to the diet with helpings of the corn cereal produced at the Sanatorium became the best-selling product still popular today, Kellogg's Corn Flakes. The cereal product line expanded and Kellogg's of Battle Creek Michigan became a household name across the country and world. One of the many guests at the Sanatorium was a fellow entrepreneur, CW Post. Corporate espionage was suspected as someone broke into Mr. Kellogg's office and stole plans for a new cereal. Shortly thereafter Post's Grape-Nuts came to market claiming additional health properties over the competing Kellogg's products. The fierce competition between Post Cereals and Kellogg's is a case study in corporate and industry lore.

CW Post became a titan of the cereal industry with their main facilities in Battle Creek as well, just a few miles from Kellogg's. Post had a number of health setbacks and when thought that he might have appendicitis had his private train take him from his California residence to Rochester Minnesota to see the famed Mayo Brothers who established the Mayo Clinic. The diagnosis was not favorable, surgery was not performed and he returned to California where he committed suicide. His only child Marjorie Meriwether Post inherited his enormous wealth, married E. F. Hutton, and had a remarkable life that has been chronicled in the media of her day, books, and film.

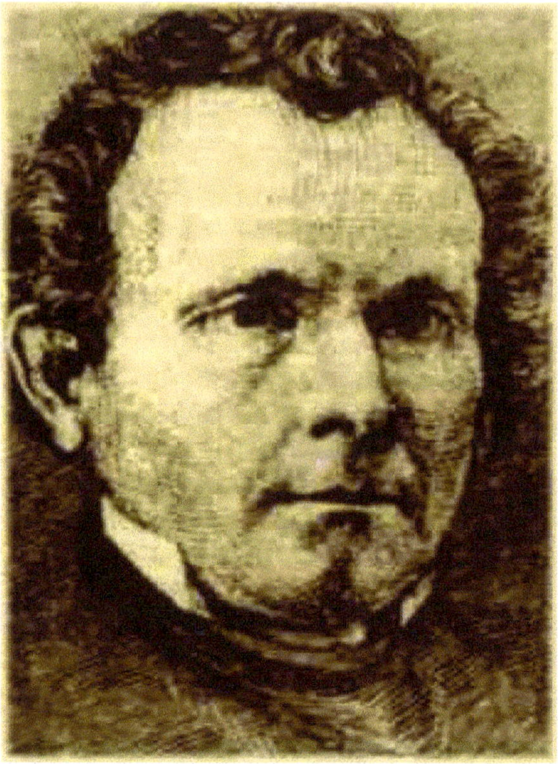

Sylvester Graham

Presbyterian minister Dr. Sylvester Graham (1794 - 1851) was born in Boston, Massachusetts the youngest of seventeen children. He studied anatomy, physiology and general health, was a very gifted orator and influential health teacher. He invented the Graham cracker wafer in 1829, and to this day it remains a very popular food product, but most people are completely unaware of its original purpose.

It was made from wheat with finely ground unbleached flour finely ground and the bran and germ coarsely ground. He was quoted as saying that "bread should be baked in such a way that it will...require and secure a full exercise of the teeth in mastication" . Although the words mastication may sound a lot like masturbation it is simply a fancy way of describing the act of chewing. Graham crackers were marketed as a bland product to suppress self-abuse, as masturbation was referred to at that time, and carnal urges both of which he believed led to poor health.

Health Boards in 1830's sometimes prohibited sale of vegetables, due to the dangers of cholera and other communicable diseases. People were advised to restrict themselves to meat, potatoes, wine, milk, tea and coffee. The medical profession, even into the twentieth century, strongly discouraged eating fresh fruit and uncooked vegetables, which were described as reeking with disease germs.

Graham's first observations of diet on health were made in 1820 in Philadelphia. A small sect of Bible Christians who abstained from all animal foods, all condiments and used no tea, coffee, tobacco or alcohol were unaffected by the cholera epidemic. In 1830 Graham started to lecture and write articles on the Graham System advocating a vegetarian diet, preferably raw, even a fruitarian diet.

Graham warned against drug remedies, stimulants, and overworking. He emphasized sleep, rest, and education in sex hygiene. He soon had a large following with books, restaurants, the world's first health food stores, and Graham boarding houses. Strong opposition also developed immediately from physicians, butchers, bakers, tobacconists, brewers, distillers, and saloon keepers – all of who saw their business threatened from the new doctrines.

Enemas and colonics remain popular today and have many advocates. Many simple enema preparations are available over the counter and the Fleets Company, a market leader, has advertised them prominently with the Fleets Naturals product. The advertisement reads, "Keep your backcountry clean, ... Mild enough for daily use." Apparently it is a popular product for those engaged in anal intercourse.

Others use colonics for constipation, bowel management, and sense of personal hygiene. Those with klismaphilia derive sensual pleasure from the experience. As long as the equipment and fluids are clean and sterile the risk of injury is very slight. Canonic hydrotherapy equipment improvements and hydrotherapist professional standards have enhanced their safety even further. Remaining concerns would be related to individuals using the wrong product, such as enemas with high phosphorus and salt contents leading to toxicity and electrolyte imbalances, and overutilization disrupting the normal gut microbiome flora.

<u>Enema - Coffee Enema</u>

Coffee enemas use coffee as the irrigating fluid, often times at a stronger concentration than a typical coffee beverage, for therapeutic enema purposes. The use of such an approach has been advocated as a cancer treatment and to remove 'toxins' but there is no scientific evidence for either its theoretical or practical benefit. Adverse reactions that have been reported include infections, severe electrolyte imbalance, inflammation, internal burns, perforation, pleural effusions, pericardial effusions, heart failure and death.

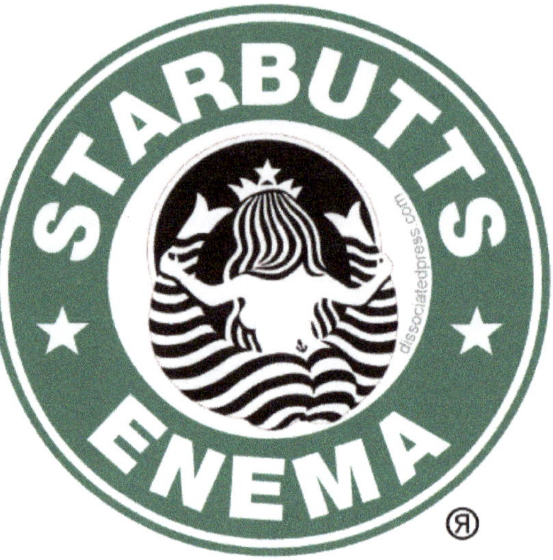
STARBUTTS
ENEMA
dissociatedpress.com

www.DissociatedPress.com. Used with permission.

For those who survived, the long-term use of coffee enemas also led to reports of malabsorption of fat, vitamins, and calcium. If there were anything humorous about such adverse events and the activity that generates them it would be that there are no reports comparing sleep patterns with regular vs. due caffeinated enemas, nor espresso or cappuccino. I suspect that if there were any validity to the concept, with popular variations on the theme of coffee enemas, we would have seen a Starbutts franchise take hold.

Enema - Hatha Yoga Hygienic Practices

Dhauti, the yogic practice of internally washing the digestive tract, is one of the six body cleansing and purification acts of Hatha Yoga known as Shatkarma. According to Gheranda Samhita, one of the three classic texts of hatha yoga, it is divided into four parts: Antar (internal) dhauti, Danta (teeth) dhauti, Hrid (cardiac or chest region) dhauti and Moola shodhana (rectal cleansing). Many practices of Hatha Yoga require intense personal training and expert guidance. This is particularly true of the cleansing and purification techniques briefly described below.

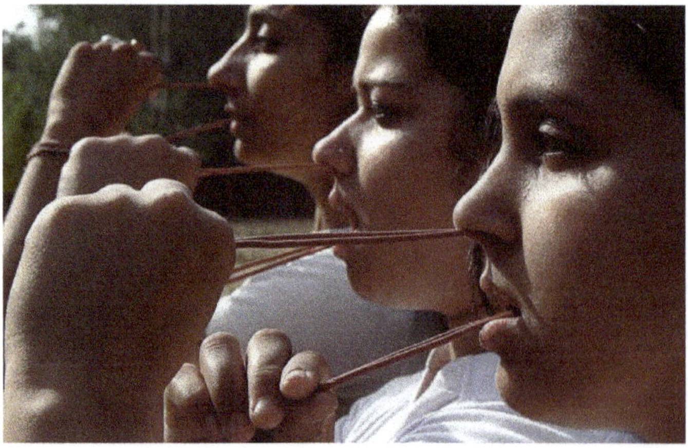

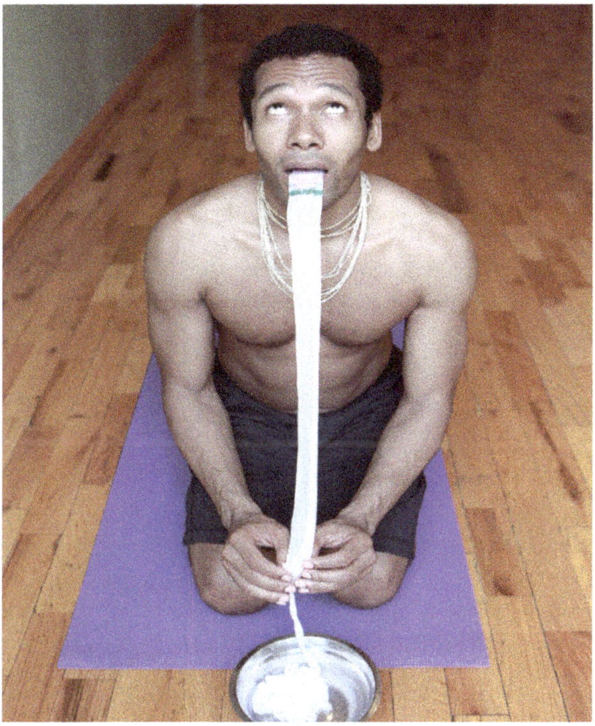
Dhauti www.hotashtanfa.blogspot.com

The performance of dhauti involves the swallowing of a damp cloth approximately four inches wide and five feet long and its subsequent withdrawal. Adherents believe it rids the body of unhealthy impurities and may cure a variety of conditions such as coughs, enlarged spleen, lymphatic afflictions, and leprosy.

Another yogic exercise called jala basti draws water into the rectum for colonic irrigation via a bamboo tube placed in the anus. With practice adherents no longer need the rectal tube and using sphincter control alone are able to suction up water into the colon for self-irrigation colonics. Sthala basti is the advanced practice after jala basti has been mastered without the tube. This is a dry form of basti where air is suctioned into the colon without water. Joseph Pujol who used this skill to become a performer called Le Pétomane on the Moulin Rouge in Paris in the late nineteenth and early twentieth centuries apparently accidentally discovered this ancient yogic practice.

Sutra neti involves a dampened waxed string inhaled through one nostril into the back of the throat. The string is grasped through the mouth and with gharshana-neti the string is rubbed back and forth with a flossing type action. For most people a trial of nasal irrigation with sea salt solution using a neti pot is the extent of their interest in nasal hygiene and other body cleansing techniques.

Enema - Yogic Air Enema

Sthala Basti, also called Vata Basti, Air Basti, Air Enema, is an advanced Hatha yoga technique that is best learned from an expert teacher. There are a number of different approaches and techniques but mastery of anal sphincter control is a challenging practice. Once you master this technique you may not become as famous as Le Pétomane of the Moulin Rouge but you will certainly be able to entertain your soon to be former friends.

Sthala Basti starting from Paschimottanasana:
Sit with your legs stretched out in front of you and then bend forward halfway. You do not fully place your upper body on your legs, but only bend forward halfway. Perform Uddiyana Bandha by exhaling completely and then taking a false inhalation while holding the breath. This flattens and pulls in the abdomen under the rib cage as if the chest was suctioning it. The process is repeated many times followed by relaxation of the anal sphincter muscles to allow air to be drawn in with the Uddiyanna Bandha maneuver. The air suctioned in is released as flatus.

Sthala Basti in lying Position:
Lying on the back bend the knees up towards the chest and raise the buttocks. Practice developing control of the anal sphincter muscles by contraction and relaxation of the sphincter. When the sphincter is relaxed air suctioned into the colon is released as flatulence.

Sthala Basti in Utkatasana:
Sit in Utkatasana, also called the chair or lightning bolt pose, by squatting while standing with the knees bent 90 degrees backwards to thighs. The back and upright arms form a forward facing 90 degree angle from the thighs. If necessary, until sphincter control is mastered, a hollow tube like bamboo or a catheter is placed in the anus and Uddiyama Bandha is performed. Air is sucked into the colon and released as flatus.

Enema – Klismaphilia

Klismaphilia refers to sexual arousal from introducing liquids into the rectum and colon via the anus. Klismaphilia is usually practiced secretly by both heterosexuals and homosexuals, and by women, and more commonly by men. They may receive pleasure from the pressure and distension of the colon and may try to get others to administer enemas under the pretense of being constipated. The Diagnostic and Statistical Manual of Mental Disorder classifies klismaphilia under the diagnosis of "Paraphilias, Not Otherwise Specified."

Enema - Proctoclysis

Prior to the development of convenient means of access for intravenous administration, fluids and medication were commonly administered by proctoclysis or rectoclysis. This was also known as the Murphy drip after its developer, American surgeon John Murphy. The rationale for its use, particularly when oral intake could not be accomplished, remains valid although it is rarely used today.

The colon is the primary organ for the absorption of fluids and electrolytes. It's rich blood supply and absorptive capacity makes it a suitable route for the administration of fluids and medicines. Proctoclysis is an easy, safe and effective way to provide fluid replacement. It does not require sterile fluids, specialized equipment, or advanced training, and it is very useful when alternative routes are not available such as remote locations away from access to medical care. Suppositories have the additional advantage of avoiding the portal circulation and bypassing metabolism in the liver. Hypodermoclysis, the subcutaneous administration of fluids, was also used as an alternative, and continues to be popular in veterinary medicine.

Enteric Nervous System

The enteric nervous system is often referred to as "the second brain" and is a part of the peripheral nervous system and a division of the autonomic nervous system, which controls the gastrointestinal tract. This system is complex and integrated with afferent and efferent connections with the central nervous system. It is also capable of autonomous function and can control the digestive system both from the context of the physiological state locally to the body as a whole.

The enteric nervous system is embedded within the wall of the digestive tract and extends from the esophagus to the anus. Thousands of ganglia reside within the walls of these areas and the number of neurons contained in the enteric nervous system is approximately four-hundred-million, more than any other peripheral organ and about the same number of neurons as the spinal cord. The nerve fibers within the walls of the gastrointestinal tract consist of enteric axons, extrinsic axons projecting to the gut wall, and glial cells.

The concept of the gut being a secondary brain is partly based on the remarkable concentration of neurotransmitters, as well as the fact that the enteric nervous system has its own reflexes and pathways that can function independently of the brain and spinal cord. Historically the concept of 'gut feelings' and 'gut instinct' are tied into the folk tradition that the gut is a sentient organ in its own right.

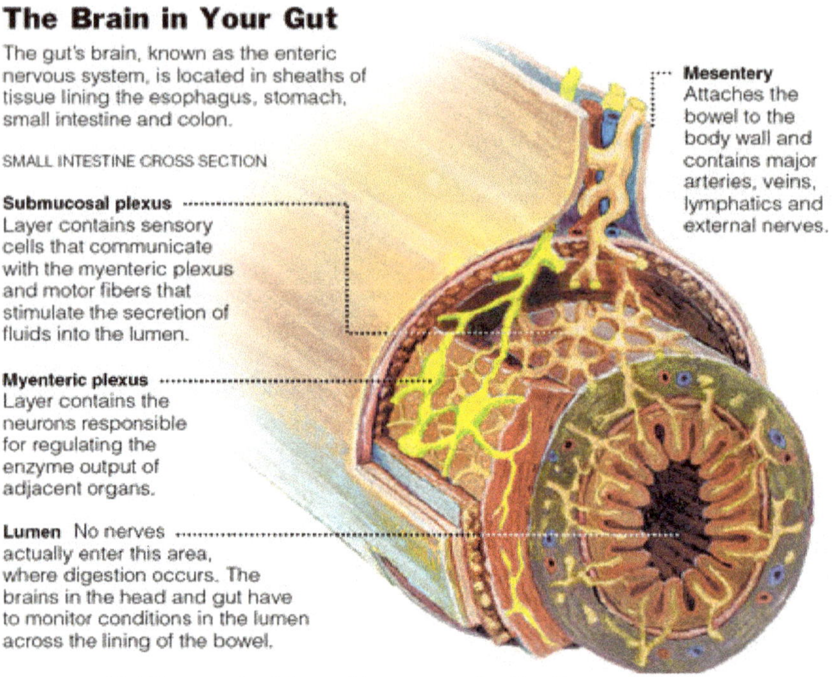
The Brain in Your Gut
The gut's brain, known as the enteric nervous system, is located in sheaths of tissue lining the esophagus, stomach, small intestine and colon.
SMALL INTESTINE CROSS SECTION
Submucosal plexus
Layer contains sensory cells that communicate with the myenteric plexus and motor fibers that stimulate the secretion of fluids into the lumen.
Myenteric plexus
Layer contains the neurons responsible for regulating the enzyme output of adjacent organs.
Lumen No nerves actually enter this area, where digestion occurs. The brains in the head and gut have to monitor conditions in the lumen across the lining of the bowel.
Mesentery
Attaches the bowel to the body wall and contains major arteries, veins, lymphatics and external nerves.

kin450-neurophysiology.wikispaces.com Creative Commons License

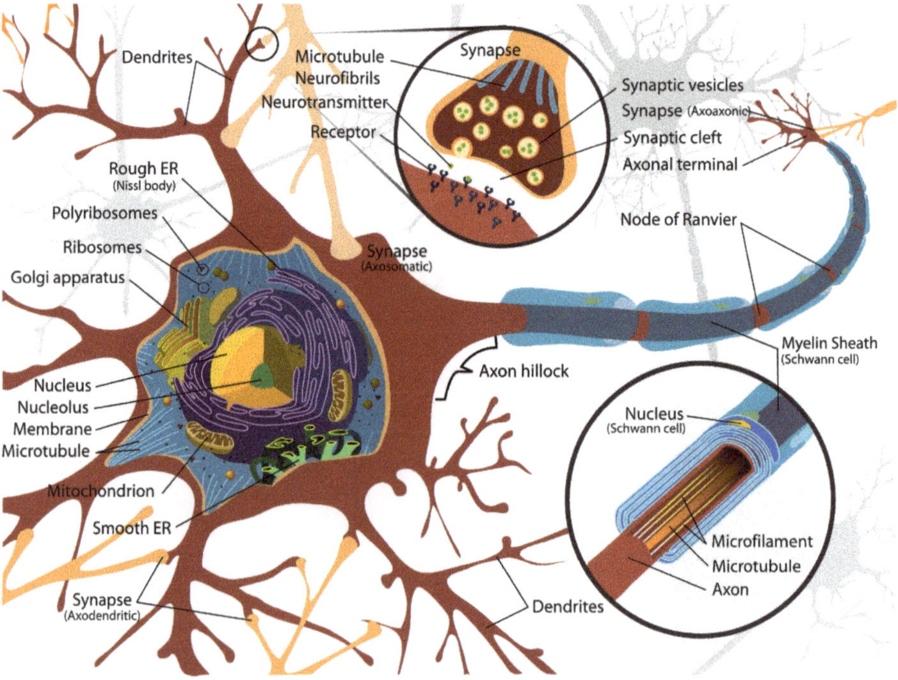
Dendrites
Microtubule
Neurofibrils
Neurotransmitter
Receptor
Synapse
Synaptic vesicles
Synapse (Axoaxonic)
Synaptic cleft
Axonal terminal
Rough ER
(Nissl body)
Polyribosomes
Ribosomes
Golgi apparatus
Synapse
(Axosomatic)
Node of Ranvier
Myelin Sheath
(Schwann cell)
Axon hillock
Nucleus
Nucleolus
Membrane
Microtubule
Mitochondrion
Smooth ER
Nucleus
(Schwann cell)
Microfilament
Microtubule
Axon
Synapse
(Axodendritic)
Dendrites

Nerve cell anatomy. Creative Commons License

Gut intuition, know it in your gut, gut wrenching experience, gut wrong, gut check, butterflies in the stomach, gut instinct, gut reaction, listen to your gut, go with your gut, are all common expressions to describe the common experiences of intuition most commonly known as gut feelings. The gastrointestinal tract is sensitive to stress and emotion. Anger, anxiety, sadness, fear, elation are all among the many feelings that can trigger symptoms in the gut ranging from mild spasm to intense nausea, vomiting, cramps, diarrhea, and fecal incontinence.

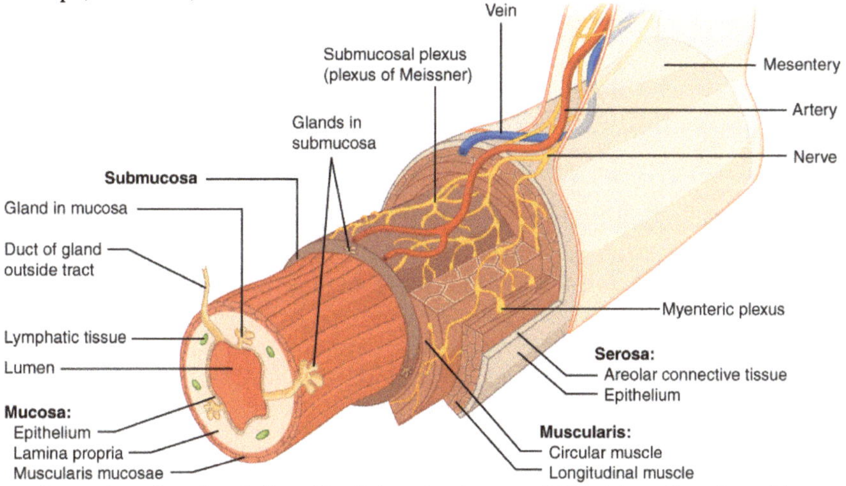
Vein
Submucosal plexus
(plexus of Meissner)
Mesentery
Artery
Nerve
Glands in submucosa
Submucosa
Gland in mucosa
Duct of gland outside tract
Myenteric plexus
Lymphatic tissue
Lumen
Serosa:
Areolar connective tissue
Epithelium
Mucosa:
Epithelium
Lamina propria
Muscularis mucosae
Muscularis:
Circular muscle
Longitudinal muscle

Connexions, OpenStax College, Rice University, Anatomy & Physiology, Overview of the Digestive System Creative Commons License

These major ganglia can be of two plexuses: the myenteric plexus and the submucosal plexus, also referred to as Auerbach and Meissner plexuses, respectively. The myenteric ganglia are located deep between the external muscle layers and form a continuous network around the stomach. It extends upward to the upper esophagus and downward to the internal anal sphincter. Myenteric ganglia exert control primarily over digestive tract motility.

The stimulation of the ganglia causes increased tone of the gut wall, increased intensity and frequency of the rhythmical contractions in the gut, and increased rapid movements of peristaltic waves. It also inhibits muscles that can impede the movement of food between segments of the gastrointestinal tract. The submucosal ganglia are located in the submucosa, which is below the mucosal membrane in the small and large intestine. The submucosal plexus helps to control local intestinal secretion, absorption, and contraction of the submucosal muscle.

The enteric nervous system involves over thirty neurotransmitters many of which play a central role in the central nervous system such as acetylcholine, dopamine, and serotonin. More than ninety percent of all of the serotonin in the entire body and approximately fifty percent of the body's dopamine is found in the enteric nervous system.

The enteric nervous system includes efferent sensory neurons, afferent motor neurons, and interneurons. The sensory neurons report on mechanical and chemical conditions such as distention and pH. Through intestinal muscles the motor neurons control peristalsis, inter-digestive phase activity, mass movements and the mixing churning of intestinal contents. Other neurons control the secretion of enzymes, hormones, and neurotransmitters.

Epigenetics

Once thought to number 80,00 separate genes, the human genome project scientists were flabbergast to discover that the number of human genes numbered only 22,000. Many of these are nonfunctional. Many others have been retained through the process of evolution, some from the very earliest forms of life, others more recent and yet still many millions of years ago. Some genes were transferred laterally from one form of life to another. Previously independent life forms evolved to become an integral part of larger life forms, much like today's Portuguese man-of-war is actually a symbiotic colony of a multitude of independent life forms. The energy centers of the modern cell, the mitochondrion, evolved from a unicellular independent organism and brought along with it its own distinct genetic material, which in humans is inherited solely through the maternal lineage.

Even more amazing is that the genes of other life forms may play an active role in the metabolism, function, and life of independent organisms with which they are in a shared environment and in previously unrecognized communication. Humans with 22,000 genes may be influenced by the 2,000,000 and counting genes present within the gut microbiome alone. The human genome represents less than one percent of the genes, which can affect the human organism. As each gene can lead to the production of a specific protein, hormone, neurotransmitter, metabolite, or other product new fields of discovery are rapidly developing and expanding. Besides genomics, new disciplines already recognized include proteomics, metabolomics, microbial endocrinology, microbial neuroscience, microbial immunology, and others.

Deoxyribonucleic acid, most commonly known by its initials DNA, is a molecule, which serves as the primary means of transmitting genetic information. Most DNA molecules are in the form of complementary strands that form a spiral structure known as a double helix. Each nitrogen containing nucleotide base is attached to helix backbone of a monosaccharide sugar called deoxyribose alternating with a phosphate group. The bases of adenine with thymine, and guanine with cytosine, are bonded as pairs with hydrogen bonds. The matching pairs allows any single strand of DNA to duplicate its matching strand, which is the process by which DNA is transmitted to the next generation with cell division. The double helix structure of DNA was identified by Nobel Laureates James Watson & Francis Crick, who relied on the experimental work and data collected by Rosalind Franklin and Maurice Wilkins.

The DNA on chromosomes of cells is often billions of base pairs long, and each three-letter sequence of base pairs may code for a specific amino acid that must be assembled in the proper sequence to manufacture a protein with a specific function. A mutation of a single letter in the sequence of base pairs may result in a defective or inactive protein that may have major consequences for the health or survival of the cell. There are a variety of mechanisms for self-repair of DNA, and with the astronomical number of cell divisions and duplications of DNA the efficiency and accuracy of the system is remarkable.

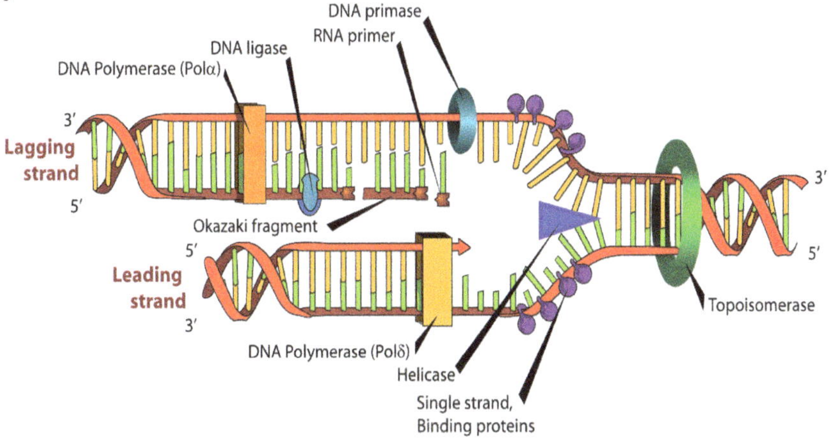
DNA primase
RNA primer
DNA ligase
DNA Polymerase (Polα)
3′
Lagging strand
5′
Okazaki fragment
5′
Leading strand
3′
3′
5′
Topoisomerase
DNA Polymerase (Polδ)
Helicase
Single strand, Binding proteins

DNA replication. Creative Commons License

The vast majority, over 98% of DNA does not code for genes. Science presumed these non-genomic coding regions were simply filler, an enormous quantity of useless gibberish, which science labeled as 'junk DNA'. 'Junk DNA' is beginning to reveal its mystery, and as would be expected of Mother Nature it would not invest so heavily in transcribing millions of base pairs as an exercise in futility. Yesterday's junk remains a great mystery, but without a doubt is not only not junk, but it appears to be on the verge of becoming today's treasure.

In the nineteenth century the theory of evolution was a cauldron of controversy, and Darwin's 'survival of the fittest' was just one of many completing theories. With the general acceptance of Darwin as being correct, the other theories were relegated to the dust heap of history and false conjecture. Genes were described as destiny, sealing one's fate by the random coupling of myriad genetic strands consisting of billions of base pairs in the sprawling double helix of the DNA on the chromosomes. The countless permutations ensured that all but identical twins would be unique in the universe. As destiny would often have it, declarations of destiny are often proven wrong.

What science has only recently discovered is that genes are not the static sealed destiny as initially thought. Genes are actually actively manipulated, modified, and turned on and off by a host of variables described as the new field of epigenetics. Variables beyond the base genetics include diet, sleep, exercise, meditation, stress, climate, pharmaceuticals, infections, parasites, radiation exposure, altitude, nutrients, trace minerals, and a host of others yet to be identified or discovered. What is even more remarkable is the recognition that one of Darwin's contemporaries, Charles Lamarck, will need to be rehabilitated from the dustbins of genetic theorists, because he was right after all. Just as he predicted, when opposing Darwin's theory, epigenetic changes can be transmitted to future generations. The ability for epigenetics to change the inheritable genetic program offers opportunity to design interventions to enhance wellness, vitality, and longevity, and to avoid or minimize illness and aging.

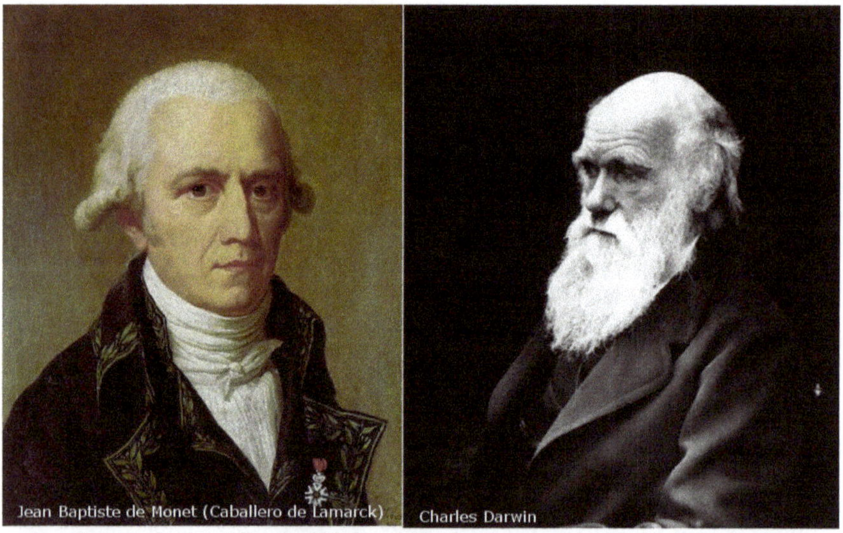
Jean Baptiste de Monet (Caballero de Lamarck)
Charles Darwin
Jean Baptiste de Monet (Lamarck) left and Charles Darwin right. File by Alejandro Porto Creative Commons License

An example of epigenetics is the experiment utilizing baby mice in utero. The mouse is usually attracted to the aroma of vanilla, however when pregnant mice were continually shocked when exposed to vanilla aroma they developed anxiety and an avoidance behavior. Their offspring, who normally would have a 'natural' attraction to vanilla were exposed to the vanilla scent and showed the avoidance behavior that had been conditioned in their mothers. This experiment shows the power of environmental conditions and how it impacts genes and can cause genetic modifications in what was previously thought to be inherited and genetically pre-determined traits.

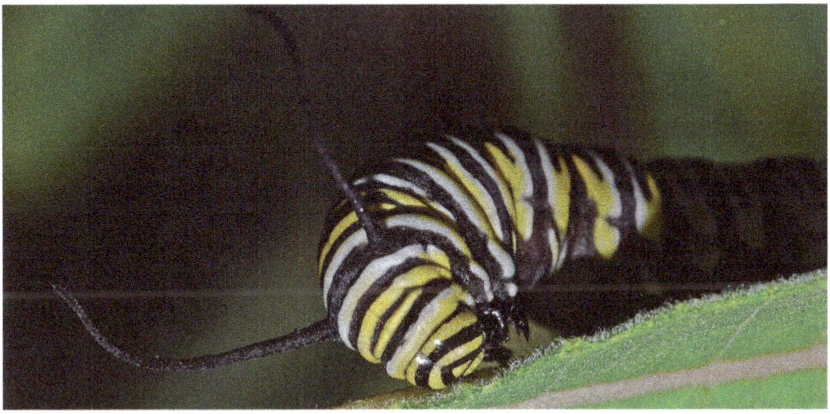

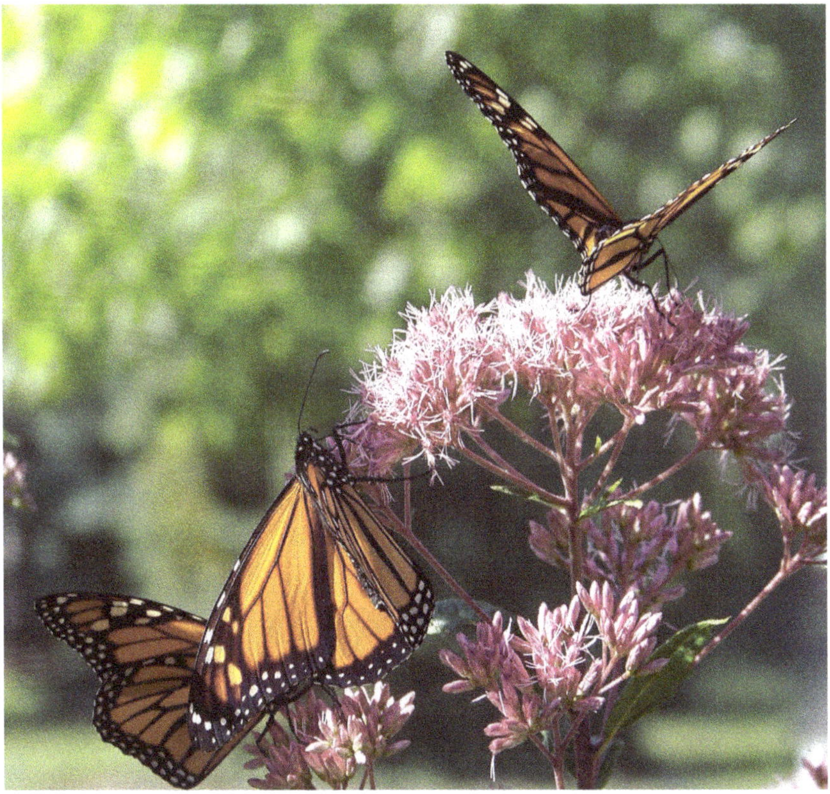

Eproctophilia

Eproctophilia is a fart fetish, the receiving of sexual pleasure and arousal from the fart of another. The famous author James Joyce describes this fetish in letters published after his death. His writing and other aspects of farts in literature, art, culture, and history are covered in the companion volume *Artsy Fartsy, Cultural History of the Fart* referenced in the afterword of this book.

Euphemisms, Feces (see Appendix B)

Evacuative Dysfunction

Evacuative dysfunction, also known as obstructed defecation syndrome, is difficulty in evacuation of the rectum in the presence of normal stool consistency and a normal colonic transit time. Obstructed defecation syndrome is one of the causes of chronic constipation.

Causes of evacuative dysfunction may include functional outlet obstruction, short-segment Hirschsprung disease, Chagas disease, pelvic floor dysfunction, internal anal sphincter spasm, anal stenosis, fecal impaction, anorectal cancer, anismus, multiple sclerosis, spinal cord lesions, mechanical outlet obstruction, enterocele, rectocele, descending perineum syndrome, rectal prolapse, impaired rectal sensitivity, megarectum, and others.

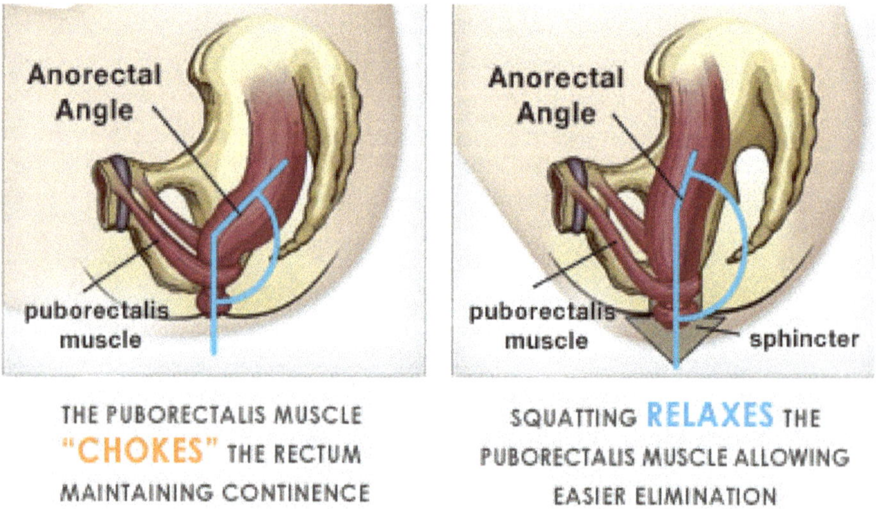
Anorectal Angle
puborectalis muscle
Anorectal Angle
puborectalis muscle
sphincter
THE PUBORECTALIS MUSCLE "CHOKES" THE RECTUM MAINTAINING CONTINENCE
SQUATTING RELAXES THE PUBORECTALIS MUSCLE ALLOWING EASIER ELIMINATION

www.squattypotty.com Creative Commons License

Symptoms may include excessive straining with prolonged episodes on the toilet, the required use of enemas and/or laxatives, finger insertion into the vagina or rectum to aid defecation, rectal pain, tenesmus (sensation of urgent need to defecate), dyschezia (painful defecation), abdominal discomfort and/or pain. It may also lead to an incomplete evacuation, which is defined as the evacuation of less than ninety percent of the rectal contents. Incomplete evacuation may contribute to tenesmus and fecal leakage.

Excrement (see Manure)

Excrement, also known as feces, shit, and dozens of euphemisms, is the excreted waste product from the digestive tract expelled through the anus during defecation. Although the digestive tract has extracted and absorbed many of the nutrients of the food ingested the fecal matter often has fifty percent of its energy value remaining. This is a vital resource for organisms such as bacteria, fungi, and insects such as the fly and dung beetle.

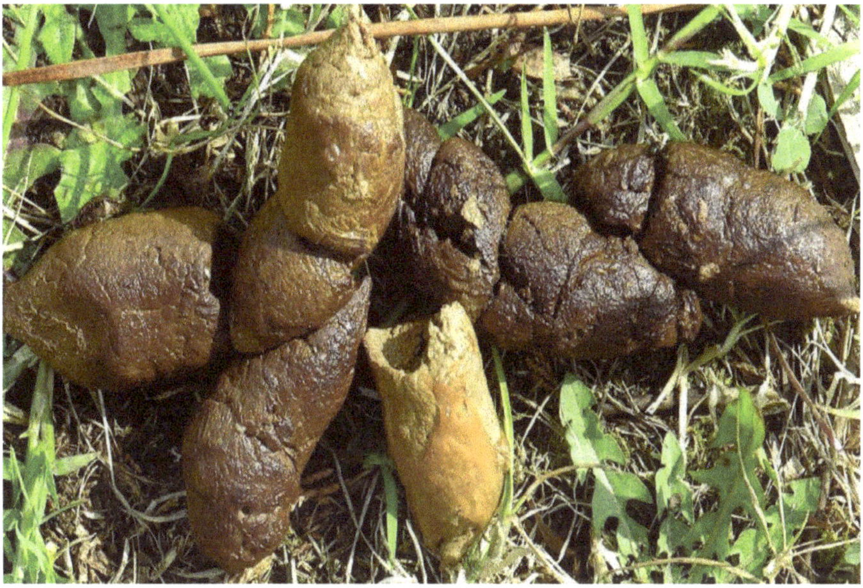

Feces on grass. Curezone.com Creative Commons License

Human fecal matter varies significantly in appearance, depending on diet and health. A sticky gummy texture is often noted with substantial internal bleeding, which also often presents as black tarry stool called melena. Feces are often used as fertilizer, both manure and guano becoming large commercial enterprises. Historically human waste, euphemistically called night soil, was used as a major source of fertilizer. Animal feces, especially those of the camel, bison, oxen, yak, water buffalo, and cattle can be used as fuel or building material when dried. Terms such as dung, scat, spoor, manure, castings, spraint, fewmets, guano, frass, and droppings are used to refer to specific animal feces.

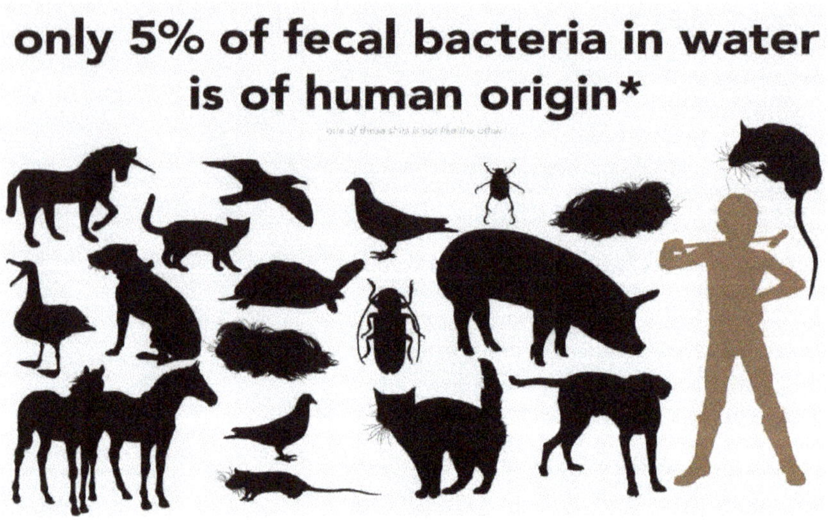
only 5% of fecal bacteria in water
is of human origin*

Public Domain

Common animal dropping names include:
bat: guano
cattle: tath
otter: spraints
cow: bodewash, cowpies, buffalo chips
seafowl: guano
earthworm: wormcast
dinosaur: coprolite
hart and deer: fewmets
hare: crotiles, crotisings
boar, bear, and wolf: lesses
fox: billitting
insects: frass
vermin: fuants
hawk: mutes
dog: scumber

See the entry under Fecal Waste Management for contemporary approaches to managing animal and human waste. Feces waste management has been a concern from pre-Biblical times. "And thou shalt have a paddle upon thy weapon; and it shall be, when thou wilt ease thyself abroad, thou shalt dig therewith, and shalt turn back and cover that which cometh from thee: For the LORD thy God walketh in the midst of thy camp, to deliver thee, and to give up thine enemies before thee; therefore shall they camp be holy: that he see no unclean thing in thee, and turn away from thee." (Deuteronomy 23:13-14)

Exercise

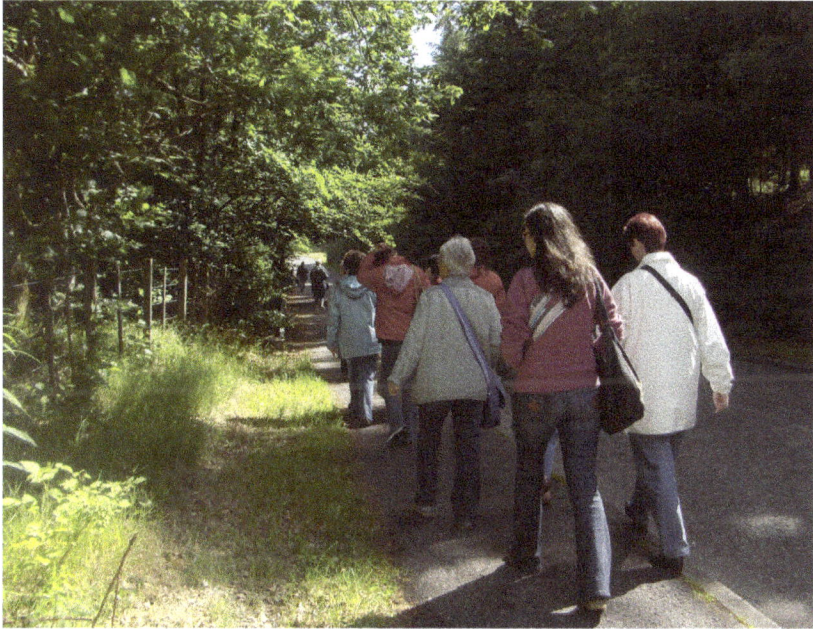

Walking is an excellent exercise Photo: marydoll1952 flic.kr/p/4ALdGG Creative Commons License

Physical activity and exercise enhance bowel motility. The extreme example of intense exercise leading to diarrhea is seen in the condition known as 'runner's trots'. Even gentle exercise such as walking can enhance bowel motility and prevent constipation. The term constitutional is often used to refer to something that enhances good health, and was a common euphemism for walking as a form of exercise. Because the walk would often lead to enhanced bowel motility and a subsequent bowel movement the phrase 'daily constitutional' or 'morning constitutional' entered the lexicon as one of several euphemisms for bowel movement.

Fart

The word fart is the correct word to use in the English language, and indeed is one of its oldest words. The alternative words used, such as flatus and flatulence are not original English words as they have been borrowed from the Latin. There is controversy as to the derivation of the word fart. It is thought to have Indo-European roots in the Germanic language word 'farzen'. One thought is that it originated as an onomatopoeia, a word that phonetically imitates the sound of the event it describes. Another thought is that it was related to the term for partridge, as the bird makes a fart like sound when it is disturbed in its natural habitat and takes flight.

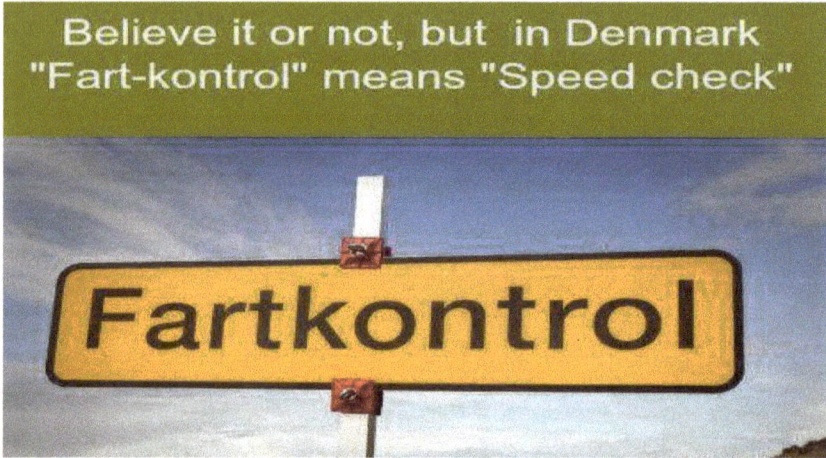
Believe it or not, but in Denmark "Fart-kontrol" means "Speed check"
Fartkontrol
onpasture.com

Farts are ubiquitous, all living creatures generate gas from their cellular respiration, and humans are no exception. The bacteria in your colonic flora generate microscopic farts, and these microfarts collect into larger bubbles of gas in the human and animal bowel. They are intermixed with the atmospheric air swallowed throughout the day and particularly at meals, as well as swallowing saliva at rest, chewing gum or tobacco, or smoking other recreational products.

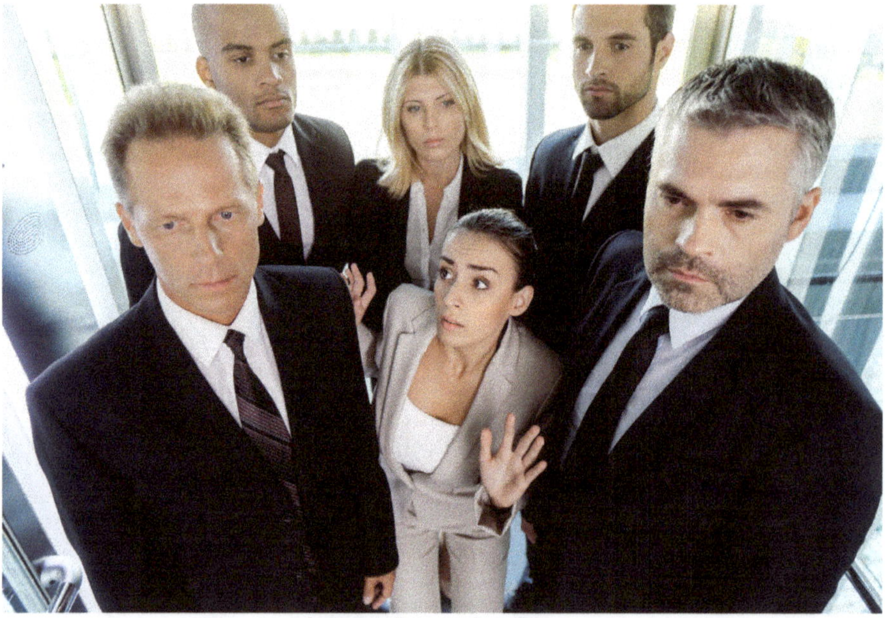
shutterstock/g-stockstudio

Other behaviors that may increase the amount of air swallowed include drinking from a straw, bottle or can, talking while eating and drinking, and tilting the head back when drinking. Eating or drinking foods that have a high air content, such as bread, ice cream, whipped foods, etcetera also increases the amount of air in the gastrointestinal tract. Aerophagia is universal and we swallow on average three to five cubic centimeters (one teaspoonful) of air with every swallow. Now add into the mixture the gasses produced during the enzymatic digestive processes, as well as the neutralization of gastric hydrochloric acid and pancreatic and duodenal bicarbonate, and the result is a large volume of gasses transiting the bowel that may be eliminated as a fart

Fortunately the vast majority of the gasses produced are absorbed by the gut, then into the bloodstream through diffusion and as a solution, finally being exhaled when they reach the alveoli of the lungs. In the alveoli they are released into the atmospheric air and oxygen enters the circulation bound to hemoglobin in the red blood cells. The component gasses have very different properties of diffusion through the bowel wall and into the bloodstream. Carbon dioxide readily diffuses and enters solution and is readily exhaled. Although it is the largest volume of gas generated within the digestive tract it is only a temporary contributor to distention and postprandial (after meal) discomfort. Carbon dioxide is the easiest gas to eliminate from the bowel because of its ease of absorption into the circulation and release via the lungs. Because of these properties it is only a minor contributor to flatulence.

The volume of gasses in the gastrointestinal tract is dependent on the quantity and nature of the foods ingested, the body's ability to synthesize and utilize specific enzymes for the various food types, and the nature and quantity of the bacteria in the gut flora. It is also affected by the speed of gastrointestinal transit, which may be influenced by drugs, hormones, food product and illness. Other factors include the absorptive capacity and health of the mucosal lining, and the physical length of the gastrointestinal tract.

The often-quoted figure of twelve farts per day is a reasonable approximation of the average number of farts passed but there is a very wide range of what is considered normal. There are so many variables that what is normal for an individual can only be determined over a longer period of time than a single day. For those who are curious to know more about the physiology and science of the digestive process and intestinal gas there is an informative and entertaining companion volume to this book available: ***To 'Air' is Human, Everything You Ever Wanted to Know About Intestinal Gas.*** A second companion volume is ***Artsy Fartsy, Cultural History of the Fart*** a fascinating and factual review of the common fart through human culture and history.

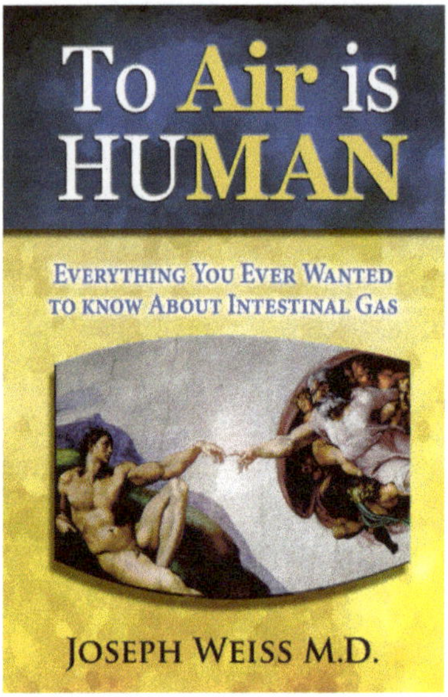
To Air is HUMAN
EVERYTHING YOU EVER WANTED TO KNOW ABOUT INTESTINAL GAS
JOSEPH WEISS M.D.

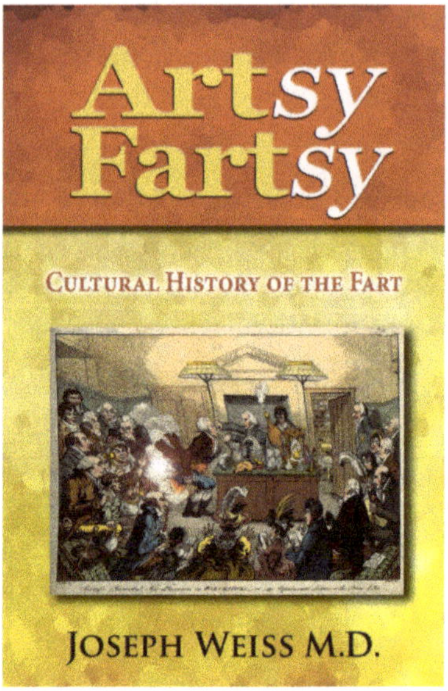
Artsy Fartsy
CULTURAL HISTORY OF THE FART
JOSEPH WEISS M.D.

Fecal Impaction

A fecal impaction is a hard of bolus human feces that cannot be eliminated by defecation. Symptoms typically include chronic constipation. Pain, discomfort, sensation of rectal fullness, distention, and tenesmus may also be noted if there is no underlying neuropathy. A fecal impaction may result in constipation that becomes a self-promulgating condition. As the stool remains in the colon for an extended time period, the colonic mucosa continues to remove moisture. As the stool continues to harden the constipation itself becomes more severe and a vicious cycle takes hold.

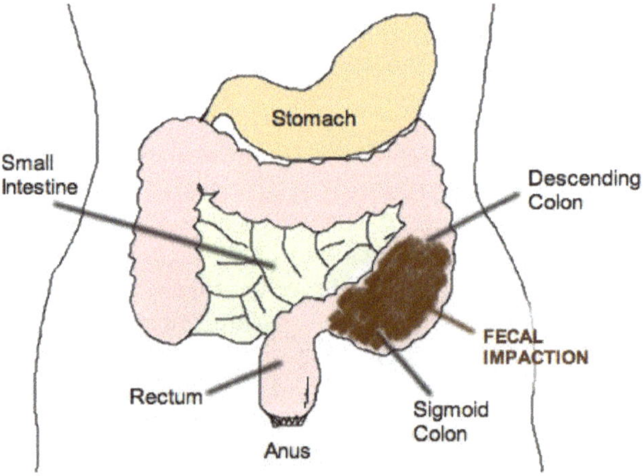
Stomach
Small Intestine
Descending Colon
FECAL IMPACTION
Rectum
Sigmoid Colon
Anus

www.constipation-remedies-for-all.com Creative Commons License

A fecal impaction can also result from unresolved constipation related to narcotic and opioid use, either prescribed or illicit. Morphine and the narcotics derivatives including codeine, heroin, oxycodone, and others may induce profound constipation that may ultimately result in fecal impaction. In addition to the usual treatment of constipation, the offending narcotic or opioid must be discontinued.

Naloxegol (Movantik) may help to restore bowel function in patients who have chronic illness and receive opioids or narcotics for pain relief. This prescription product recently approved by the Food & Drug Administration (FDA) is a mu-opioid receptor antagonist and decreases the constipating effect of the opioids or narcotics on the gut. Because naloxegol is a pegylated derivative of naloxone, it has limited ability to cross the blood-brain barrier so it does not interfere with the central analgesic effect desired. Another product available for managing chronic severe pain with an opioid or narcotic is marketed as Targin, Targinact, or Targiniq ER an extended release combination of oxycodone and naloxone. The naloxone is a narcotic antagonist and reduces the risk of dependence and constipation by its effect on the gut after absorption, but before its metabolism in the liver.

Overflow fecal incontinence may occur as liquid stool passes around the obstruction. Complications may include bowel obstruction, stercoral ulcer, abscess, and perforation from pressure necrosis and ulcers of the colon mucosal tissue. Abdominal pain and bloating could also be present depending on the length of time the condition has been ongoing. Stool softeners, enemas, colonic irritation, osmotic laxatives, or mineral oil may be effective. Digital disimpaction using a gloved finger to fragment the mass of stool may be required and can be successful with time and persistence as long as the bowel is not totally obstructed. If complete bowel obstruction or complications such as a stercoral ulcer or abscess occur surgery may be necessary.

An unusual cause of fecal impaction is Hirschsprung disease also known as congenital aganglionic megacolon. In this condition there is a failure to complete fetal development of the innervation of the enteric nervous system. This involves both the Auerbach plexus and the Meissner plexus, and may involve variable lengths of the intestinal tract. In a newborn infant failure to pass meconium, the first stool, is a sign that Hirshsprung disease may be the cause. The most common form involves a short segment just proximal to the anus.

Without the proper ganglions and nerve activity the bowel cannot relax to allow the passage of stool and fecal impaction ad obstruction results. Surgical resection of the segment of bowel affected is necessary. The bowel proximal to the involved segment is often distended because of the blockage and is known as a megacolon. Another condition caused by a parasite can mimic Hirschsprung disease and is more common in certain Latin American countries where the parasite and its vector are found. This condition is known as Chagas disease and is caused by the parasite *Trypanosoma cruzi*.

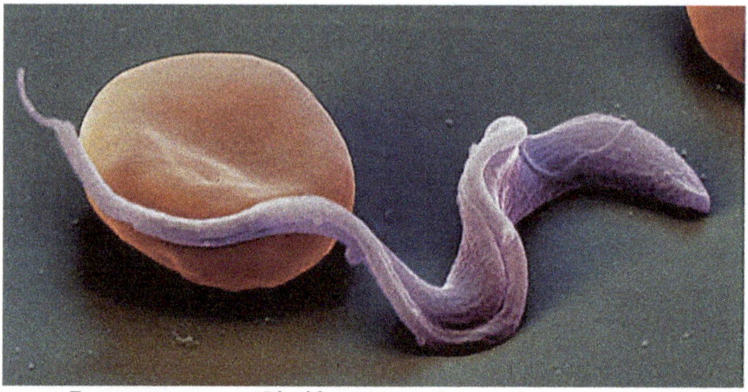

Trypanosmoma cruzi 2.bp.blogspot.com Creative Commons License

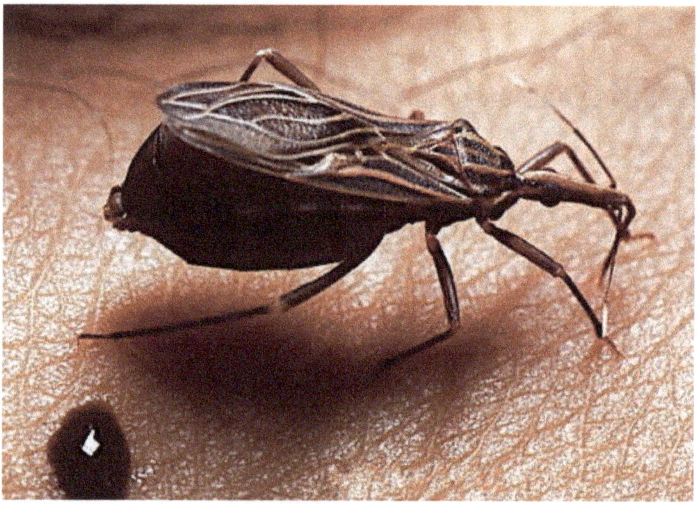

Reduviid bug is the vector for *Trypanosoma cruzi* 1.bp.blogspot.com Creative Commons License

The parasite is transmitted by the reduviid bug, also known as the kissing bug. The insect bites the victim on the face usually while they are sleeping. The infection is not transmitted by the bite itself. It is that the reduviid bug then defecates on the bite wound, and the itching and scratching of the wound allow the parasite to enter the body of the victim. The parasite destroys the nerve ganglion cells of a number of organs including the colon, esophagus, and heart.

Fecal Incontinence

Fecal incontinence is a lack of control over defecation leading to involuntary loss of bowel contents. The most common causes are damage to the anal sphincter from childbirth, complications from prior anorectal surgery, and altered bowel habits. An estimated 2.2% of adults are affected. The primary symptom is a lack of control over bowel contents, which may worsen without treatment. Secondary symptoms are the result of leakage and include the intense itching of pruritus ani, the irritation and inflammation of perianal dermatitis, and urinary tract infections.

There is often reduced self-esteem, depression, humiliation, and avoidance of enjoyable activities. Unfortunately it is an easily and mistakenly stigmatized genuine medical condition where people may be too embarrassed to seek medical help and unsuccessfully attempt to deal with the frustrating symptoms in secrecy. It is generally very treatable with a variety of dietary, pharmacologic, or surgical options.

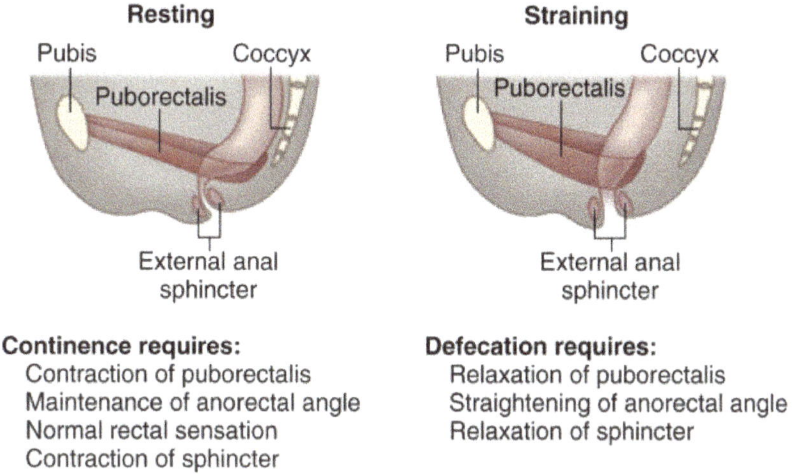
Resting
Pubis
Coccyx
Puborectalis
External anal sphincter
Straining
Pubis
Coccyx
Puborectalis
External anal sphincter
Continence requires:
Contraction of puborectalis
Maintenance of anorectal angle
Normal rectal sensation
Contraction of sphincter
Defecation requires:
Relaxation of puborectalis
Straightening of anorectal angle
Relaxation of sphincter

The evaluation of incontinence is multifactorial. Some of the factors that are considered in evaluation and treatment include the nature and magnitude of the incontinence. It may be limited to or include the passage of flatus, mucus, liquid stool, or solid stool. The volume passed may be minor staining of underwear, increasing to soilage, seepage, or full bowel movements. There may be tenesmus, a sensation of urgency and impending passage, implying that the sensory pathway is intact and the message can be detected, or passive release without sensation. There may be a reduction in the ability of the rectum to distend normally to store and accommodate stool prior to evacuation. The internal anal sphincter, external anal sphincter, or both may be impaired.

The description of incontinence may not be incontinence at all. It may be a rectal discharge of mucus and blood from various causes ranging from inflammatory bowel disease and local infections to radiation proctitis and rectal stercoral ulceration. There may be a perianal fistula such as is frequently seen in the inflammatory bowel disease of Crohn Disease, a perianal abscess, or rectal prolapse which can cause drainage mistaken for incontinence.

Anal fissures, hemorrhoids, anal warts, anal cancer, hemorrhoids, abscess, and fistula may also prevent complete and continent closure of the anus. There may be a condition causing diarrhea, which is harder to maintain continence of compared to solid stool. Constipation as well as fecal impaction can cause an overflow incontinence. There are a number of interrelated mechanisms and factors that contribute to normal continence. In up to eighty percent of patients with continence issues there is more than one contributing factor. The puborectalis sling forming the anorectal angle is responsible for gross continence of solid stool.

The internal anal sphincter is an involuntary muscle that contributes about fifty-five percent of the resting anal pressure. Together with the hemorrhoid vascular cushions the internal anal sphincter maintains continence of flatus and liquid during rest. The external anal sphincter is a voluntary muscle, doubling the pressure in the anal canal during contraction. The rectoanal inhibitory reflex is an involuntary internal anal sphincter relaxation in response to rectal distention. This allows a sampling of some of the rectal contents to descend into the anal canal. Here it is brought into contact with specialized sensory mucosa to detect consistency. The rectoanal excitatory reflex is an initial semi-voluntary contraction of the external anal sphincter and puborectalis, which returns tone following the rectoanal inhibitory reflex.

Other factors include the specialized anti-peristaltic function of the last part of the sigmoid colon, the sensory ability of the lining of the rectum and the anal canal to detect the consistency and quantity when of stool present, and the normal rectoanal reflexes and defecation cycle that completes evacuation. Problems affecting any of these mechanisms and factors may be contributing to incontinence. Reduced rectal storage capacity with either a reduction in rectal volume or rectal compliance for distention may lead to urge incontinence. It may be caused by surgery such as a lower anterior resection, radiation therapy of the rectum, or inflammatory bowel disease all of which may cause scarring and reduced compliance. Tumors and strictures also may impair reservoir function. A rectocele may cause an incomplete evacuation of the rectum with post defecation leakage.

Caffeine can contribute by relaxing the anal sphincter tone.

Pharmaceuticals that can reduce sphincter tone pressure and contribute to incontinence include nitrates, calcium channel antagonists, beta-adrenoceptor antagonists (beta-blockers), sildenafil, selective serotonin reuptake inhibitors (e.g. fluoxetine, Prozac) antibiotics, topical drugs applied to anus including glyceryl trinitrate ointment, diltiazem gel, and bethanechol cream. Botulinum toxin A injection, vitamin C, magnesium, phosphorus, calcium, and a large number of others may also relax the anal sphincter

Beyond a thorough history and physical examination, including close examination of the anorectal area, additional studies may be undertaken. Anorectal physiology tests assess the functioning of the anorectal anatomy. Anorectal manometry records the strength and tone of the anal sphincters and puborectalis during rest and during contraction. Anal electromyography tests for nerve damage which is often associated with a difficult obstetric delivery.

Pudendal nerve terminal motor latency tests for damage to the pudendal motor nerves. Dynamic pelvic MRI is replacing defecography as the most informative study of the anorectal anatomy and defecation function. Proctosigmoidoscopy of the anal canal, rectum and sigmoid colon inspects for inflammation, tumors, or scar tissue. Endoanal ultrasound evaluates the structure of the anal sphincters, and may detect occult sphincter tears.

Historically, bowel management has been a practical approach to manage fecal incontinence or constipation. The definition of fecal incontinence is the inability to voluntarily hold feces in the rectum. This can lead to significant disruption in social activities and reduction in the quality of life. Bowel management is the purposeful clearing of colonic contents on a schedule that prevents uncontrolled bowel movements. Daily enemas, laxatives, and a controlled diet may be components of a bowel management regimen.

For those dependent on a daily enema as part of the regimen a creative approach has been the development of an operation to convert the appendix to an access port for the administration of fluid into the colon. Called a continent appendicostomy or Malone procedure a catheter to administer the enema fluid is inserted into a small orifice usually located near the belly button. This allows full control of the enema process to be in the hands of the individual to maintain independence. Even more dramatic advances have taken place in both the surgical techniques and technology widening the therapeutic options.

There have been very significant advances in the diagnosis and management of fecal incontinence. A clear and accurate diagnosis of the underlying contributing factors leads to the proper treatment and management, which generally provides considerable improvement. Conservative measures are always the preferred approach but there have been great advances in the surgical management as well. Dietary modifications, avoidance of caffeine, checking for contributing medications are a basic first step. Drug treatment, anal and pelvic floor exercises, biofeedback, and perineal hygiene and pads or plugs may be used during the course of treatment.

Nerve stimulators may be helpful in increasing sphincter tone and are available in a variety of approaches ranging from intra-anal to sacral implants. The injection of material that closes the anal opening at rest has shown promising results and continues to be refined and improved. Newer pharmacologic agents to enhance sphincter tone are being investigated. If necessary surgical procedures ranging from sphincter repair to replacement with a neosphincter or artificial anal sphincter have been successfully developed.

Perhaps the most remarkable advance is leaving the realm of science fiction and getting closer to reality, the use of a person's stem cells to repair or create a new sphincter. Successful replacement of a number of human tissues has already been accomplished including the replacement of the trachea in several different medical centers. Additional organs successfully regenerated and transplanted into humans include tear ducts, vagina, and urinary bladder. Regenerated nose, ear, coronary artery, urethra, and bile duct are now ready for clinical trials. The work on anal sphincters has already taken place in animal models, and holds great promise.

Pseudo incontinence or overflow incontinence is actually due to underlying constipation and fecal impaction with liquid stools bypassing the blockage. When the impaction and constipation are corrected continence can once again be achieved. Can you really 'scare the shit out of someone'? This common phrase actually has a physiological basis and can be taken literally; yes you can scare the shit out of someone, including yourself. It is part of the survival response to stress called the fight-or-flight response. It occurs in response to a perceived threat to survival, and results in the generalized discharge of the autonomic and sympathetic nervous system and the hormonal releases of adrenaline (epinephrine), norepinephrine, and other catecholamine.

The heart rate races, the pupils of the eye dilate, your breathing quickens, you become super alert with a discharge of cortisol and glucose into the bloodstream, increased blood flow to the muscles and away from digestion, and yes the anal sphincter and urinary sphincters can suddenly give way to a mass evacuation of feces and urine to lighten your load if you needed to sprint to safety. The generalized body shaking and knocking of knees is also reality, not fiction.

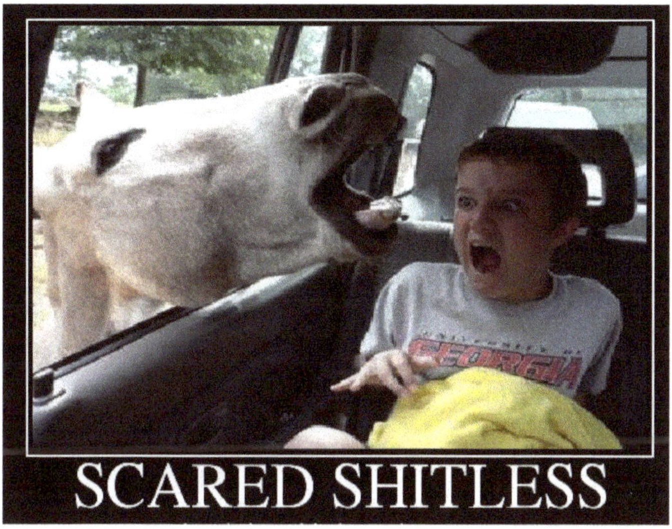
SCARED SHITLESS

The story of hanging victims losing bowel and bladder control could either be the fear factor if it occurs just prior to hanging, or the consequence of decerebrate posturing with the broken neck and quadriplegia that results from the hanging action. In states where capital punishment is carried out by hanging, the victim is provided with rubber pants and diapers so as not to embarrass him or herself and to give the procedure a more civilized veneer.

The Far Side cartoonist Gary Larson had one of his early cartoons rejected for publication by his syndicate because they considered it in poor taste. A spider with a paper bag over its head approaches another spider in the web that has just released his entire internal supply of web silk into a large pile on the ground underneath the web. The caption reads: "Did I scare you, or what?"

Runner's Diarrhea, often termed "runner's trots" is a condition that often affects long distance runners and is characterized by an extremely urgent need for a bowel movement. It also can occur to a lesser degree in other endurance sports like long distance bicycling. The cause is uncertain although mechanical trauma from the vigorous running is suspect. Another theory ascribes it to mesenteric ischemia from reduced blood flow to the intestines with the increased cardiovascular demands of the body musculature.

There have been many instances of fecal soiling accidents in mid race or other sporting events. Dramatically demonstrating the immediate need to have a bowel movement, several sports figures have either soiled themselves or defecated in public on live television at internationally broadcast sporting events.

Fecal Occult Blood

Fecal occult blood refers to blood in the feces that is not visibly apparent. A fecal occult blood test checks for hidden (occult) blood in the feces. Fecal Immunochemical Test (FIT) and occult blood tests such as Hemosure utilize specific antibodies to detect human hemoglobin and are used as a screening test for detection of colorectal cancer.

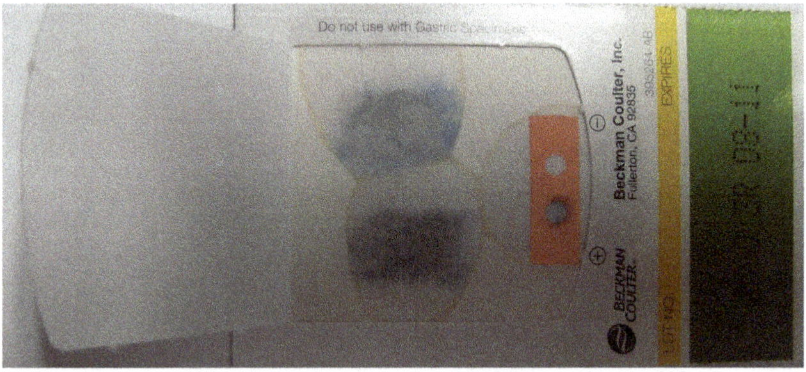
Beckman Coulter, Inc.
Fullerton, CA 92835
BECKMAN COULTER
EXPIRES

Occult gastrointestinal bleeding is when the presence and degree of internal bleeding are not visible to gross inspection of the feces or toilet bowl water, but only by testing the stool for blood. A positive occult blood test may use one of several testing modalities, the one illustrated turns blue in the presence of hemoglobin. Author James Heilman Creative Commons License

The stool guaiac test involves detecting the peroxidase effect of heme in a sample of feces. This may be helpful in determining an upper gastrointestinal bleed because the heme is less likely to be broken down in the upper gastrointestinal tract than globin. This test is less sensitive and can be false positive by reacting with animal blood from a meal such as a rare steak, as well as by certain vegetables such as horseradish and cauliflower.

Fecal DNA test- Cologuard and the PreGen-Plus test extracts human DNA from the stool sample and tests it for alterations that have been associated with cancer. The test looks at twenty-three individual DNA alterations, including twenty-one specific point alterations in the APC, KRAS and p53 genes, as well as testing BAT26, a gene involved in microsatellite instability. The DNA based PreGen-Plus was four times more sensitive than fecal blood testing, including detection of early stage disease, when treatment is most effective.

Gastrointestinal bleeding has many potential sources. Typical screening of large populations has up to five percent with a positive fecal occult blood test. Of these less than ten percent have cancer, while another twenty to thirty percent have adenomas, which increases the risk of future cancer development. The removal of these adenomas while they are smaller, safer and easier to remove, and benign significantly reduces the future risk of cancer development. A positive fecal occult blood test can result from either upper or lower gastrointestinal bleeding. Endoscopy of the upper and lower gastrointestinal tract is often performed to identify the source of the often asymptomatic bleeding. Common causes include colon adenomas or polyps, colon or gastric cancer, gastritis, esophagitis, peptic ulcer, and angiodysplasia of the colon amongst other conditions.

Gastrointestinal complaints and low intensity GI bleeding may occur in marathon runners. Strenuous exercise may cause heartburn, nausea, vomiting, abdominal pain, diarrhea and gastrointestinal bleeding. Approximately one-third of long distance runners experience exercise limiting symptoms, and the gastrointestinal bleeding occasionally causes iron deficiency anemia.

Fecaloma, Fecalith

A fecaloma or fecolith is a lump of feces so hardened by the absorption of its water content by the colon lining that it becomes stone like in character. Anything that delays the transit of stool through the colon can predispose to it. At times stool can remain trapped in the appendix and a fecolith formed in this location is referred to as an appendicolith. On occasion this may present with appendicitis. Diverticulosis may also see feces trapped in a diverticulum become a fecolith over time and it may present as diverticulitis.

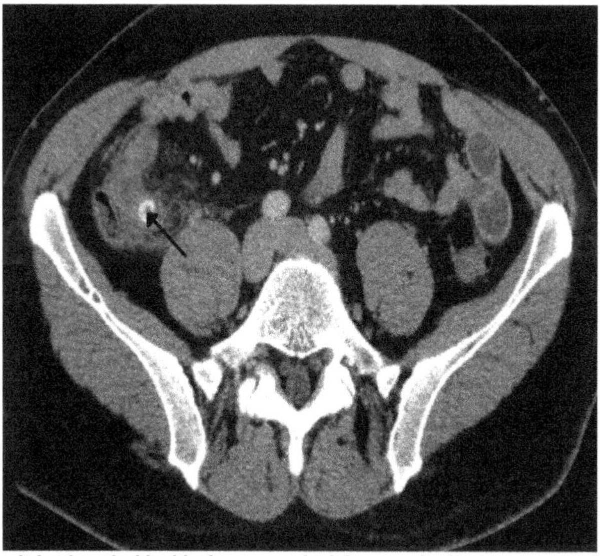

A calcified fecalith, identified by black arrow, which has resulted in acute appendicitis. Author James Heilman, MD Creative Commons License

Most commonly chronic constipation is responsible. Partial colonic obstruction, Chagas disease, Hirschsprung disease and others conditions that damage the colons neuromotor physiologic elimination process can lead to very large fecalomas. These may lead to fecal impaction and bowel obstruction.

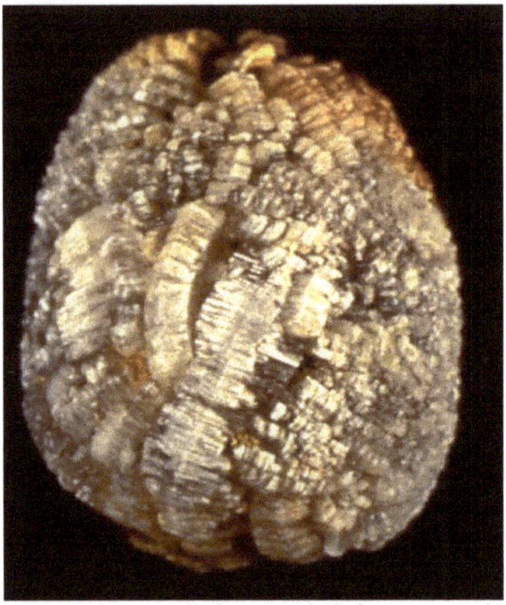

Fecalith, inspissated feces in the appendix, became calcified over time and became a stone like mass that led to appendicitis. With the calcium deposition it can become visible on radiographic studies and be identified prior to surgery . Creative Commons License

Fecal Oral Contamination Route

Fecal oral route (fecal oral contamination) is the transmission of a disease pathogen via feces particles that are ingested by the newly infected host. The process of transmission may be by gross contamination as described by the term coprophagia, but much more often the transmission is less visible or microscopic (although it technically remains coprophagia). Examples may include a scenario where a fly that had been feeding on feces lands and feeds on open food at a picnic, which it contaminates by the feces residue on its feet. Swimming in a pool that had an undisclosed recent toddler 'accident' may lead to fecal oral contamination. Poor hand washing after a bowel movement with toilet paper wiping, then eating finger foods such as potato chips or popcorn from a common bowl is a common route of transmission.

Rotavirus is transmitted by the fecal oral route and is the most common cause of severe diarrhea among infants and young children. Nearly every child in the world has been infected with rotavirus at least once by the age of five. If is estimated to cause about forty per cent of all hospital admissions due to diarrhea among children under five years of age worldwide leading to 100 million episodes of acute diarrhea that result in 350,000 to 600,000 child deaths each year.

Most transmission of pathogens is via the fecal to oral route is usually accomplished by way of the hands. The average human stool contains three trillion microorganisms. Wiping with toilet paper nearly guarantees that the hands will come into contact with fecal microorganisms. After wiping it is not uncommon to find brown streaks on underwear because of inadequate anal hygiene. The average man's underwear contains one tenth of a gram of feces at laundering.

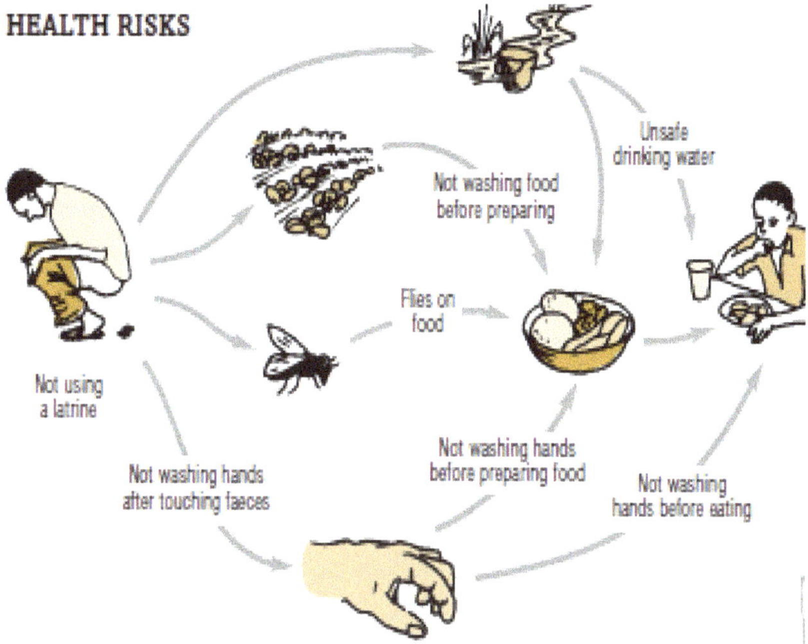
HEALTH RISKS
Unsafe drinking water
Not washing food before preparing
Flies on food
Not using a latrine
Not washing hands after touching faeces
Not washing hands before preparing food
Not washing hands before eating

www.infonet-biovision.org/res Creative Commons License

The degree of fecal-oral contamination that takes place on a daily basis in even the most sophisticated and highest levels of socioeconomic achievement are sobering. An illness that is easily transmitted by purely fecal oral contamination will infect nearly all members of any closely living household within a matter of days. The number of infectious particles we are exposed to each and every day is astronomical.

The number of infectious viral particles in one gram (less than 1/30 of an ounce) of feces from a child with rotavirus is more than ten trillion (10,000,000,000,000). One child in a household has more than enough viral particles in a thimble of stool to infect every human on the planet Earth and another 10,000 planets with the same population.

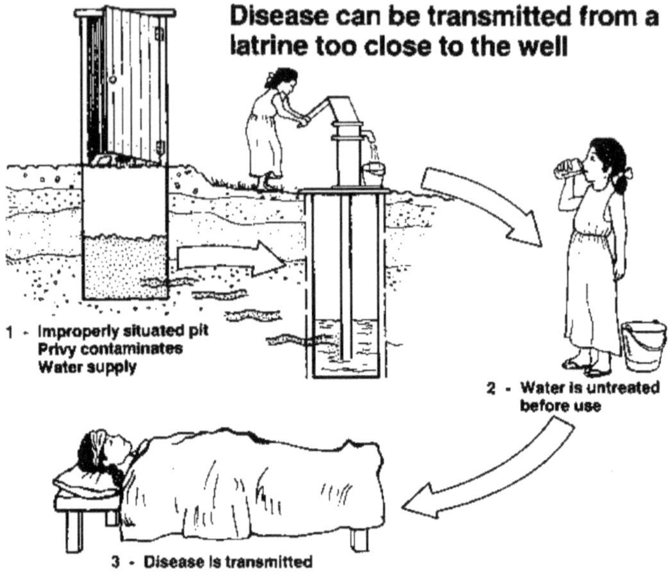
Disease can be transmitted from a latrine too close to the well
1 - Improperly situated pit Privy contaminates Water supply
2 - Water is untreated before use
3 - Disease is transmitted

www.nzdl.org/gsdl Creative Commons License

Some of the diseases that can be passed via the fecal-oral route include poliomyelitis, norovirus acute gastroenteritis, giardiasis, hepatitis A, hepatitis E, rotavirus, shigellosis (bacillary dysentery), typhoid fever, *Vibrio parahemolyticus* infections, enteroviruses, cholera, *Clostridium difficile,* cryptosporidiosis, ascariasis, and many others.

Fecal (Microbiota) Transplant

Fecal transplant is the treatment of choice for antibiotic associated colitis, also known as pseudomembranous colitis. The causative organism, *Clostridia difficile,* often does not respond to intensive antibiotic treatment, and fecal transplants of stool from a healthy donor have been successfully utilized. Much akin to blood banks, banks of healthy stool are being established as more conditions, such as inflammatory bowel disease, and irritable bowel syndrome, appear to benefit from fecal transplants in selected cases.

Bedouins have used consumption of fresh, warm camel feces as a remedy for bacterial dysentery for ages. Its efficacy may be attributable to the antibiotic subtilisin from *Bacillus subtilis* or the wholesale substitution of the gut flora. German soldiers in North Africa confirmed the effectiveness of the camel feces during World War II to whom it was administered when they had dysentery. Another possibility is that a number of the 'cured' did not get better but refused to admit it in order to avoid another dose of a 'medicine' that literally tasted like shit.

Feces (see Manure)

Feces (Latin fæx "dregs") are the excreted waste product from the digestive tract expelled through the anus during defecation. Feces is also known as excrement, dung, ordure, manure, droppings, scat, shit, poop, and dozens of other words and euphemisms. Although the digestive tract has extracted nutrients, the fecal matter often has fifty percent of its energy value remaining. This is a vital resource for organisms such as bacteria, fungi, and insects such as the fly and dung beetle.

Human fecal matter varies significantly in appearance, depending on diet and health. A sticky gummy texture is often noted with substantial internal bleeding, which also often presents as black tarry stool called melena.

Brown Stool - Human feces ordinarily has a light to dark brown coloration, which results from a combination of bile and bilirubin that is derived from the breakdown products of dead red blood cells.

Yellow Stool - Stool that is yellow may suggest presence of undigested fat in the stool. The stool containing the undigested fat may appear yellowish in color, greasy, and also may smell foul. Yellowing of feces may also be caused by an infection that may also cause diarrhea, such as from *Giardia lamblia*, a protozoan parasite.

Black Stool (Melena) - Feces can be black due to the presence of red blood cells that have been broken down by digestive enzymes. This is known as melena, and is typically due to bleeding in the upper digestive tract, such as from a bleeding peptic ulcer. The same color change can be observed after consuming foods that contain a substantial proportion of animal blood, such as black pudding or tiết canh.

Black feces can also be caused by a number of medications containing bismuth products (such as Pepto-Bismol and the newer formulation of Kaopectate in the United States), iron supplements, or foods such as beetroot, black licorice, or blueberries.

Red Stool - Hematochezia is similarly the passage of feces that are bright red due to the presence of undigested blood, either from lower in the digestive tract, or from a more active source in the upper digestive tract. Ingestion of red beets will also color the stool and can be easily misinterpreted as a sign of internal bleeding. Besides the dramatic blood red color of beets, a similar red color may also come from natural or artificial coloring such as red gelatin, popsicles, Kool-Aid, and dragon fruit

Blue Stool - Prussian blue, used in the treatment of radiation, cesium, and thallium poisoning, can turn the feces blue. Substantial consumption of products containing blue food dye, such as blue curaçao or grape soda, can have a similar effect.

White (Acholic) Stool - Acholic stools, which are pasty white in color, are characteristic of complete biliary obstruction.

Silver Stool - Silver or aluminum feces color results when biliary obstruction of any type (acholic or white stool) combines with gastrointestinal bleeding from any source that would normally present as black stools or melena.

Green Stool - Feces can be green due to having large amounts of unprocessed bile in the digestive tract. When stool passes through the intestines rapidly (diarrhea) there may be little time for bilirubin to undergo its usual chemical changes. Green feces may occasionally be the result from eating liquorice candy, as it is typically made with anise oil rather than liquorice herb and is predominantly sugar. Excessive sugar consumption or a sensitivity to anise oil may cause loose, green stools.

Medical students are taught the significance of stool color. A pediatric colleague, Richard Buchta, shared the story of a professor quizzing medical students about the significance of different colored stools. The group was asked what question they should ask if a young lady told them she was passing golden stools. A witty medical student quickly responded that the question to be asked was 'Will you marry me?'

Feces are often used as fertilizer, both manure and guano becoming large commercial enterprises. Historically human waste, euphemistically called night soil, was used as a major source of fertilizer. Animal feces, especially those of camel, bison, oxen, yak, water buffalo, and cattle can be used as fuel or building material when dried. Terms such as dung, scat, spoor, manure, castings, spraint, fewmets, guano, and droppings are used to refer to specific animal feces..

Feces, Aroma

Olfaction, the sense of smell, is a form of chemoperception that in humans occurs when odorant molecules bind to olfactory receptors. Cloning of olfactory receptor proteins and identifying that odor molecules that bind to specific receptors led to the 2004 Nobel Prize being awarded to Linda B. Buck and Richard Axel.

Feces and farts have a characteristic aroma that most people find offensive. Females have greater olfactory sensitivity than males, particularly at the time of ovulation. More than pheromones is involved, and females can detect by olfaction potential mates that have a genetic diversity that would be beneficial for their offspring. Odor information is retained in long-term memory and the olfactory system is anatomically associated with the regions of the brain associated with emotion. It has been long recognized that odors can trigger memories and emotions from remote times.

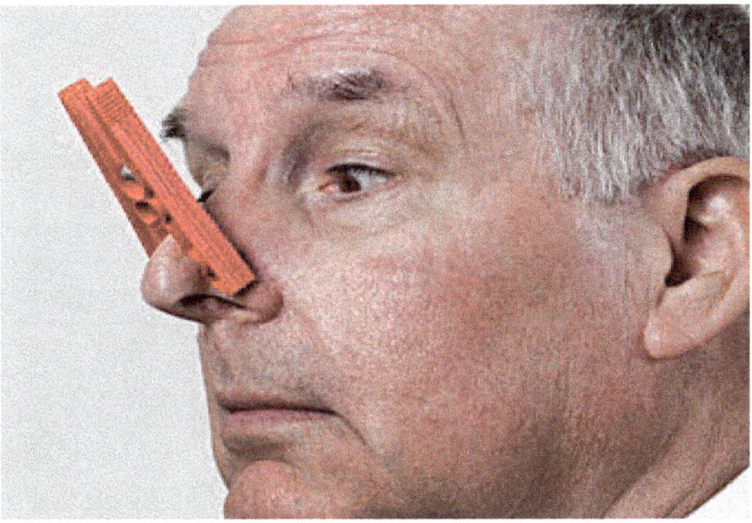

www.theguardian.com

The sense of olfaction is the most sensitive of all human senses. The nose can identify a single scented molecule hiding amongst two billion unscented ones. To use a visual analogy, paint one single square sheet of a toilet paper roll the color red. Now wrap that unlimited length roll of toilet paper around the twenty-five thousand mile long equator of the planet earth, and go around a second time, a third, a fourth, and a full fifth time. Your nose can instantaneously identify the single red square of a one-hundred-and-twenty-five-thousand mile roll of toilet paper. Are you impressed with the human sense of smell? Just like wealth and beauty, there is always someone who has more to keep us from being number one.

The human olfactory epithelium is less than ten percent of the surface area of olfactory epithelium of the dog. The dog also has one hundred times more receptors per square centimeter. Bloodhounds have olfactory receptors up to one hundred million times the sensitivities of humans and are trained to track a human trail several days old. North American grizzly bears have the keenest sense of smell, seven times greater than the bloodhound.

Salmon utilize their keen sense of smell in ocean waters to locate the stream from which they emerged as hatchlings many years earlier. This keen sense of smell allows them to return instinctually to the stream of their origin to spawn. Much like there are colors that the human eye cannot see (such as ultraviolet and infrared), there are 'odorless' compounds, which we cannot smell, but are not necessarily odorless to others. An example is the mosquito smelling the 'odorless' carbon dioxide that mammals exhale to locate their next blood meal. The keen olfactory sensitivity of the mosquito is located on their antennae.

The aromas generated by intestinal gas are normally considered unattractive or offensive. There is a surprising percentage of the presumably normal population (predominantly males) who profess enjoyment and pleasure with the olfactory stimulation generated by their own farts, but not those of others.

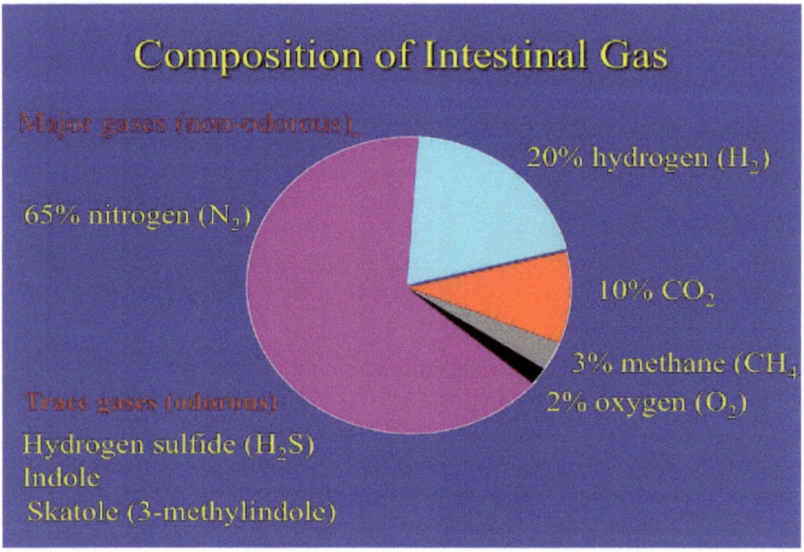
Composition of Intestinal Gas
Major gases (non-odorous)
20% hydrogen (H_2)
65% nitrogen (N_2)
10% CO_2
3% methane (CH_4)
2% oxygen (O_2)
Trace gases (odorous)
Hydrogen sulfide (H_2S)
Indole
Skatole (3-methylindole)

Perhaps even more surprising is the fact that the vast majority of the components of intestinal gas are odorless. Nitrogen, hydrogen, carbon dioxide, methane, and oxygen comprise 99.9% of intestinal gas by volume, and each of these individual gasses are odorless to humans. So what on earth is in that other miniscule but powerful fraction of one percent?

<u>Indole</u>

Indole is an organic compound known as an aromatic heterocyclic because it consists of a six-membered benzene ring fused to a five-membered nitrogen-containing pyrrole ring. Indole is often used as a component of fragrances and is used in the production of a number of pharmaceutical products. The amino acid tryptophan is the precursor of the neurotransmitter serotonin and is an example of an indole derivative.

Tryptophan is one of the twenty-two amino acids, and is also considered an essential amino acid. Essential amino acids are those amino acids that cannot be synthesized by humans, and therefore must be obtained through the diet. Because of its importance as an essential amino acid, tryptophan is a common constituent of most protein foods and supplements. A diet rich in tryptophan can contribute to the fecal aroma of intestinal gas.

Indole occurs naturally in human feces and contributes to the characteristic fecal odor. Surprisingly, at very low concentrations it has a flowery smell and is a constituent of many perfumes. The name indole is a portmanteau created from the words indigo and oleum. Indole was first isolated by the dye industry in treatment of the deep blue indigo dye with oleum.

Indole is widely distributed in the natural environment and can be produced by a variety of bacteria as a degradation product of the amino acid tryptophan. tryptophan is an indole derivative and the precursor of the hormone melatonin, the neurotransmitter serotonin, and the plant hormone auxin. As an intercellular signal molecule, indole regulates various aspects of bacterial physiology, including spore formation, plasmid stability, resistance to drugs, biofilm formation, and virulence. It takes several million jasmine blossoms to make one pound of natural jasmine oil, which is two-point-five percent indole. It is priced over one thousand times as much as synthetic jasmine, which takes advantage of the commercial production of indole.

Skatole

Skatole (from the Greek το σχατος = feces), or methylindole, is a mildly toxic organic compound belonging to the indole family. It is the primary source of the odor of feces and is produced from the breakdown of the important amino acid tryptophan, the precursor of the neurotransmitter serotonin. Surprisingly, in low concentrations skatole has a very pleasant flowery smell and is found in orange blossoms, jasmine, and other flowers and essential oils. It is used as a fragrance in many perfumes.

Skatole is attractive to males of various species of bees, who gather the chemical to synthesize pheromones. It is also an attractant to gravid (pregnant) mosquitos. The U. S. military has used skatole as a non-lethal malodorant weapon. The German physician Ludwig Brieger, who also identified cadaverine and putrescence, discovered skatole in 1877. His neighbors were probably not pleased with the smell coming from his laboratory as the names he gave his discoveries were derived from their source material.

Skatole also plays a major role in the aroma of pork obtained from mature male pigs (boars). After puberty, under the influence of the male hormone androstenone, the gut microbiome of the male pig generates skatole. This odorant is deposited in the fat and muscle giving it an offensive smell and taste known as taint. Because it cannot be sold at market, male pigs are typically castrated at a young age or slaughtered before puberty. The male of the human species, under similar hormonal influence is also a larger producer of skatole contributing to the enhanced offensive potency of male farts after puberty.

Of particular interest to some scientists is that androstenone, and its effect on skatole, appear to have a pheromone like effect on the human female. Much like color-blindness, there appear to be some odors that cannot be smelled by all people. Initial studies suggested that about thirty percent of human females could not sense androstenone. Further studies revealed that the majority of the non-scenters could be trained to identify it, yet there remained a small proportion of less than five percent who could not perceive the scent. The ability to sense androstenone was found to be genetic and the gene responsible was identified.

The sense of smell in the human female is intimately tied to the menstrual cycle. The height of olfactory sensitivity peaks at the time of ovulation. The androstenone and skatole scents are perceived to be less offensive or more attractive at the time of ovulation. The androstenone skatole connection also explains why the feces and flatus of males is considered more powerful or offensive than that of females.

Diet also plays a role in that the ingestion of more meat and fat also leads to more skatole production than a diet with higher fiber content. This is partly due to the diet containing more tryptophan, the amino acid precursor of skatole, as well as the diet induced change in the microbiome. Androstenone also occurs naturally in some plants, including celery, parsnip, and truffle. The celery has long had a reputation as an aphrodisiac dating from Greek and Roman times.

<u>Thiol, Sulfhydryl, Mercaptans</u>

The sulfur hydrogen functional group may also be referred to as a thiol group or a sulfhydryl group. Thiols are also referred to as mercaptans. The term mercaptan (Latin mercurium captans 'capturing mercury') is used because the thiolate group bonds so strongly with mercury compounds. Hydrogen sulfide is known for its characteristic odor of smelling like rotten eggs. Surprisingly women tend to produce more hydrogen sulfide then men. Diet certainly plays a role as cruciferous vegetables such as broccoli, cabbage, cauliflower, and Brussels sprouts are common offenders. Dried fruits such as apricots are often treated with sulfur products that create odiferous gasses. Red meat, beer, garlic, and aromatic spices are other significant contributors. The offensive smell of sulfur products led to religions ascribing an association between the devil and sulfur.

Hydrogen sulfide is a toxic substance in high concentrations yet very valuable and beneficial on a cellular level when present in minute quantities. The human nose is exceptionally sensitive to this toxin and can identify in in minute concentrations, such as in a fart. When present in very high concentrations the olfactory cells are overwhelmed and can no longer sense it. This has led to a sever hazard for farmers and workers in animal waste manure pits and sewage treatment facilities. A worker collapses on exposure to the high concentration of hydrogen sulfide and fellow workers coming to their aid are likewise stricken because there was no olfactory warning. With a toxic potency equivalent to cyanide workers in such hazardous occupations are urged to use self-contained breathing apparatus to avoid exposure.

Volatiles may have distinctive and strong garlic like odor. The spray of skunks consists mainly of thiols and derivatives. These compounds are detected by the human nose at concentrations as low as ten parts per billion. Human sweat contains methyl-sulfanylhexan (MSH), found in higher concentrations in females, and has a fruity onion-like odor. Not all thiols have unpleasant odors. The aroma of roasted coffee is due to thiols as is the characteristic scent of grapefruit. Dimethyl sulfide has an aroma that is often described as sweet. Natural gas distributors were required by law to add odorants such as thiols to odorless natural after a tragic school explosion in New London, Texas, in 1937.

Most natural odorant additives used today contain mixtures of mercaptans and sulfides. T-butyl mercaptan is often utilized as the main odorant constituent. The characteristic and pungently offensive odor of animal flesh decay is caused by putrescence and cadaverine. Putrescence and cadaverine are the breakdown products of the amino acids ornithine and lysine, respectively. Cadaverine and putrescence were also used as odorant additives for natural before improved odorants became commercially available.

<u>Methanethiol</u>

Methanethiol (methyl mercaptan) is a flammable, colorless with a powerful smell like rotten cabbage or decomposing vegetables. It is a natural substance found in certain foods such as some nuts and cheese, and is released from decaying organic matter. Methanethiol is also a byproduct produced by the metabolism of asparagus. The change in the odor of urine may be apparent within thirty minutes of eating asparagus. It is one of the main chemicals responsible for bad breath and the smell of feces and flatus. Natural gas and propane are colorless and odorless, and an undetected leak can lead to tragic consequences. To serve as a odorous marker that a leak is occurring small amount of methyl mercaptan or ethyl mercaptan may be added as an odorant. The addition of an odorant is often required by law to prevent the danger of natural leaks going undetected.

Fatty Acids

A fatty acid is a saturated or unsaturated carboxylic acid with a long aliphatic tail (chain). Fatty acids with carbon–carbon double bonds are known as unsaturated, and those without such double bonds are known as saturated fatty acids. Fatty acids are derived from triglycerides or phospholipids and when unattached to other molecules are described as 'free'. Fatty acids are an important cellular fuel and yield large quantities of adenosine triphosphate when metabolized. Adenosine triphosphate is one of the major energy transport molecules that fuels cellular metabolism. Energy of a phosphate bond is made available to the cell when adenosine triphosphate (ATP) is reduced to adenosine diphosphate (ADP).

Many cell types can use either glucose or fatty acids for this purpose. Heart and skeletal muscle prefer fatty acids although most cells can use glucose interchangeably. The brain has the ability to use fatty acids, glucose, or ketone bodies as a fuel. Fatty acids that must be obtained via the diet because humans cannot synthesize them are called essential fatty acids. Fatty acid chains are categorized by their length. Short-chain fatty acids (SCFA) have aliphatic tails of fewer than six carbons. Medium-chain fatty acids (MCFA) have tails of six to twelve carbons in length and can form medium-chain triglycerides. Long-chain fatty acids (LCFA) have tails of thirteen to twenty-one carbons, while very long chain fatty acids (VLCFA) are longer than twenty-two carbons.

Short- and medium-chain fatty acids are absorbed by the intestines directly into the blood stream. Long-chain fatty acids are absorbed into the cells of the intestinal villi and converted into a triglyceride cholesterol compound known as a chylomicron. These enter lymphatic capillaries called lacteals and are transported via the thoracic duct of the lymphatic system. They eventually enter the circulatory system via the left subclavian vein.
Fatty acids and chylomicrons in the blood circulation may be processed in the liver and subsequently circulate as very low-density lipoproteins (VLDL), low-density lipoproteins (LDL), and high-density lipoproteins.

Aromatic Amino Acids

Aromatic amino acids are amino acids that include an aromatic ring. Examples include phenylalanine, tryptophan, histidine, and tyrosine. Phenylalanine, histidine, and tryptophan are essential amino acids in that animals cannot synthesize them and they must be obtained from the diet. Tyrosine is semi-essential in that it can be synthesized but only if phenylalanine is ingested. The disorder phenylketonuria occurs when there is an absence of the enzyme phenylalanine hydroxylase, which is required for tyrosine synthesis.

All plants and microorganisms synthesize their aromatic amino acids, unlike animals, which obtain them through their diet. Animals have lost these energy intensive metabolic pathways, since they obtain aromatic amino acids through their diet. Herbicides and antibiotics inhibiting enzymes involved in aromatic acid synthesis, are toxic to plants and microorganisms dependent on this pathway, but not to animals which do not utilize these enzymes.

Volatile Organic Compounds

The term volatile refers to the ability of a substance to evaporate or readily vaporize at room temperature. Most instances of vaporization refer to evaporation where a liquid becomes a gas, such as liquid water boiling into gaseous steam and water vapor. Some solids vaporize from the solid state directly without entering an intermediate liquid phase, a process is known as sublimation. One example would be dry ice, frozen carbon dioxide, which leaves the solid state and is immediately transformed into a gas.

Vaporization also has another form that is not evaporation, but is the scattering or diffusing of molecules or particles through the air. The particles have so little mass that they can remain airborne for extended periods of time, and become airborne again upon being disturbed or moved even by a gentle gust of air. This is frequently noticed when a bright beam of light enters a darkened room and the dust particles circulating in the air become visible.

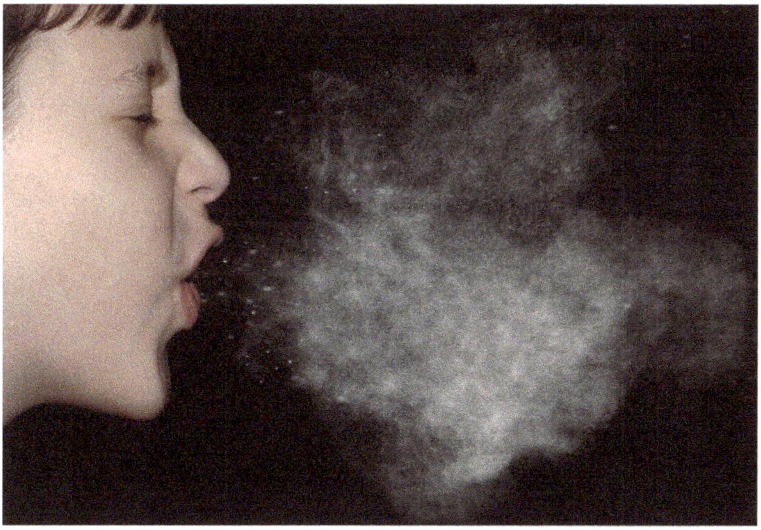

Mold, spores, pollens, viruses, bacteria, fecal matter of mites, volatile organic compounds and others can circulate and spread through large open spaces. Allergies, acquiring viral or bacterial infections from the sneeze or cough of others even hours earlier, occur because of this aerosolization. The ability to detect the aroma of certain compounds, and volatile organic compounds are the result of this form of vaporization as well as they can vaporize at room temperatures.

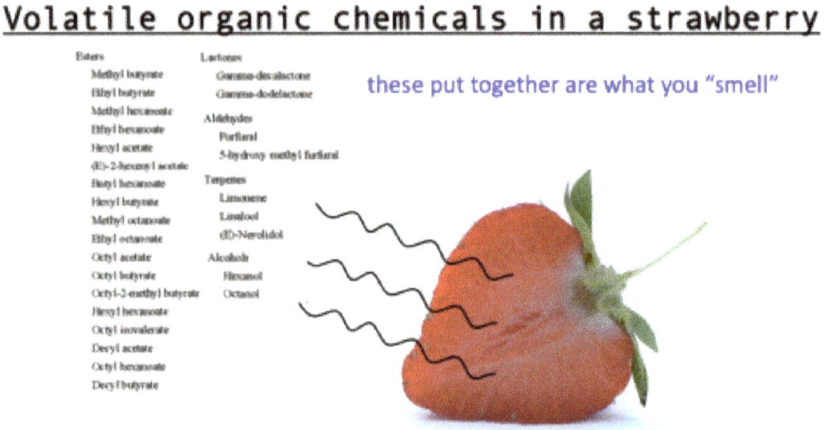
Volatile organic chemicals in a strawberry
Esters
Methyl butyrate
Ethyl butyrate
Methyl hexanoate
Ethyl hexanoate
Hexyl acetate
Butyl hexanoate
Hexyl butyrate
Methyl octanoate
Ethyl octanoate
Octyl acetate
Octyl butyrate
Hexyl hexanoate
Decyl acetate
Octyl hexanoate
Decyl butyrate
Lactones
Aldehydes
Furfural
Terpenes
Limonene
Linalool
(E)-Nerolidol
Alcohols
Hexanol
Octanol
these put together are what you "smell"

from Kafkas and Paydas, *World Journal of Agricultural Sciences* 3(2) 191-195 (2007)

clearscience.tumblr.com/post/610596286/a-list-of-the-volatile-organic-compounds-found-in

A list of the volatile organic compounds found in strawberries includes approximately two dozen chemicals including methyl butyrate, octyl acetate, hexanol, and others. Since these compounds are volatile they may vaporize and if they reach your olfactory receptors you may detect them and identify them as coming from a strawberry.

Therapeutic Options

Many individuals have issues with unpleasant fecal odors, and unfortunately it is not as easily remedied as flushing or walking away. The fecal aroma generated by the gut microbiome that smells in defecated feces is the identical aroma that may be discharged with intestinal gas, fecal incontinence, fistula, ostomies, diarrhea, inflammatory bowel disease, after gastric bypass surgery, and a host of other conditions. The numbers of individuals affected is in the millions in the United States alone. Unfortunately, the majority of the general public remains uninformed and impose a social stigma on a medical condition over which they have limited or no control.

Fortunately there are a number of effective therapeutic options available, but too many sufferers are not aware of or have access to them. They range from external appliances and clothing, to external and internal deodorants and suppressants. Of course there are also tongue-in-cheek suggestions, such as getting a dog to blame as the source of the fart odor. The Merck Manual a few years back suggested working on perfecting one's glare, just glare at someone else as if they were the source.

More direct references to farts have been employed in the advertising campaign of air-freshener company Poo-Pourri. Although the advertising campaign received a nomination as one of the worst ads by a national newspaper, it was a major hit on social media with over thirty million views. For a holiday themed advertisement Santa Claus is farting on the toilet while an attractive model sings a parody of a seasonal tune.

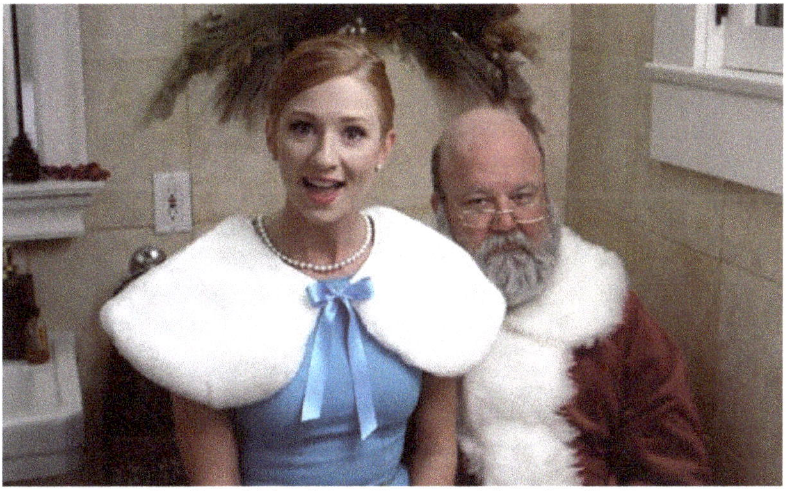

Poo-Pourri Advertising video www.ninjamarkweting.it

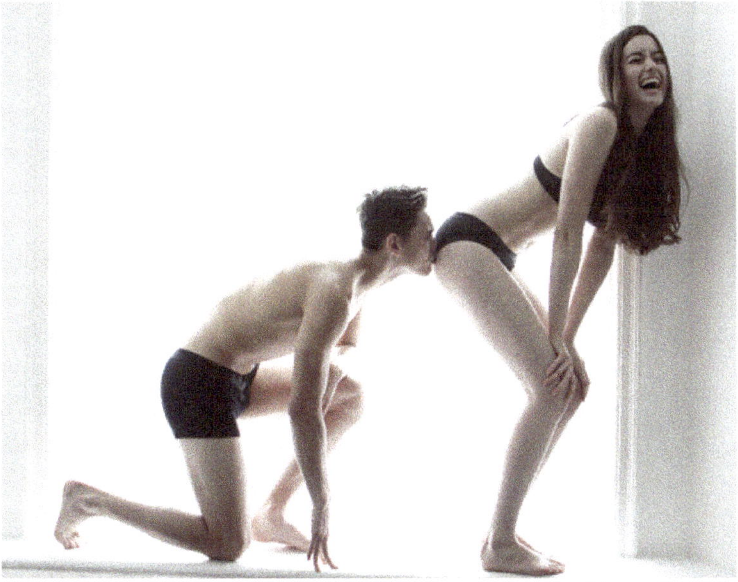

Shreddies advertising campaign for activated charcoal odor adsorbing underwear
myshreddies.com

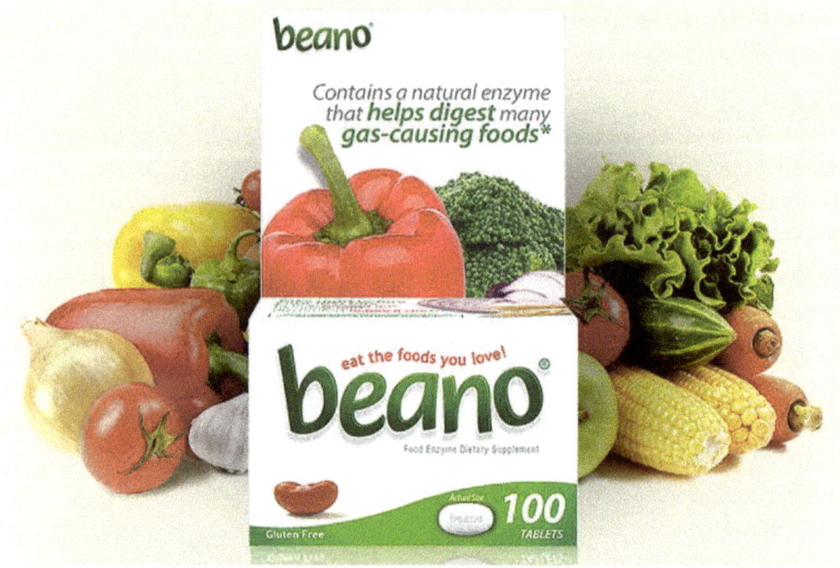
beano
Contains a natural enzyme that helps digest many gas-causing foods*
eat the foods you love!
beano
Food Enzyme Dietary Supplement
Gluten Free
100
TABLETS

Beano was one of the first products to advertise a product designed to reduce intestinal gas. Its ad first appeared in Vegetarian Times

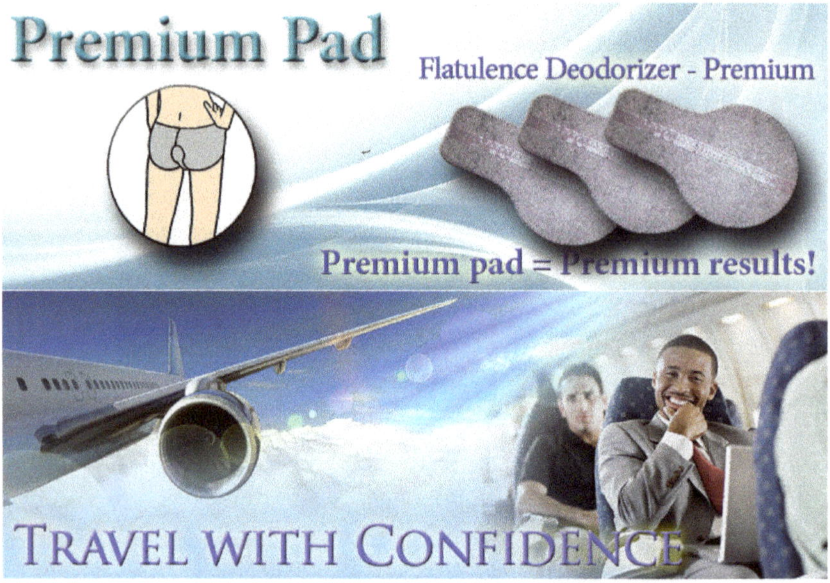
Premium Pad
Flatulence Deodorizer - Premium
Premium pad = Premium results!
TRAVEL WITH CONFIDENCE

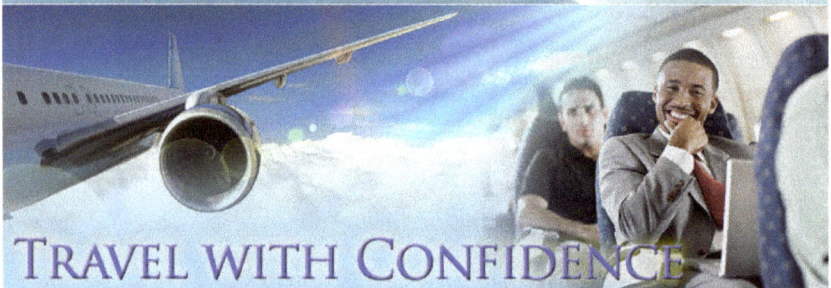

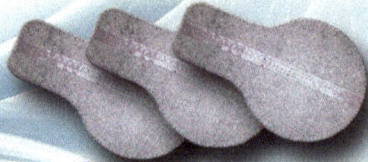

Flat-D advertises and markets a wide variety of activated charcoal products to adsorb the aroma of flatus and other body odors. www.flat-d.com

Surprisingly where it can provide relief and comfort to many sufferers, some media outlets refuse to place advertisements for products dealing with flatulence and ostomy odors. Deodorants, feminine hygiene douches, tampons, sanitary napkins for menstruation, diapers for adults with incontinence, erectile dysfunction prescriptions, etcetera have been seen by the public and the country still stands. Devrom, an effective internal deodorant that suppresses fecal odor was not allowed to place their advertisement in Reader's Digest or AARP (Association for the Advancement of Retired People) because it contained the word stool and smelt flatulence. Somehow the publications did not see the irony in that their policy did not pass the smell test.

Devrom is an over the counter preparation of bismuth subgallate and has been marketed for over fifty years as an internal deodorant. Bismuth does have antibacterial properties it may change the microbiome by reducing the organisms that contribute to offensive flatulence. Another bismuth product that has been popular in the marketplace is Pepto-Bismol, which is a bismuth subsalicylate. Bismuth subsalicylate is related to aspirin (salicylic acid) and does not appear to provide as significant relief from the unpleasant odors as has been reported with Devrom.

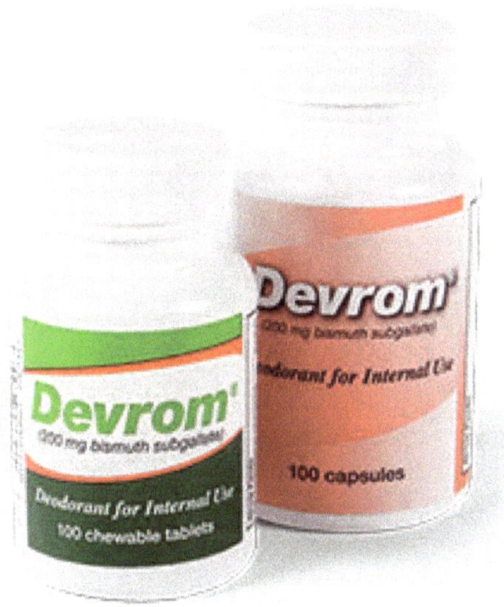
Devrom
100 capsules
Devrom
100 chewable tablets

It has been particularly popular for individuals who have undergone gastric bypass surgery, inflammatory bowel disease, as well as those with ostomies and others. With advances in surgery, and the ability to preserve sphincters or create artificial sphincters, ostomies are seen less frequently. This is where the intestinal discharge exits the body through an artificial opening, the ostomy, created at surgery. Because the bowel is diverted from the colon less moisture is absorbed and the feces may be semi-formed or liquid. The more liquid form allows for the more rapid vaporization of volatile organic compounds and gasses that give rise to the feculent odor. In spite of being in otherwise excellent health, many individuals with these issues find themselves socially restricted in their activities because of concern about embarrassment or offending others. Safe and effective products are available, but many individuals are unaware and suffer unnecessarily because of the lack of information and understanding.

Bismuth is a chemical element, number eighty-three on the periodic table, which has a long history of being used in preparations designed to treat gastrointestinal complaints. It is a heavy metal with a low level of toxicity. Its various compound have also been used historically to treat syphilis and the severe diarrhea from cholera. Bismuthinite is a mineral consisting of bismuth sulfide (Bi_2S_3) and is an important ore for bismuth mining.

The mechanism of action is unknown and may be related to its known antimicrobial activity, perhaps inhibiting the microbes that generate some of the more offensive gasses that are usually contain sulfur as well as aromatic and volatile organic compounds. Bismuth also reacts directly with sulfur generating bismuth sulfide, a dark black insoluble compound. This can cause darkening or blackening of the tongue if sulfur is found in high concentrations in the saliva. It will also cause blackening of the stool as it binds with the sulfur that would otherwise give rise to hydrogen sulfide and other offensive sulfur gasses. The dark black color of the stool may be mistaken for melena, a sign of internal bleeding that results from the digestive process on blood cells and hemoglobin. The black coloration is not a health concern and is temporary clearing with cessation of bismuth intake.

Activated carbon is used to treat oral poisonings by binding to and preventing the poison from being absorbed by the gastrointestinal tract. Charcoal biscuits were marketed in the early 19th century as an antidote to flatulence, and are still marketed today for diarrhea, indigestion, flatulence, and as a pet care product. Unfortunately orally ingested charcoal pills are not effective in appreciably reducing intestinal gas. This may be because the adsorptive capacity of the activated charcoal is fully utilized before it finally gets to the colon where its gas adsorbing properties are needed. Fortunately, bismuth products do provide a significant advantage by binding to the sulfur compounds and eliminating them without producing offensive gas.

Feces, Density

For some unknown reason many people are fixated on the difference between shit that floats and shit that sinks. It is entirely dependent on whether its density is lighter or heavier than water. It used to be thought that a high roughage, high plant fiber diet led to floating stools. It was discovered that was not the case it the secret of floating or sinking stools was related to their methane gas content. Gas being lighter than water, the methane containing stools floated.

Oils and fats are also lighter than water and those with steatorrhea and keriorrhea from fat malabsorption will have not only floating stools, but stools that are considered more foul smelling. This is partly because the stool as it is floating is exposed to the air and can release more odiferous volatile organic compounds and gasses that can then be sensed by the olfactory nerves. Animal fats in particular generated odiferous gases and volatile organic compounds.

Feces Waste Management

In Western society human feces waste management is usually a matter of indoor plumbing, a toilet, and a sewer or septic system. Animal waste, especially of dairy herds, cattle, pig farms, poultry houses, domestic pets, are a source of challenges and often commercialized solutions. Human feces waste management, especially outside of but even within Western society, is a major health and public safety concern. Anal cleansing after defecation was historically accomplished with sticks, leaves, stones, clay, corncobs, water, or literally whatever was available at hand. The ancient Greeks used clay and stone. Romans used a water soaked sponge on a stick. The first recorded use of toilet paper was in China in the sixth century. In France the invention of the bidet in the 1710's made water cleansing popular.

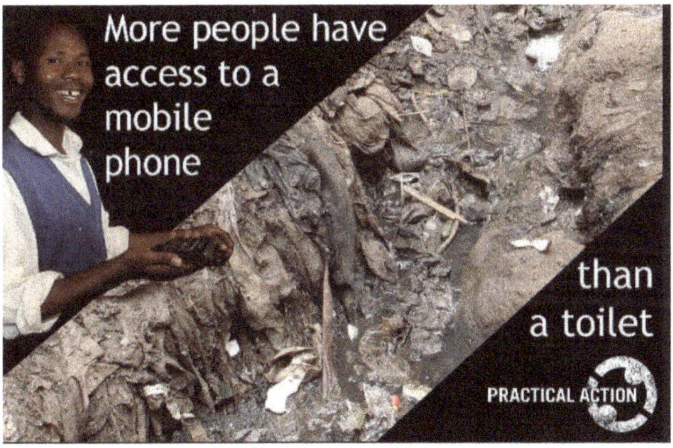
More people have access to a mobile phone
than a toilet
PRACTICAL ACTION
Creative Commons License

Worldwide there are approximately two million fatalities every year due to diarrhea. The majority of these are in children under five years of age. Routine hand washing with soap and water could reduce diarrhea by almost fifty percent and respiratory infections by nearly twenty-five percent. Hand washing also reduces the incidence of skin diseases, eye infections, and intestinal worms and parasites.

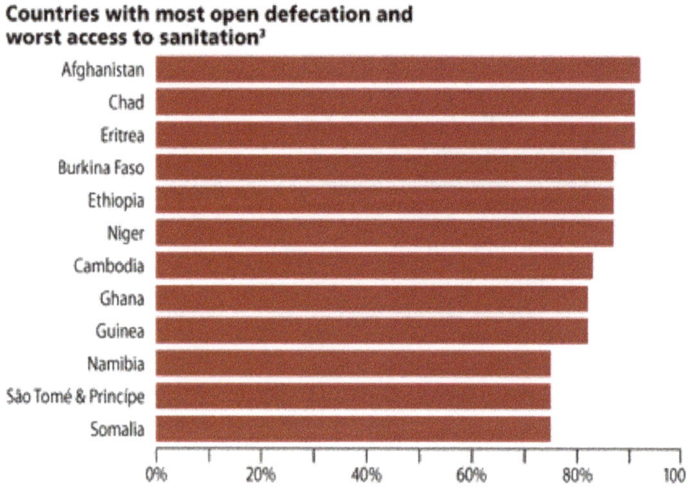
Countries with most open defecation and worst access to sanitation³
Afghanistan
Chad
Eritrea
Burkina Faso
Ethiopia
Niger
Cambodia
Ghana
Guinea
Namibia
São Tomé & Príncipe
Somalia
0%
20%
40%
60%
80%
100

New Internationalist Magazine State of the World's Toilets, WaterAid, 2007, based on data from WHO/UNICEF Joint Monitoring Programme.

Composting Toilet

A composting toilet is a dry toilet that uses managed aerobic decomposition to treat human waste. They are an alternative to flush toilets where there is a limited water supply or no waste treatment facility is available. The human excrement is normally mixed with sawdust, coconut coir, or peat moss to support aerobic processing, absorb liquids, and to reduce odor. The decomposition process is typically faster than the anaerobic decomposition used in wet sewage systems such as septic tanks.

Urine can contain ninety percent of the nitrogen, fifty percent of the phosphorus, and seventy percent of the potassium present in human excreta. In healthy individuals the urine is sterile and thus pathogen free. Undiluted urine may contain inorganic salts and organic compounds toxic to plants. The requirement critical for aerobic microbial action is sufficient oxygen. Some units require manual methods for periodic aeration of the solid mass. Significant reductions in the volume of waste occur through the process with only ten percent of the inputs coming out as a humus-like material, which can be used as a soil amendment.

Pit Toilet

A pit toilet is a dry toilet system, which collects human excrement in a large container and can range from a simple slit trench to a more elaborate outhouse with a ventilation pipe. They are used in rural and wilderness areas as well as in much of the developing world. When the pit is improved with a small enclosed structure with a roof for shelter and a seat with a hole in it is commonly known as an outhouse.

The ventilated improved pit latrine, or VIP, is a pit toilet outhouse with a ventilation pipe and a screen at the top outlet. VIP latrines are an improvement over simple pit latrines by reducing odors, flies, and mosquitoes. nuisance and unpleasant odors. The ventilation pipe also removes the explosive danger of accumulated methane gas from the decomposition of the human waste in the pit.

Sewers

A sewage system may convey the wastewater by gravity, pumping, or vacuum to a sewage treatment plant. Pipelines range in size from six inches (150 mm) to tunnels of up to thirty feet (10 m) in diameter. Although sewer systems are intended to transport only sewage and not storm runoff all sewer systems have some degree of infiltration of groundwater, which can lead to sewer overflows.

The first sanitation system has been identified in prehistoric Ruins near Zabol, Iran. The ancient cities of Harappa and Mohenjo-Daro of the Indus Valley civilization developed networks of brick-lined sewers around 2600 BC and also had outdoor toilets that were flushed with water from reservoirs. Ancient Minoan civilization also had stone sewers that were flushed with water. Roman towns and garrisons in the United Kingdom between 46 BC and 400 AD had sewer networks sometimes constructed out of hollowed-out logs.

In the developed world sewers are usually pipelines from buildings to larger underground trunk mains, which transport the sewage to sewage treatment facilities. Vertical pipes, called manholes, connect the mains to the surface and are used for maintenance and to vent sewer gases. Sewers are generally gravity powered although pumping stations may be necessary. For decades sanitary sewer cracks or other damage could be repaired only by the expensive operation of digging up the damaged pipe and replacing it. In the mid-1950's technology advanced where a special cement mixture coated the inside of the pipe sealing all cracks and breaks.

Many cities built sewer systems to control outbreaks of disease such as typhoid and cholera. Initially these systems discharged sewage directly to surface waters such as rivers and lakes without treatment. As pollution of water bodies grew cities added sewage treatment plants to their systems to chlorinate and filter the water and sewage discharged. The institution of sewerage systems was a great public health advance.

Dung Beetle

Dung beetles are beetles that feed partly or exclusively on feces. All the species belong to the superfamily Scarabaeoidea, which alone comprises more than five thousand species. Many dung beetles known as 'rollers' roll dung into round balls, which are used as a food source or brooding chambers. They can roll up to ten times their weight and some species can pull up to one thousand times their weight. Other dung beetles, known as tunnelers, bury the dung wherever they find it. A third group, the dwellers, neither roll nor burrow: they simply live in manure. Dung beetles are currently the only animals, other than humans, known to navigate and orient themselves using the Milky Way.

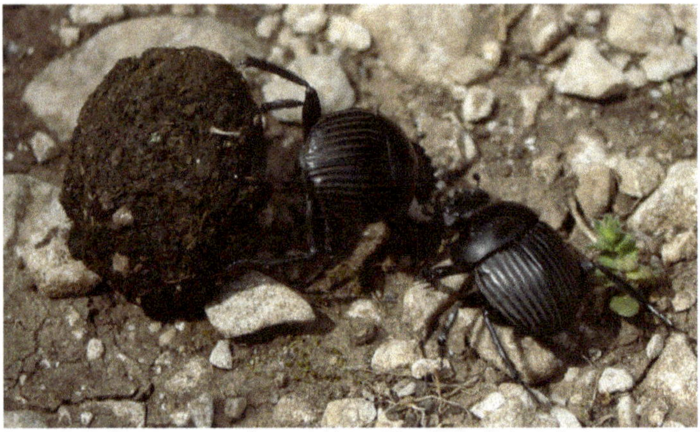

Scarabaeus iaticollis near a nuraghe near Monte Tiscali, Sardinia, Italy Author Rafael Brix
Creative Commons License

Dung beetles play an important role in agriculture. By burying and consuming dung they improve nutrient recycling and soil structure. They also protect livestock such as cattle by removing the dung, which if left in the open could provide habitat for pests. Many countries have introduced the dung beetles for the benefit of animal husbandry and as a means of improving standards of hygiene and public health.

Chamber Pot

A chamber pot (French: pot de chambre) is a pit like receptacle for receiving human waste. It was usually kept in the same chambers and under the sleeping bed, and since the sixteenth century often enclosed in a stool with a lid. Chamber pots were used in ancient Greece at least since the 6th century BC and remained in common use in many parts of the world until the mid-twentieth century. In rural areas lacking indoor plumbing they are still in use today. They have also been modified to serve as bedpans for the ill and disabled. The affectionate term 'potty' is often used with children especially during toilet (potty) training. The term potty is also used to describe the child size chamber pot type toilets that are at the appropriate height for a child. Importantly, they also have a child size opening to sit on.

Regular adult toilets have an opening that is too large and frightening for a child who could accidentally fall in if not assisted. To remind you that their fear is not unjustified American adults suffer 40,000 toilet related injuries per year. Falling off a toilet directly contributed to the death of King George II of Great Britain. The height of the adult toilet does not allow their feet to touch the ground to assist in the squatting maneuver that assists defecation. A footstool to give their feet a place on which to rest can assist squatting, which eases the initiation of a bowel movement and can accelerate toilet training.

Close (Night) Stool

A close stool, also called a necessary or night stool, was in popular use for nearly five hundred years from the sixteenth century until the advent of indoor plumbing. It was an enclosed cabinet at chair height with an opening in the top often covered by a lid. It contained a pewter or earthenware chamber pot. In the nineteenth century it was referred to as a night commode, and in the twentieth century the commode euphemism was extended to the flush toilet.

Gong Farmer

Gong farmer was a term used in Tudor England for the worker who removed human excrement from outhouses, privies, cesspools, and cesspits. 'Gong' is derived from the Old English gang, which means 'to go', and since the eleventh century has been used to refer to a toilet facility, or privy, and its contents. They were only allowed to work at night and later became known as 'night soil men' or 'night man'. The human feces they collected were known as 'night soil' and were used as fertilizer. The emptying of cesspits today is usually accomplished with mechanical suction, by specialized tankers or trucks referred to by the euphemism Honey Truck or Honey Wagon.

Towns usually provided public latrines, known as houses of easement. Cesspits were often placed under cellar floors some of which had wooden chutes to convey the excrement. Cesspits allowed the liquid waste to drain leaving only the solids. Besides the offensive odor, cesspits were a continual problem as the accumulation of solid waste required the services of gong farmers to dig out and remove the excrement. Perhaps to avoid overfilling their cesspit it was not uncommon for the contents of chamber pots to be thrown into the streets from upstairs windows. Despite being well paid, being a gong farmer was not considered an enviable occupation. They were only allowed to work between 9 PM and 5 AM and were permitted to live only in certain areas. Besides the occupational hazard of infectious diseases, concentrations of noxious and toxic gasses sometimes led to fatalities due to asphyxiation.

Gong farmers often employed young boys to fill and lift buckets, known as a form of honey buckets, of excrement out of the pit because of the confined spaces. The excavated solid waste was removed in large barrels, which were loaded onto a horse-drawn cart called the honey cart or wagon. It was not an infrequent event to discover the corpse of an unwanted infant during the clearing of cesspits.

The job is still commonplace in India where it has estimated that up to 1.3 million Indians work with the collection of human waste. These workers are considered the lowest of the untouchable caste. They confine marriage to within its members leading to a waste-collecting caste passing the profession and caste burden on to the next generation. The film *Slumdog Millionaire* showed a brief glimpse of their existence, although the faux waste was actually made of chocolate and peanut butter.

Honey Bucket & Honey Wagon

A honey bucket is a bucket that is used as a toilet in locations that do not have more advanced facilities available. It often has a frame with a toilet seat lid and may be lined with a plastic bag for ease and convenience of disposal. A cover material such as sawdust may be used to reduce the odors from collected waste. Honey buckets are common in the far northern Arctic type climates especially where permafrost makes the installation of septic systems or outhouses impractical. They are seen throughout the world, especially in rural and undeveloped areas.

A honey wagon is a cart, wagon or truck for collecting and carrying excrement or manure. The term is often applied to the trucks that service septic tank systems as well as the bathroom on commercial aircraft. A recent news incident of a motor home bungled burglary was reminiscent of a honeywagon. The police were called to investigate what was presumed to be an attempt to siphon off and steal the gasoline from a parked vacation motor home. They found several empty gasoline transport containers, a length of rubber tubing, along with a pool of fecal material and vomited food.

The nighttime would be fuel thieves opened the flap door, removed the cap, and put the siphon hose in an applied oral suction to start the flow of what they assumes would be gasoline. The thieves opened the cap and valve to the septic system by mistake, got a mouthful of sewage, which they vomited up and fled the scene leaving their paraphernalia behind.

Night Soil

Night soil is the common name used for human fecal waste collected at night from cesspools and outhouses. It is often used as a fertilizer in developing countries where it contributes to the higher risk of acquiring parasites. This is not unexpected because the feces may well be contaminated and contain large quantities of parasite eggs, such as is commonly seen in the roundworm *Ascaris lumbricoides*. Rarely diseases have been transmitted into developed countries by the importation of vegetables with contaminated soil.

The use of night soil as fertilizer was common in Japan. The feces of rich people were sold at higher prices because their diet was better and it was thought that there would be more nutrients remaining in their waste. It brings a new level of understanding to the common phrases "filthy rich" and the "rich get richer".

Selling night soil as fertilizers became less common after World War II for sanitary reasons as well as the increased availability of chemical fertilizers. Modern Japan still has some areas with ongoing traditional night soil collection and disposal. The Japanese name for the 'outhouse within the house' style toilet, with the night soil collected, is Kumitori Benjo (汲み取り便所). China, Singapore, and Hong Kong also had extensive use of night soil collection, especially from urbanized areas where open honey buckets were carried through the streets. Hong Kong has a euphemism called 倒夜香, which literally means "pour night fragrant".

<u>Septage</u>

The partially treated waste in a septic tank that does not drain into the soil or is decomposed by the bacteria in the tank is called septage. This term should not be confused by a septuagenarian who in their 70's may occasionally feel like a septagenarian. It can be transported to local wastewater treatment centers or stored to be used as fertilizer. The septage in a septic tank is usually considered in one of three categories. Scum which floats to the top generally harbors the greatest concentration of bacteria. The layer below is called the effluent and is a semi-treated liquid. The layer of solids at the bottom of the tank is called sludge. A septage pump truck removes the septage material from septic tanks, portable toilets, recreational vehicles such as motor homes, and boats. In commercial aviation and other industries, this type of vehicle may also be called a honey wagon, a reference to sewage collection of ages past.

<u>Open Defecation</u>

This is the terminology used when the feces deposited are left at the site untreated and uncovered. In many impoverished areas this is the unfortunate routine, with contamination of drinking water and public health hazards being the primary concern, with odor and appearance secondary. Some outdoor activity such as hunting, camping, exploring, may also lead to occasional open defecation if the opportunity to bury or cover the feces is not possible. One extreme example is mountaineering or polar expeditions, which bring another risk to open defecation

Frostbite is a real risk for mountaineers, and for Mount Everest climbers the comforts of base camp at an altitude of 17,590 feet may be the last chance they have for a protected bowel movement without exposing their behinds to the extreme winds and weather approaching the summit. Frozen poop stays permanently frozen and does not decompose at that altitude, so there is a growing collection from the open defecation of earlier expeditions that is of concern. Climbers are having a more challenging timed finding ice that has not been contaminated for melting into drinking water. Drinking contaminated water and developing diarrhea would increase the exposure to frostbite dramatically. I propose a new term for the medical malady of frostbite of the buttocks from open defecation in extreme cold, 'frostbutt'.

<u>Outhouse</u>

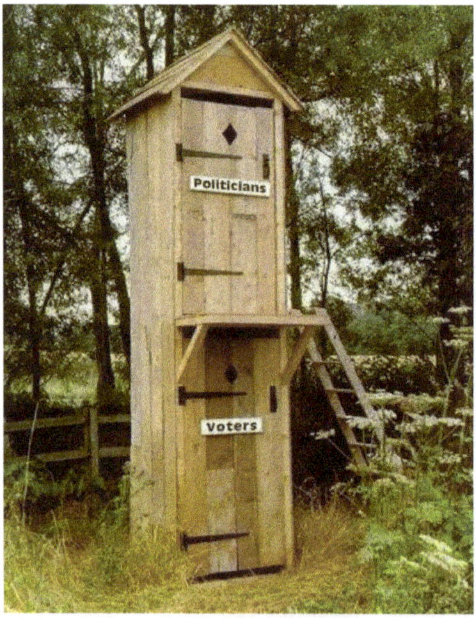
Politicians
Voters

A two-story outhouse with a political satire message. Creative Commons License

Many outhouses are simply holes in the ground, once the capacity is reached a new site is selected and the outhouse structure moved. To avoid the unpleasant odors, outhouses were usually kept a minimum of fifty feet away from a residence. Keeping the waste site away from the source of drinking water is very important from a disease prevention and hygiene perspective. Many of the deaths attributed to military campaigns were actually caused by poor sanitation and waste management. The lack of hygiene and contaminated drinking water frequently led to more deaths and incapacitation of soldiers than those injured or killed in battles.

Toilet Gods

Deities associated with defecation and elimination have an ancient history preceding Babylonian times. They were worshiped in Roman times and still have a role in folk beliefs of indigenous peoples of Japan, China, New Zealand and other parts of the world. Such deities have been associated with bowel health, as well as general well-being and fertility because of the use of human waste as a fertilizer for agriculture.

Ancient Rome had three gods involved in the passage of human waste. The sewer goddess Cloacina (Latin sewer) had her origins in Etruscan beliefs and was the protector of the Cloaca Maxima, Rome's sewage system. Titus Tatius, who ruled early Rome with Romulus, built a shrine to her in his toilet and she was appealed to if sewers backed up. She was also the Goddess protector of sexual intercourse in marriage and her worship was later combined with that of Venus. Her image was placed on Roman coins.

Crepitus was described as the Roman god of flatulence but probably was a fiction created to denigrate Roman theology. He appears as a god in several works of French literature by Voltaire, Baudelaire, and Flaubert as well as material promoting Roman Catholicism as the true faith. **S**tercutius (Latin stercus 'excrement') was the god of dung who was particularly important to farmers when fertilizing their fields with manure. Worshipping the porcelain god, or ceramic throne, is a jocular reference to past toilet worship when heaving into the toilet bowl during vomiting.

Fiber (see Dietary Fiber, Soluble Fiber, Insoluble Fiber)

Flora, Gastrointestinal

Fetuses do accumulate a mass of sterile and odorless greenish feces called meconium, in their intestines. Fetuses usually pass meconium after birth but approximately twelve percent of pregnancies have yellow or green bile pigmented meconium stained amniotic fluid. The risk increases with the length of the pregnancy. In births occurring after forty-two weeks, described as post term, the rate of meconium staining approaches fifty percent. Fetuses have amniotic fluid in their lungs until they take their first breath of air after birth. In a minority of meconium stained amniotic fluid cases potentially fatal meconium aspiration syndrome occurs.

If the newborn fails to pass meconium, a congenital abnormality of the colon needs to be excluded. Hirschsprung disease may involve failure of fetal development of the ganglions of the enteric nervous system. When it involves the colon, the bowel may not relax to allow the passage of meconium or feces and surgery may be required to remove the affected segment of bowel.

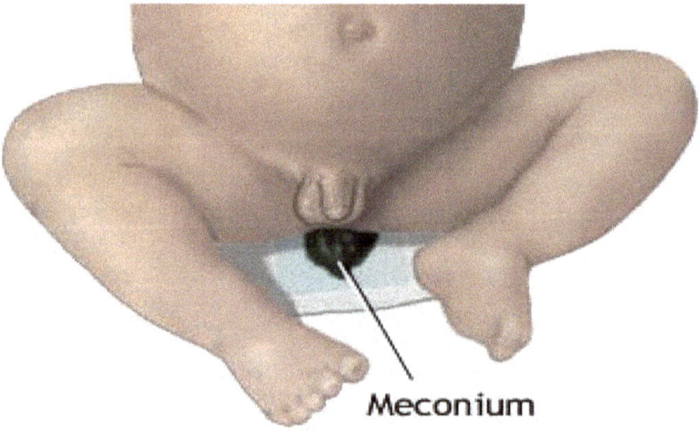
Meconium

www.healthcentral.com Creative Commons License

Since the digestive tract of the newborn is sterile, there are no microorganisms generating gas through cellular metabolism. All of the gas the newborn infant begins to pass is swallowed air. If an infant is bottle fed rather than breast fed they are much more likely to swallow even more air. Baby bottles are a common cause of aerophagia in infants as they suck in and swallow air if the formula does not always cover the nipple. Burping the baby after a feeding is the means of allowing the swallowed air to escape otherwise it will cause distention and discomfort. Some bottles are designed to use an internal plastic sleeve to prevent air from reaching the nipple when the formula is depleted the sleeve forms a vacuum so the infant is not sucking in air.

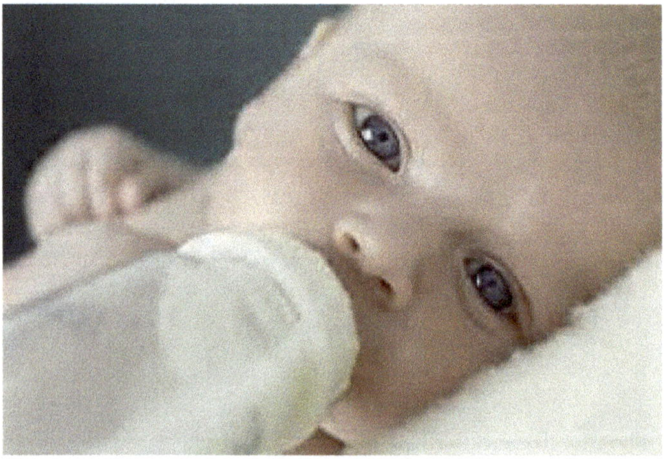

Baby bottles are a common source of aerophagia in infants. If the milk or formula does not completely cover the nipple of the bottle the baby will suck in and swallow air.
www.deltadentaliblog.com Creative Commons License

The first exposure to microorganism that will be swallowed and begin to colonize the infant digestive tract are from the birth mother if the delivery is vaginal and breast-feeding is initiated. The microorganisms that colonize the infant become its microbiome and play a major role in its ongoing health and wellness. The initial gut flora of the infant if born via a vaginal delivery and breast-feeding is identical to the vaginal and skin microbiome of the mother. This initial flora changes over the next few months especially if formula and other milks and foods are introduced. At about three months of age the gut flora is well established, and although changes will occur it is similar to the gut flora it will have as an adult.

The gut flora helps to set the infant's immune system, and it recognizes and tolerates microorganisms that are beneficial known as commensals. One of the theories why breast-feeding is preferable, as well as why a vaginal delivery is preferable to Caesarean section, is the natural microbiome exposure has advantages. The immunity of infants who did receive the natural microbiome from the mother is at a disadvantage. Some experts are advocating exposing the newborn to the mother's vaginal secretions and microbiome if the birth is via a Caesarean section.

The microbiome is established rapidly upon exposure to the environment. Most people think that the digestive tract is an internal organ because it is located inside the body. They are often surprised to find out that that the digestive tract is actually considered an organ exposed to the external environment. It is a long hollow tube exposed to the external environment at both ends, and is transited by material that for the most part comes from outside of the body.

The results of cell division and multiplication are similar between cells of the body, and cells of the microbiome. Mathematically this growth pattern is described as exponential or logarithmic growth. For those more familiar with finance, it is more akin to compounding interest instead of simple arithmetic addition. If a single cell divides into two cells, those cells divide into four cells, those into eight cells, and the numbers increase rapidly.

The colonization and establishment of the microbiome is extremely rapid. The limitation of cellular division and growth of human cells are controlled by genes, hormones, neurotransmitters, and a variety of other feedback control mechanisms. The microbiome is also under the influence of these mechanisms, as well as competition for habitat and nutrition. The gut flora is the gastrointestinal microbiome. The gut microbiome is much more important than most people give it credit for. The microbes of the body far outnumber the number of human cells. The vast majority are commensals or are engaged with us in a symbiotic relationship from which we both benefit.

The normal flora is site specific so that the microbiome of the stomach is different from the small intestine, which is different again from the colon. The appendix serves as a reservoir of the normal large intestinal bacteria flora. It represents the healthy gut microbiome from which the gut flora can be replenished after a bout of intestinal dysentery.

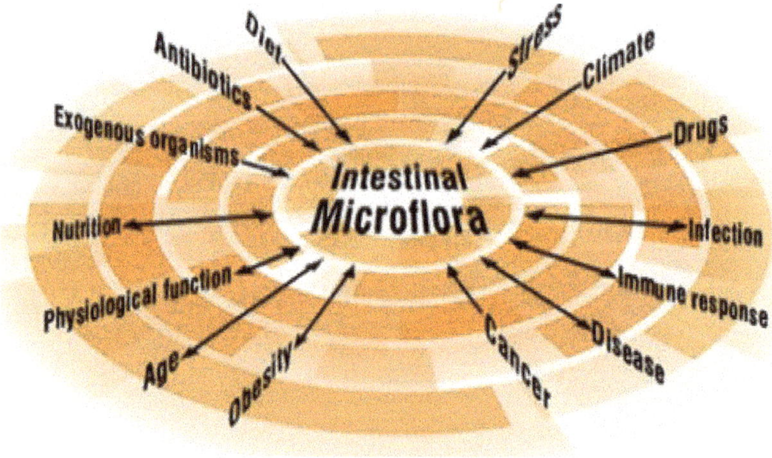
Intestinal
Microflora
Diet
Antibiotics
Exogenous organisms
Nutrition
Physiological function
Age
Obesity
Cancer
Disease
Immune response
Infection
Drugs
Climate
Stress

www.vitahealthstores.ca Creative Commons License

The effect of the microbiome includes microbes, their genomes, and their environmental interactions. Gut flora consists of the microorganisms that live in the digestive tract and are the largest component of the human flora. The gut flora contains approximately one-hundred-trillion microorganisms in the intestinal tract, a number much greater than the ten-trillion cells of the human body. The gut flora has approximately one-hundred times as many genes as the human genome.

The human genome has twenty-three thousand genes and the human microbiome genome exceeds over one-million genes and still counting. Any one or combination of these genes, human and/or microbial, can play a very important role in health and disease. Alterations in an individual's flora may occur with changes in lifestyle, diet, illness, and age. The National Institutes of Health has embarked on the Human Microbiome Project to identify the organisms present in the human microbiome and their role in health and disease.

Anaerobic bacteria make up most of the microbial flora of the colon and up to sixty percent of the dry mass of feces. These micro-organisms perform a variety of metabolic activities that benefit the host, so much so that some scientists refer to it as the 'forgotten organ'. Their metabolic activity includes extracting energy from undigested carbohydrates by fermentation and absorption of short chain fatty acids. They also synthesize vitamin B and vitamin K, as well as metabolizing bile acids and lipids.

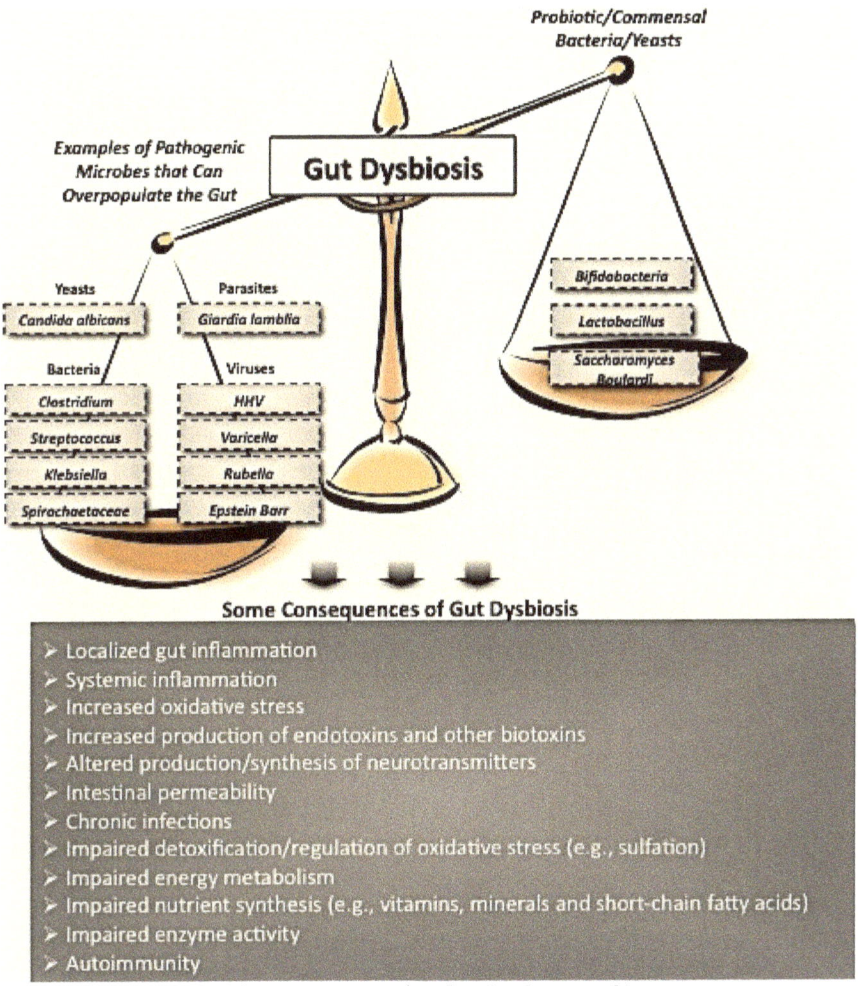
Probiotic/Commensal Bacteria/Yeasts
Examples of Pathogenic Microbes that Can Overpopulate the Gut
Gut Dysbiosis
Yeasts
Candida albicans
Parasites
Giardia lamblia
Bacteria
Clostridium
Streptococcus
Klebsiella
Spirochaetaceae
Viruses
HHV
Varicella
Rubella
Epstein Barr
Bifidobacteria
Lactobacillus
Saccharomyces Boulardi
Some Consequences of Gut Dysbiosis
Localized gut inflammation
Systemic inflammation
Increased oxidative stress
Increased production of endotoxins and other biotoxins
Altered production/synthesis of neurotransmitters
Intestinal permeability
Chronic infections
Impaired detoxification/regulation of oxidative stress (e.g., sulfation)
Impaired energy metabolism
Impaired nutrient synthesis (e.g., vitamins, minerals and short-chain fatty acids)
Impaired enzyme activity
Autoimmunity

www.epidemicanswers.org/wp Creative Commons License

The gut flora also prevents pathogens from colonizing the intestines through competitive exclusion, also known as the 'barrier effect'. The bacteria stimulate the immune system lymphoid tissue to produce antibodies to pathogens, and to recognize and not develop an immune response to beneficial flora.

One of the major advances in the understanding of microbial life has come about with the recent advances in genomics technology. This technology now allows the rapid and precise identification of organisms that could not be identified because they were too fastidious and difficult to culture from stool specimens. These advances include the discovery of extremophiles, organisms that can live in extreme environments, and represent a previously undiscovered form of life called Archaea. This has prompted a reevaluation of the biological system of taxonomy, the categorizing of life forms. Most scientists now recognize six separate kingdoms: Animals (Animalia), Plants (Plantae), Fungi, Bacteria, Protozoan (Protista), and Archaea.

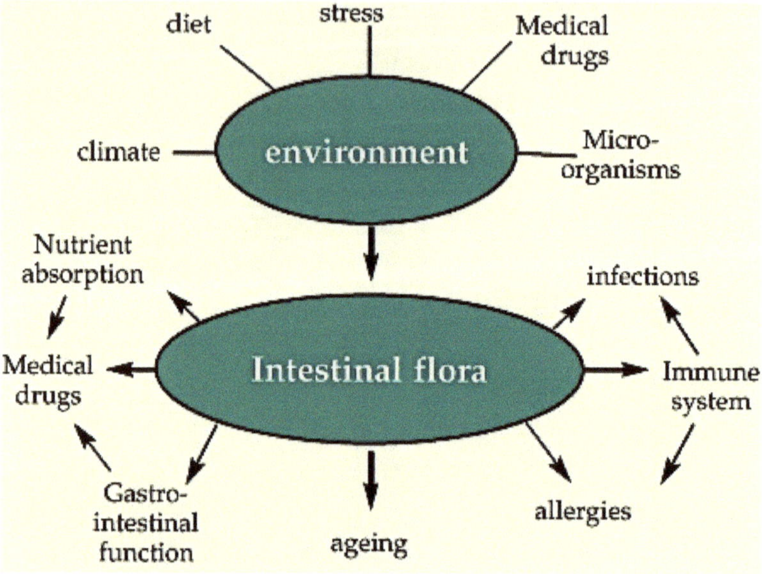
diet
stress
Medical drugs
climate
environment
Micro-organisms
Nutrient absorption
infections
Medical drugs
Intestinal flora
Immune system
Gastro-intestinal function
ageing
allergies

www.positivehealth.com Creative Commons License

Significant portions of the human microbiome are not bacteria at all and are actually Archaea. In fact, the methane produced in flatus comes from the methanogenic Archaea of the colon's microbiome. There will undoubtedly be major advances in the understanding of human health and diseases as the microbiome is explored and understood. The hygiene hypothesis proposes that a lack of early childhood exposure to infectious agents, parasites, and symbiotic microorganisms in the gut flora suppresses the development of the immune system. It is proposed that allergies, autoimmune disorders, and diseases seen at higher rates in the developed world may be due to excessive hygiene preventing the exposure necessary for optimal health. The hygiene hypothesis is supported by epidemiological data, yet the topic remains controversial with extensive research ongoing.

As a result of the hygiene hypothesis, helminthic infections emerged as a possible explanation of the low incidence of immunological disorders and autoimmune diseases in less developed countries. Helminthic therapy is the treatment of autoimmune diseases and immune disorders by means of deliberate infestation with a roundworm parasite. It is currently being studied as a promising treatment for several (non-viral) autoimmune diseases including Crohn disease, multiple sclerosis, asthma, and ulcerative colitis.

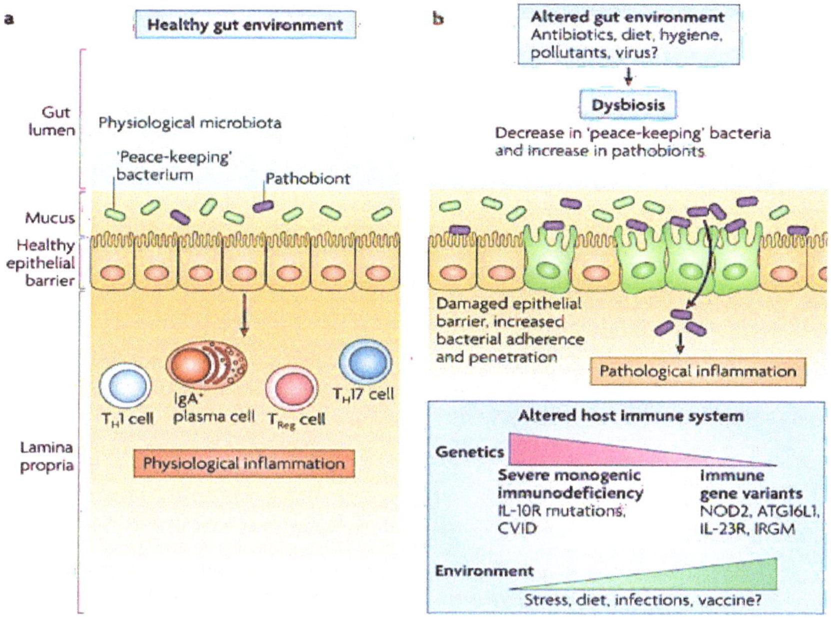
a
Healthy gut environment
Gut lumen
Physiological microbiota
'Peace-keeping' bacterium
Pathobiont
Mucus
Healthy epithelial barrier
IgA+ plasma cell
T_H1 cell
T_Reg cell
T_H17 cell
Lamina propria
Physiological inflammation
b
Altered gut environment
Antibiotics, diet, hygiene, pollutants, virus?
Dysbiosis
Decrease in 'peace-keeping' bacteria and increase in pathobionts
Damaged epithelial barrier, increased bacterial adherence and penetration
Pathological inflammation
Altered host immune system
Genetics
Severe monogenic immunodeficiency
IL-10R mutations, CVID
Immune gene variants
NOD2, ATG16L1, IL-23R, IRGM
Environment
Stress, diet, infections, vaccine?

mikemutzel.com/wp Creative Commons License

The anti-inflammatory effects of helminth infection are also prompting research into diseases that are not currently considered to have an immune basis. For example, heart disease and arteriosclerosis both have similar epidemiological and inflammatory profiles to the autoimmune diseases. Presently the two versions of helminthic therapy being studied are *Trichuris suis* ova and *Necator americanus* larvae.

Dysbiosis (dysbacteriosis) refers to a condition with microbial imbalances on or inside the body. Dysbiosis is most prominent in the digestive tract or on the skin, but can also occur on any surface or mucous membrane exposed to the environment such as the vagina, lungs, mouth, nose, sinuses, ears, nails, or eyes. It has been associated with different illnesses, such as inflammatory bowel disease, as imbalances in the intestinal microbiome may be associated with bowel inflammation and chronic fatigue syndrome.

Microbial colonies found on or in the body are normally benign or beneficial. These beneficial and appropriately sized microbial colonies carry out a series of helpful and necessary functions, such as aiding in digestion. They also protect the body from the penetration of and infection with pathogenic microbes. These beneficial microbial colonies compete with each other for space and resources. When this balance is disturbed by any of a variety of causes, such as antibiotic exposure, the balance of the microbial populations becomes disturbed. This can lead to an overgrowth of one or more of the organisms, which then may have a negative effect on some of the beneficial organisms. The imbalance and negative impacts can initiate a vicious cycle with further disruption from the normal flora.

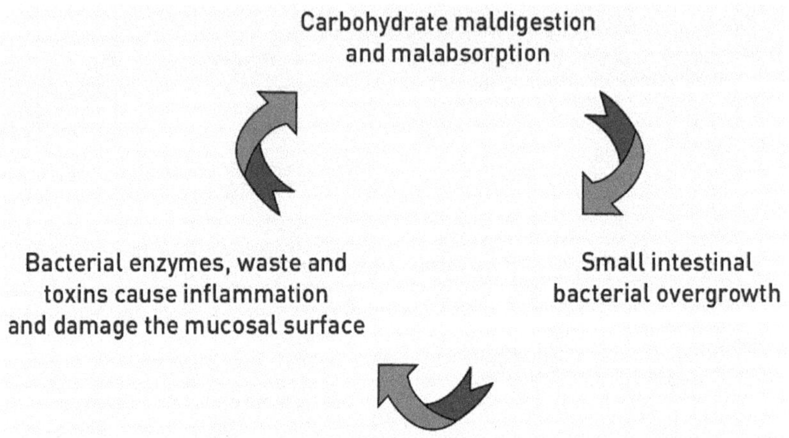
Carbohydrate maldigestion
and malabsorption
Small intestinal
bacterial overgrowth
Bacterial enzymes, waste and
toxins cause inflammation
and damage the mucosal surface

digestivehealthinstitute.org/wp Creative Commons License

Small intestinal bacterial overgrowth (SIBO) is a disorder of excessive bacterial growth in the small bowel. Risk factors included decreased motility or anatomical changes that lead to stasis, immune deficiencies, and reflux of bacteria from the colon into the small bowel such as the surgical removal of the ileocecal valve. The symptoms of bacterial overgrowth may include nausea, vomiting, bloating, flatus, chronic diarrhea, constipation, abdominal discomfort, weight loss, malnutrition, and anemia from vitamin B_{12} deficiency.

Irritable bowel syndrome (IBS) may have an association with small intestinal bacterial overgrowth with some studies showing improvement after treatment. Rosacea, a dermatological condition, also appears to have an association with improvement after treatment. Small bowel bacterial overgrowth syndrome is treated with antibiotics, and if retreatment is required, various antibiotics may be given in a cyclic fashion.

Continued in Volume Two

Afterword

To 'Air' is Human, Everything You Ever Wanted to Know About Intestinal Gas is a uniquely informative, entertaining, and well-illustrated. It covers everything you ever wanted to know about the fart, burp, and bloat but were too embarrassed to ask. Intestinal gas has been produced and released by virtually every human who has ever lived, yet very few people have been provided with the knowledge that can offer comfort and relief. This volume is overflowing with practical information, fascinating facts, surprising trivia, and tasteful humorous insight about this universal phenomenon. Extensive knowledge about the physiology and science of the digestive process and intestinal gas is clearly explained. The knowledge gained will contribute to your enhanced health and comfort, and sharing this wisdom with others can leave a lasting impression on friends and family.

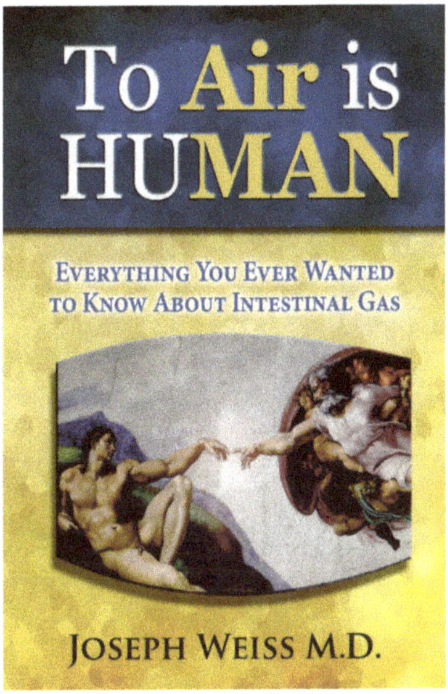
To Air is HUMAN
Everything You Ever Wanted to Know About Intestinal Gas
Joseph Weiss M.D.

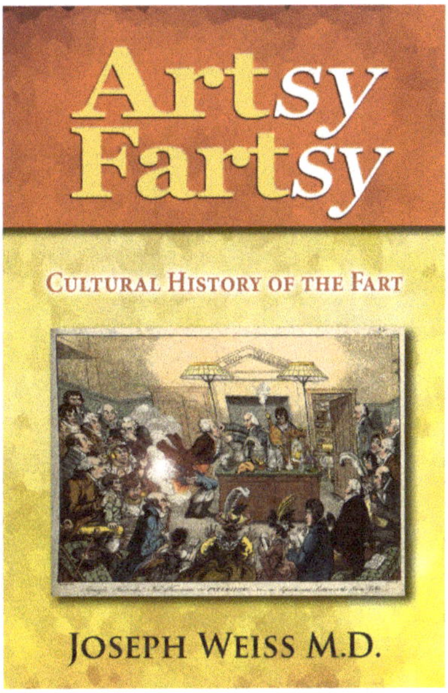
Artsy Fartsy
Cultural History of the Fart
Joseph Weiss M.D.

Artsy Fartsy, Cultural History of the Fart is a fascinating and factually correct review of the common fart through human culture and history. The cough, sneeze, hiccup, stomach rumble, burp, belch, and other bodily sounds simply cannot compete with the notoriety of the fart. Whether encountered live and in person or through the medium of literature, television, film, art, or music it may leave a powerful and lingering memory. The intent of the book is to demonstrate that the ubiquitous fart has a more illustrious story to share than just lowbrow humor. The societal standards and cultural acceptance of this normal physiologic event have evolved over the years, and it is currently popular as a point of humor even in sophisticated circles. The history of the fart in culture and society is a seldom told but fascinating tale.

How Do You Doo? Everybody Pees & Poops! A delightfully informative, entertaining, and colorfully illustrated volume with valuable practical insights on toilet training. Tasteful color photographs of animals answering the call of nature allows the child to understand that everybody does it! Additional informative relevant content to entertain the adult while the child is 'on the potty' is included.

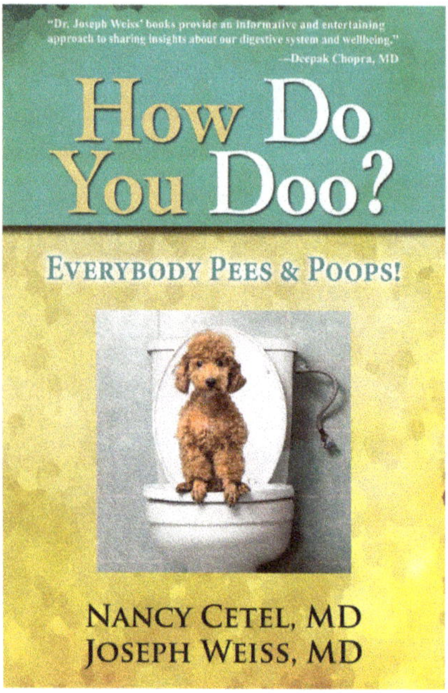
"Dr. Joseph Weiss' books provide an informative and entertaining approach to sharing insights about our digestive system and wellbeing."
—Deepak Chopra, MD
How Do You Doo?
Everybody Pees & Poops!
Nancy Cetel, MD
Joseph Weiss, MD

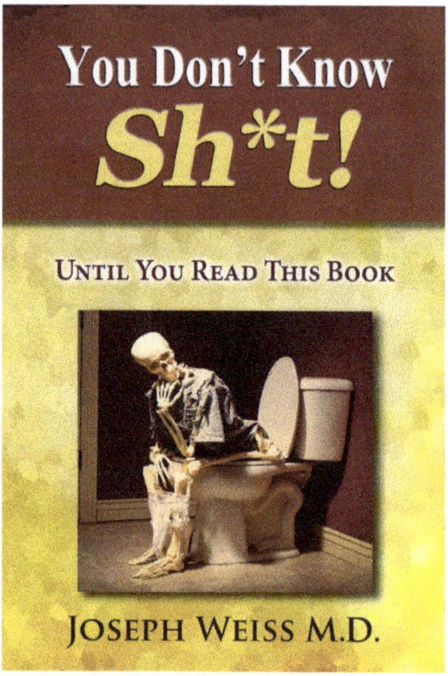
You Don't Know Sh*t!
Until You Read This Book
Joseph Weiss M.D.

The identical content of ***The Scoop on Poop, Flush with Knowledge*** has been provocatively and cheekily retitled as ***You Don't Know Sh*t! Until You Read This Book***. This volume is an informative, entertaining and colorfully illustrated fountain of knowledge that is full of valuable information, including eccentricities and peculiarities, about the remains of the digestive process. Although this end result is politely described as feces or excrement, it is more commonly known by one of oldest words in the English language, shit. The book covers everything you ever wanted to know about this subject. Whether you disdain it, or appreciate it, it is part of the human (and animal) experience. The purpose of this volume is to share rarely discussed but very important knowledge about poop. The information ranges from the potentially life-saving to the sidesplitting descriptions of the eccentricities and peculiarities of human behavior on the subject matter. The wealth of information and trivia can sustain a long social conversation, or cut it short abruptly!

AirVeda: Ancient & New Medical Wisdom, Digestion & Gas covers the remarkable advances in the understanding of digestive health and wellness. New information about the critical role of genomics, epigenetics, the gut microbiome, and the gut-brain-microbiome-diet axis are opening new avenues to optimal whole body health and wellness. An appreciation of the ancient wisdom of Ayurveda and other disciplines shows that they had advanced insights into the nature of the human body and the holistic approach. Although intestinal gas, basic bodily functions, and feces have been topics culturally suppressed, knowledge and understanding are needed to achieve and maintain optimal health. This volume, and others in the series, provide an informative and entertaining in depth look at the amazing world of human health and digestion.

"Ayurveda is a 5,000 year old system of natural healing that reminds us that health is the balanced and dynamic integration between our environment, body, mind and spirit. In Dr. Joseph Weiss' book, AirVeda, he provides an informative and entertaining approach to sharing insights about our digestive system and wellbeing by applying the ancient wisdom of Ayurveda to everyday life." **Deepak Chopra, MD**

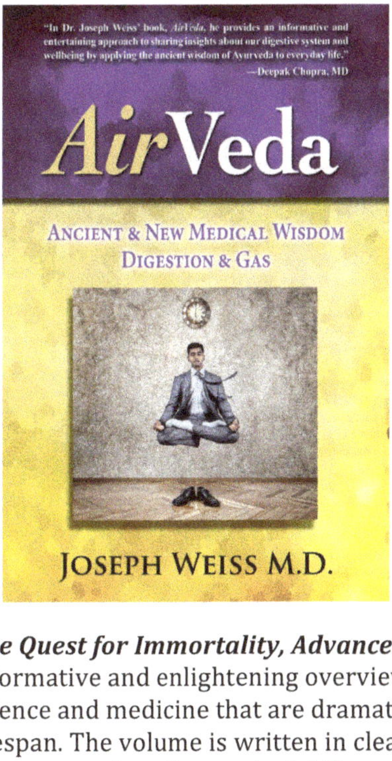
"In Dr. Joseph Weiss' book, AirVeda, he provides an informative and entertaining approach to sharing insights about our digestive system and wellbeing by applying the ancient wisdom of Ayurveda to everyday life."
—Deepak Chopra, MD
AirVeda
ANCIENT & NEW MEDICAL WISDOM
DIGESTION & GAS
JOSEPH WEISS M.D.

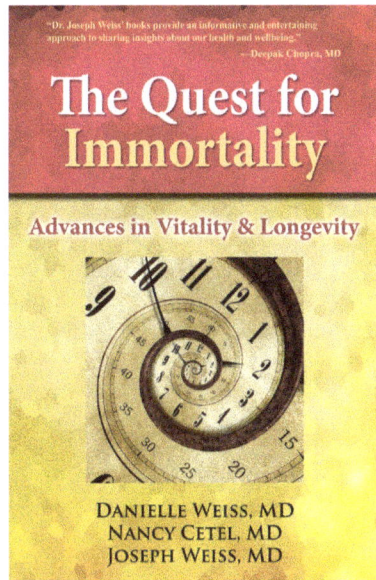

"Dr. Joseph Weiss' books provide an informative and entertaining approach to sharing insights about our health and wellbeing."
—Deepak Chopra, MD
The Quest for Immortality
Advances in Vitality & Longevity
DANIELLE WEISS, MD
NANCY CETEL, MD
JOSEPH WEISS, MD

The Quest for Immortality, Advances in Vitality & Longevity provides an informative and enlightening overview of the remarkable advances in science and medicine that are dramatically enhancing human health and lifespan. The volume is written in clear, understandable, and engaging language with striking colorful illustrations. From groundbreaking nanotechnology to genomics and stem cells, the secrets of vitality and longevity are being uncovered along with more traditional advances and practical insights into disease prevention and health enhancement.

An even more comprehensive yet entertaining series are the extensive volumes of ***Digestive Health & Disease, An Illustrated Encyclopedia of Everything You Ever Wanted To Know About Digestion & Nutrition***. These volumes are a uniquely informative, entertaining, and lavishly illustrated compendium of alimentary knowledge and eccentricities. It covers everything you ever wanted to know about digestion and nutrition in health and disease. Volumes One through Five are available on Amazon.com.

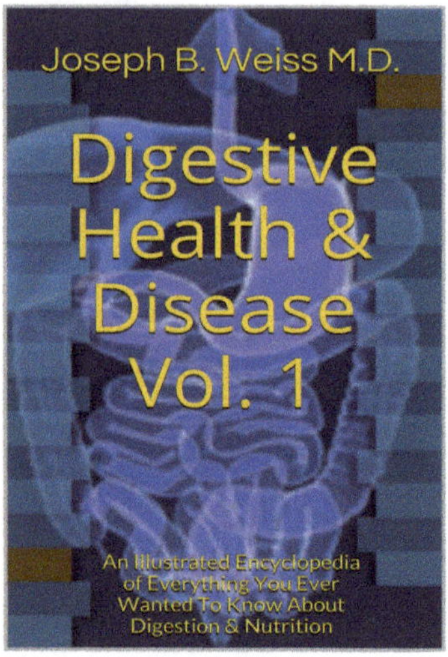
Joseph B. Weiss M.D.
Digestive Health & Disease Vol. 1
An Illustrated Encyclopedia of Everything You Ever Wanted To Know About Digestion & Nutrition

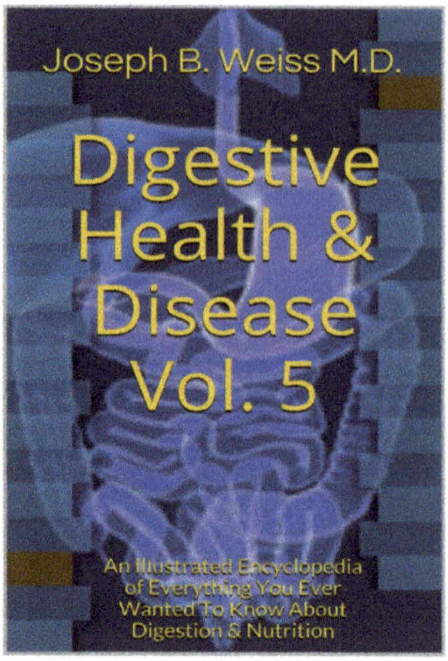
Joseph B. Weiss M.D.
Digestive Health & Disease Vol. 5
An Illustrated Encyclopedia of Everything You Ever Wanted To Know About Digestion & Nutrition

Organized as a reader friendly encyclopedia, the volumes cover over two thousand five hundred subject topics. Each volume may be utilized as an independent fully contained resource for the subjects it covers. The extensive size and scope of the series allows topics to be included that are rarely discussed in other books in the field and may be of great interest to the curious mind.

Written for the intelligent lay public, the medical and scientific terminology is translated into plain English. Practical and useful information and guidance are the primary goals, but entertaining and interesting information is included wherever possible. Designed for the visual learner as well, the clearly written text is supplemented by excellent photographs, illustrations, and charts. The reader will be informed, entertained, and the beneficiary of their newfound understanding of the universal process of digestion and metabolism that is the basis of all healthy living. The website www.smartaskbooks.com has a complete list of books and programs.

Appendix A – Feces/Shit in Foreign Languages

Afrikaans: kak, shit
Albanian: mut
Arabic: القرف, khara
Armenian: kʿakʿ
Azerbaijani: pox, pokh
Basque: kaka, shit
Bengali: হাগু, hagu
Bulgaria: лайно , lajno, podqyolite, govno
Cantonese: puk gai
Catalan: merda
Chinese (Simplified): 屁
Chinese (Traditional : 屁話
Creole: kaka, pora
Croatian: govno, sranje
Czech: hovno, sakra
Danish: lort
Dari (Farsi): برين.
Dutch: stront poep, kak, stront
English: Shit (American), shite (British)
Estonian: pask, sitt
Filipino: tae
Finnish: paska kakka
French: merde crotte
Galician: merda
Georgian: shit, mjǧneri
German: ScheiÃŸe, Scheiße, Kacke, sheisse
Greek: skata
Haitian Creole: chi
Hebrew: khara
Hind : मल
Hungarian: szar
Icelandic: skÃ-t
Indonesian: omong, kosong, eek, tahi, tai
Irish: cac, shite
Italian: merda, schifezza, escrementi, cacca
Japanese: たわごと, tawagoto, kuso, shimata,
Javanese: taek
Khmer: eih
Korean: 똥, sheeba
Latvian: sÅ«di sūds
Lebanese: Khara
Lithuanian: šūdas

Macedonia: gomna, lajna
Malay: omong, kosong, shitta, taik
Maltese: shit
Mandarin: osik, da bien
Maori: teko, tiko
Norwegian: dritt, pokker
Pakistan: tutti, tattie
Panjabi: tutti, bakvas
Persian: گه
Polish: łajno gówno, gswno
Portugese: merda, bosta, caca
Romanian: rahat căcat
Russian:дерьмó (ru) n (der'mó), говнó (ru) n (govnó), гомнó)
Samoan: ki'o, kae
Serbian: serem
Shona: duzyi, dhodi, godzva
Slovak: hovno
Slovenian: drek
Spanish: mierda
Sudanese: busiat, yaloo
Swahili: shit
Swedish: skit
Tagalog: tae
Thai: kee, òotjaará
Tibetan: kyakpa
Tongan: kasele, tae
Turkish: bok
Ukrainian: hiyno
Urdu: شٹ
Vietnamese: cứt
Welsh: cacha
Yiddish: דרעק drek
Zulu: kaka

Appendix B - Euphemisms for Feces/Shit

Bake a brownie
Bake a loaf
Bake a potato
Bake a russet
Barbarians at the gate
Big brown man knocking on the back door
Blow Mud
B.M.
Bomb the Bowl
Bowel movement
Build a dookie castle
Carpet bombing
Choke a brownie
Choke a darkie
Chop a log
Commit yourself to the dumpatorium
Conduct a movement
Cook a brown carrot
Cook a brown kielbasa
Cook a butt burrito
Cook a meat loaf in the porcelain saucepan
Cook some chocolate
Cook some fudge
Cook some sausage
Cook up a pot of anal stew
Crap
Curl some pipe
Debulk
Defecate
Disembowel
Disemfiber
Do the Royal Squat
Doo-doo
Download some brownware
Draw mud
Drill for mud bunnies
Drop
Drop Loggy Log
Drop Smokies (when camping in the winter)
Drop a bomb
Drop a brown trout
Drop a deuce
Drop a dookie
Drop a load

Drop a log
Drop a stool
Drop anchor
Drop the kids off at the lake/pool
Drop wolf bait
Drop your ordinance
Dump
Dump a stump
Eagle Shit (euphemism for U.S. military or government salary)
Enjoy a meatball sandwich
Evacuate
Fill the peanut butter jar
Float a trout
Give birth to a Marine
Give birth to a packy
Go Fecen'
Go into labor
Grow a Tail
Hatch a new boss
Hatch a new superintendent
Have a shit
Heave a Havana
Hit paydirt
Launch a Butt Shuttle
Launch a torpedo
Lay a brick
Lay a cable
Lay a log
Lay some cable
Load the crapper
Log out
Make a core dump
Make a delivery
Make a deposit
Make a deposit at the porcelain bank
Make a doo-doo
Make a log entry
Make grunt sculpture
Make mud
Make number two
Make room for lunch
Make some fertilizer
Number two
Offload some freight
Pack your underwear

Paint the bowl (especially for a really wet one)
Paint with the brown stuff
Park some bark
Park your breakfast
People who like sausages shouldn't see how they're made!!
Pinch a loaf
Plant some corn
Play at the Toilet Bowl
Poke the turtle's head out
Poop
Punish the porcelain
Put fruit in the bowl
Recycle fiber
Release your payload
Ride the hoop
Roll a Nut Log
Roll a log
Saw off a log
Seek revenge for the Brown Bomber
Shake a brown bomber
Shit a brick
Shit on a brick (euphemism for inedible food)
Sink a link
Sink a sausage
Sink the Bismark
Sit on the bowl
Sit on the can
Sit on the throne
Snap a log
Spray and wipe
Squat
Squeeze a coily
Squeeze a loaf
Squeeze one out
Squeeze the cheese
Stain the porcelain
Study at the Library
Taint the cloth
Take a Doogie
Take a dump
Take a growler
Take a load off your mind
Take a shit
Take a steamer
Test the plumbing

Visit the toilet for a poo-poo
Void your bowels
Zap the porcelain

Index (including Volume Two)

Afterword 231-234
Alimentary Canal & Tract (see Digestion)
Alli (see Orlistat)
Anal Canal 20-22
Anal Columns 23-24
Anal Expulsiveness 24
Anal Glands 25
Anal Glands, Musk 26
Anal Glands, Skunk 27
Anal Hygiene 28-40
Anal Hygiene, Toilet Contamination 41-43
Analingus 44
Anal Reflex 45
Anal Retentive 47
Anal Sex 51
Anal Sphincter, External 48
Anal Sphincter, Internal 49
Anal Stimulation 51
Anal Valves 52
Anal Wink 53
Anoscopy 53
Appendix A (Foreign Languages - Feces/Shit) 235-236
Appendix B (Euphemisms - Feces/Shit) 237-240
Archaea (see Microbiome) 310
Aroma, Feces 54-75
Aromatic Amino Acids (see Feces, Aroma) 65, 209
Asshole 74
Assume 75
Autointoxication 75
Ayurveda 75-77
Bacteria (see Microbiome) 310
Barium Enema 78
Bashful Bowel 78
Bidet 79
Bismuth 81-82
Blue Ice Fall 83
Bowel 84
Bowel Management 84
Bowel Movement 85
Bowel Sounds 88
Bristol Stool Scale 88
Bullshit 89
Carcinoid Syndrome 138, 295
Cathartic 89

Chagas Disease 181, 188, 197
Chamber Pot 91, 218-219
Chickenshit 92
Close (Night) Stool 92, 219
Clyster 161-175
Coffee, Enema 171
Coffee, Kopi Luwak 277-278
Colon 92-93, 285-286
Colonic Hydrotherapy 161-175
Colonic Hydrotherapy, Proctoclysis 94, 174
Colonography 95-97
Colonoscopy 98-102
Composting Toilet 102-103, 216
Constipation 103-107
Constitutional 108
Continence, Fecal 108-113
Coprolith 113-114
Coprographia 115-116
Coprolalia 117
Coprology 117-118
Coprophagia 118-128
Coprophilia 128
Copropraxia 128-129
Defecation 129-134
Defecation, Open 221-222
Defecography 134-135
Dentate Line 135-136
Deoxyribonucleic Acid (DNA) 136-137, 177-180
Diarrhea 137-144
Dietary Fiber 144-148
Digestion 8-18, 148-154
Digestive Health & Disease 7, 407
Dumping Syndrome 239-240
Dung 155
Dung Beetle 155-157, 217-218
Dung Fuel 157-160
Dysbiosis (see Microbiome) 223-230, 310-352
Encopresis 160-161
Enema 161-175
Enteric Nervous System 175-178, 241
Epigenetics 135-136, 178-181
Eproctophilia 182
Euphemism, Feces/Shit 237-240
Evacuatory Dysfunction 182-183
Excrement 183-184

Exercise 185
Fart 185-188
Fatty Acids 63-64, 208
Fecal Continence 108
Fecal Impaction 188-190
Fecal Incontinence 191-195, 264-268
Fecalith 197-198
Fecal Occult Blood 196-197
Fecaloma 197-198
Fecal Oral Contamination Route 198-200
Fecal Transplant 200
Feces 201-202
Feces, Aroma 202-214
Feces, Density 214-215
Feces, Euphemism 237-240
Feces, Foreign Language 235-236
Feces Waste Management 215-223
Fiber 143-147, 269-271
Flora, Gastrointestinal 223-230, 310-352
Foreign Language, Feces/Shit 236-237
Fungi (see Microbiome)
Gastrocolic Reflex 230-231
Gastroenteritis 231
Gastroenterology 232
Gastrointestinal Bleeding 195-196, 373-377
Gastrointestinal Microbiome (Flora) 223-230, 310-352
Gastrointestinal Motility 232-241
Gastrointestinal Nervous System 175-178, 241
Gastrointestinal Pacemaker Cells 233-234
Gastrointestinal Tract (see Digestion)
Gastrointestinal Transit Time 234-235
Gastroparesis 235-236
Genetics 177
Genomics 177
Gong Farmer 219-220, 241-242
Groom of the Stool 242-243
Guano 243-246
Gut-Brain-Microbiome-Food Axis 246-249
Gut Feeling 249-250
Gut Flora 223-230, 310-352
Gut Instincts 248-249
Hemorrhoid 250-253
Hirschsprung Disease 104, 181, 188, 197, 222, 298, 313
Honey Bucket & Honey Wagon 220, 253-254
Horseshit 254-256

Housefly, Coprophagia 123-124
Hydrogen 256-258
Hydrogen Sulfide 258-262
Ileum 262-265
Impaction, Fecal 187-189
Incontinence, Fecal 191-195, 265-269
Index 241-246
Indole 60, 204-205, 269-270
Insoluble Fiber 143-147, 270-272
Intestinal Fortitude 273
Intestinal Gas 184-187
Intestinal Tract (see Digestion)
Intestinal Transit Time 231-240
Intestine (see Digestion)
Introduction 5-7
Irritable Bowel Syndrome 273-274
Jejunum 275-276
Kellogg, John Harvey (see Enema, Microbiome)
Keriorrhea 276-277
Klismaphilia 277
Kopi Luwak Coffee 125-126, 278-279
Kudu Dung Spitting (see Coprophagia) 127-128
Lactose Intolerance 280-285
Large Bowel (Large Intestine) 285-286
Laxative 89, 286-291
Laxative Abuse & Dependence 290-291
Levator Ani 291-293
Malabsorption & Maldigestion 293-295
Manure 295-298
Mass Movements 236-237, 298
Meconium 298-299
Megacolon 188
Melena 299
Mercaptans (see Feces, Aroma) 61-62, 206-207
Methane 300-309
Methanethiol 62-63, 207
Microbiome, Gut 223-230, 246-249, 310-352
Mind-Body Connection 249-250, 352-353
Motilin 237, 361
Motility Disorders 232-241
Mucoid Plaque 353-355
Mucus 355-356
Murphy's Drip 94, 174, 356
Naloxegol 105, 189
Naloxone 105,189

Narcotics 105, 189
Night Soil 355-356
Night Stool 220-221, 357-358
Occult Blood, Feces 195-196
Olestra 358
Open Defecation 221-222
Opioids 105,189
Oral-Fecal Contamination 198-200
Orlistat 358-359
Outhouse 222, 359
Pacemaker Cells, Gastrointestinal 233-234
Paleofeces 114
Panchagavya 125-126, 360
Parasite (see Microbiome)
Parcopresis 77-78
Perineal Body 361
Perineal Reflex 44-45, 52
Peristalsis 238-240, 361-364
Pit Toilet 216-217, 364
Potty Training 393-397
Prebiotic 365
Preface iv
Probiotics 365-368
Proctoclysis 94, 174
Proctology 368
Proctoscopy 368-369
Prion (see Microbiome)
Protist (see Microbiome)
Pruritis Ani 369-370
Pubococcygeus Muscle 370-372
Puborectalis Muscle 372-374
Rapid Gastric Emptying 240
Rectal Bleeding 374-378
Rectal Examination 378-380
Rectoclysis 94,174, 356
Rectum 380-381
Reduviid Bug (see Chagas Disease)
Runner's Trots 381
Scat (see Shit)
Scatology 381
Scybalum 382
Septage (Septic Field & Tank) 221, 382
Sewer 217, 382-383
Shart 384
Shit 384

Shit/Feces, Euphemism 237-240
Shit/Feces, Foreign Language 235-236
Shit Stick 38-41
Shrimp, Coprophagia 123-124, 384-385
Shy Bowel 77-78
Shyster 385
Sigmoidoscopy 385-386
Skatole 60-61, 205-206, 386-387
Small Intestine 388-391
Smell (see Feces, Aroma)
Soluble Fiber (see Dietary Fiber)
Steatorrhea 391
Stinkbug 392
Sulfhydryl (see Feces, Aroma) 61-62, 206-207
Suppository 393
Thiol (see Feces, Aroma) 61-62, 206-207
To 'Air' is Human 6-7, 187-188, 406
Toilet 393-395
Toilet Gods 223, 396
Toilet Paper 27-40
Toilet (Potty) Training 396-400
Transit Time, Gastrointestinal 234-235
Transverse Folds of Houston 400
Traveler's Diarrhea 400-403
Trypanosoma cruzi (see Chagas Disease)
Ttongsul 118
Valsalva Maneuver 403-404
Villi 404-406
Virtual Colonoscopy 95-97
Virus (see Microbiome)
Volatile Organic Compounds 64-65, 209-210
Xenical (see Orlistat) 358-359
Xylospongium 38-41
Yoga 172-174

www.ingramcontent.com/pod-product-compliance
Lightning Source LLC
Chambersburg PA
CBHW051244020426
42333CB00025B/3045